The FRUGIVORE DIET

A HEALING DIET FOR WEIGHT LOSS, HEART DISEASE, CHRONIC ILLNESS, AND EVERYDAY THRIVATION.

+133 100% WHOLE PLANTS RECIPES

REYA STEELE

frugivore *(n)*: an animal whose preferred source of food is fruit and who is anatomically and physiologically equipped to thrive on a diet of fruit, shoots, roots, nuts, and seeds.

Beginning With Gratitude

My passion for preparing tasty food for people I love started at age 8 when I was given an Easy Bake Oven for Christmas. I loved making miniature multi-layered cakes and bringing them to family gatherings to share. Thank you mom for this gift which encouraged me to begin creating and sharing foods when I was a child.

Thank you to my Grandma Steele who always encouraged my cooking. When my dishes moved past Easy Bake Oven prepared-packages to more healthy and vegetarian foods, most of my other family members wouldn't even sample my creations, but Grandma always tried my food and encouraged me to keep creating. Grandma gave me my first cookbook, *A Celebration of Wellness*, when I was 16. When I first moved away to college she mailed me hand-typed recipes on 3 x 5 index cards. Her recipes for Split Pea Soup, Vegetable Soup, and Lentil Soup became some of my first go-to affordable and healthy recipes I made for myself. Even though you are no longer with us in your Earthly body, Grandma, thank you for always believing in me. I aim to carry your loving spirit onward through these recipes and my work sharing nutrition knowledge and healthy food.

Thank you to all my family and friends who have shared food with me. I always loved experimenting with recipes and creating my own. Over the years I have created many tasty dishes and have also had many failed experiments in the kitchen. I've also had many friends and loved ones sample my healthy food creations, and I owe you all great thanks. Thank you to all of you who have tasted my dishes and given me feedback—the good and the critical—which has helped me refine my recipes into ones worth repeating and worthy of sharing with you in these pages.

Thank you to Bjorn Bayer for introducing me to the Banini Smoothie when I had been stuck on banana-peanut butter for years. I include the Cinnamon Banini Smoothie in this recipe book here and variations of the Banini are a regular feature in our house.

A very special thanks to the Andrews family for welcoming me into your beautiful, loving family. When I have had no family nearby, you have welcomed me and my children in with open arms and always make us feel welcome and loved. Joining in your family gatherings has given me more excuses to make healthy salads and share my 100% plants recipes and I appreciate how you all have received me and my food creations in a way that encourages and uplifts my spirit.

Special thanks to my dear friend Miriam for always being there for me like a sister and for encouraging me to complete this book and my others with your unfailing positive perspective and loving spirit.

Thank you little Dominic for trying my foods even though it was different for you and for asking me for smoothies when you come over, it's a joy to make these for you and your mama.

Thank you to my friends who have sampled my creations, asked me for recipes, and made these recipes in your homes. Your enthusiasm for these dishes, recipes, and the encouragement you gave has helped me stay on track to complete this book! Also, a special thanks to my friend Laramie for all your loving support and encouragement on the journey!

Thank you to my fantastic editors—Miriam and Amanda. I couldn't have done this without you!

A big thank you to Carlos and Recruiting for Good for all your support of this book and Healing With Plants. You have been an angel answering my prayers for support when I most needed it.

Thank you to Kaiser Permanente and Hurst Ranch Historical Society for sponsoring the Garden Gourmets program where I have had the pleasure of working with over 1,000 students plus parents, teachers, and community members sharing nutrition science, stories, and some of the healthy recipes in this book. I love what I do!

Thank you to all the students I have had the pleasure of working with over the years sharing my healthy recipes and health and food education. You have brightened my days and given deeper purpose and drive to my life. I am so excited to complete this book to have even more recipes available to share with you!

The biggest thank you of all goes to my two children, Axel and Ayla. If not a single other person would ever see this book, I would still have made it for you. Thank you for being my most important taste-testers of these recipes and helping me perfect the dishes in this book with your always-honest feedback. Thank you for your help in the kitchen making many of these. Thank you for enthusiastically enjoying so many of the foods I prepare for you; your love and joy of these foods is the greatest motivation for me to keep creating in the kitchen. Thank you for patiently waiting for me to photograph countless meals before we eat them. Thank you for all you have taught me about our natural human diet and all the ways you have helped shaped this recipe book. I am forever blessed to have two amazing human beings as my children.

Lastly, thank you to you, reader. Thank you for picking up this book and inviting me into your kitchen. I hope you enjoy these colorful and flavorful recipes. May these foods nourish your body and help you maintain a life of wellness. May you feed yourself and your loved ones with foods that nourish your body. May you, dear reader, thrive with plants.

The FRUGIVORE DIET

...CONTENTS...

THE FRUGIVORE DIET

RECIPES

All recipes are made from 100% plants, oil-free, dairy-free, 100% vegan, nutrient-dense, whole foods.

SWEET STARTS

DIPS, DRESSINGS, & SAUCE

SUPER SALADS

SAVORY SIDEKICKS

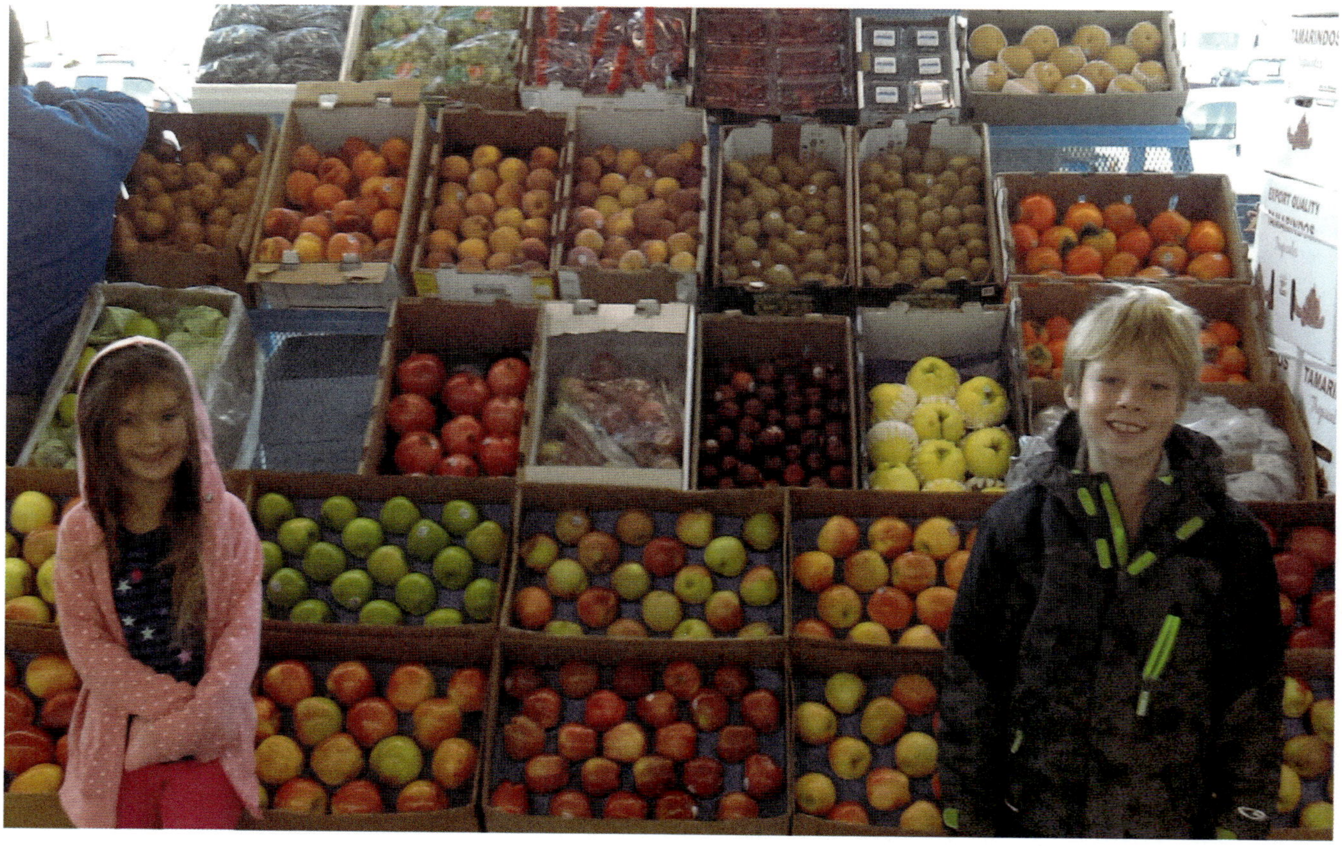

The FRUGIVORE DIET

...The Best Diet for Any Human...

People around the world are searching for answers: a better way to eat, how to take care of themselves, and how to heal chronic disease. Nutrition offers an easy fix to many of these problems that plague millions. In the United States, approximately 40% of adults over age 20 are now considered obese, and about 8% are what science and doctors consider "severely obese." Another 32% of adults are clinically overweight. This adds up to a staggering 72% of the adult population that is carrying too much weight. The extra weight is not just a cosmetic issue; science has clearly demonstrated that excess weight increases a person's risk of diabetes, heart disease, cancer, autoimmune disorders, bone fractures, sexual dysfunction, and skin disorders.

Years of poor public policy that have promoted growing and consuming the wrong sorts of foods for humans is partly to blame. Misleading food advertising and nutrition propaganda also adds to the confusion around *what's good to eat?* Many people have fallen victim to misleading propaganda from food companies and special interest groups. These corporations and groups tell people that they must eat meat, dairy, and eggs to be healthy. Many corporations push convenience foods high in processed oils and artificial chemicals. Diet gurus have sold the idea that all people are unique, and so the diet that works for one person may not work for another. People are told to watch out for chemicals on fresh fruits and vegetables, and that foods in packages are safer. The media warns about the dangers of soy or lettuce one day while promoting the virtues of butter and bone broth the next.

What's lost in all of this media madness is the simple truth that holds the key to healing and wellness for the nearly 2/3 of American adults and others around the world who struggle with weight and preventable and curable diseases. This simple truth is that there is an optimal human diet. This diet is our natural diet, the one our human biology has evolved to thrive on. The natural human diet is the one we are anatomically, physiologically, and psychologically attuned for. This diet prevents most chronic diseases that plague people today. This diet naturally and effortlessly keeps people at an ideal healthy weight. This diet can reverse and cure overweight, obesity, heart disease, Type 2 diabetes, and many types of cancer, autoimmune disorders, and skin ailments. This diet, what I call *The Frugivore Diet*, is composed of 100% whole plants.

...The Natural Human Diet...

A DIET FOR THE HUMAN BEING

If all Koala bears eat eucalyptus leaves, if all butterflies drink flower nectar, if all big fish eat little fish, then why is there not a perfect food for all humans? I wondered why, as a child, we did not eat the foods growing around us. Why did my parents prefer to feed me food ground and wrapped in plastic, enclosed in a cardboard package, with a colorful cartoon character on front. There was a mulberry tree in the backyard and wild onions and dandelions in the yard, but for dinner we'd have frozen and reheated chicken nuggets with mac n' cheese from the box.

My parents were just a product of their generation and the times that encouraged packaged, quick convenience foods. Over the course of the past 19 years studying the food system, health, and nutrition, I have come to see just how much propaganda and misinformation there is surrounding the question *what's good to eat?* I once was tricked by many of the mainstream myths about the natural human diet, which envisions humans as natural predators relying on animal flesh to survive. It has been a long road of research for me to bust these myths for myself and to prepare them in a detailed investigation I call *The Frugivore Files*.

DISCOVERING THE NATURAL HUMAN DIET

The Frugivore Files is a 3-part, nonfiction series that explores the question *What's good to eat?* from the lens of numerous scientific and academic disciplines. In these books you will find a clearly laid out case with evidence from a wide range of fields that all point to the same conclusion: human beings are frugivores, plant people molded through millenia to thrive on diets rich in ripe fruits and other plant parts. Every part of our human anatomy, physiology, psychology, natural history, and taxonomy gives away our true nature as fruit-eaters who also enjoy and benefit from the nutrition in fresh shoots, fruits, flowers, and seeds. Below I briefly summarize the evidence found in each branch of science that together illuminates that humans are biological frugivores who are designed to thrive on a diet of whole plants

...Summary of the Evidence...

Psychology: The study of the human mind, behaviors, and mental health reveals that our instincts pick fruit and other fresh plant foods, that our mental health benefits measurably from gardening and being around plants, and that killing and eating raw animal flesh goes against our human instincts and can have negative mental health effects.

Zoology: The study of animals reveals that humans are animals too, specifically, we are primates who are biologically equipped to pick fruits from trees and bushes. Most primates are correctly classified as frugivores based on their diets in nature. When fresh fruit is available, most primates select these foods first. Many primates consume more than half their calories from fruits and eat a large variety of fruits, many more species than the typical human eats today,

Archaeology: The study of fossil remains from long ago reveals that humans from the near ancient past and hominids from millions of years ago were eating a primarily plant-based diet. In recent decades, more sophisticated methods of analyzing archaeological remains has been able to determine more accurately how our ancient ancestors lived, how they died, and what they ate. This evidence has largely debunked the myth that ancient Man was primarily a hunter surviving on meat, and paints a new picture of our past as plant eaters.

Anatomy: The study of our bodily structures reveals that every part of our anatomy is perfect for picking, eating, digesting, and utilizing the energy from ripe fruits, roots, shoots, and seeds.

Physiology: The study of our body's mechanics reveals that our brains and bodies prefer to run on whole-plant foods. These are the easiest foods for our bodies to digest, and a diet of whole plant foods helps maximize our mental and physical capacities.

Epidemiology: The study of disease reveals that most of the common ailments plaguing humanity today are caused by improper nutrition. Overweight, obesity, heart disease, diabetes, and many cancers and autoimmune disorders have been linked to one common cause: eating a diet other than the one we are biologically designed for. Just as a house cat gets sick if fed a diet other than the one their carnivore biology equipped them for, a human gets sick if he or she eats a diet other than the one our frugivore biology equips us for.

Nutrition: The study of how what we eat affects the health of our body, and the nutrients we require to be healthy, reveals that whole plants are the only one-stop shop for meeting all human nutrition requirements. Humans are primates and like other primates we must get vitamin C from fresh plant foods. Whole plants contain the whole spectrum of macronutrients, micronutrients, and also contain an array of protective phytonutrients (*phyto = plant*) only found in plants. A look at basic nutrition facts reveal that plants have it all and there is absolutely zero need to include animal flesh and other animal products in the diet to obtain all of our nutritional requirements.

Gerontology: The study of aging reveals that a diet of whole plants is linked to longevity and numerous death-defying and anti-aging benefits.

Case Studies: I have personally collected nearly 500 stories of people who have cured various chronic diseases simply by eating a diet of whole plant foods. These testimonials include dozens of people who have lost weight, reversed heart disease, healed from cancer, cured an autoimmune disorder, resolved a skin disorder, and other healing stories. You can read some of these on my website www.HealingWithPlants.us and keep checking back for new ones. I will keep adding more until I have shared them all.

Cultural Anthropology: The study of human cultures, specifically of the arts, reveals that we have long had an affinity for fruit as the focus of our artistic expressions. Contrary to a popular myth that says ancient human art focused on hunting animals, a review of ancient art shows this is simply not true. The most ancient human art depicts symbols, plants, and animals that people share our world with.

Ethnobotany: The study of how plants and people interact reveals that humans have long had close relationships with plants. From cultivating forests of food to passing down knowledge of traditional medicinal plants, people have forever had close ties with the plant kingdom and depended on plants for nutrition and medicine.

Religion: The study of religions reveals ancient wisdom shared and passed on by many and systems of faith which recommend people eat primarily plants. Eating meat is strictly forbidden by some religions while others recommend consuming meat only in times of famine.

Public Policy: Studying public policy reveals how we got into the mess we are in as a society who is overfed and undernourished. Public policies that incentivize growing and consuming animal foods and processed foods has precipitated a growing obesity epidemic that is costing us our health, our savings, and time with the ones we love.

...Nutrition Science Made Simple...

Food contains substances necessary for the healthy growth and development of the human body. The two basic categories of nutrients are macronutrients and micronutrients. Macronutrients include the substances the human body requires in large amounts. Micronutrients include the substances the human body requires in relatively small amounts. The five basic macronutrients are carbohydrates, fat, protein, water, and fiber.[1] These five ingredients make up the bulk of the food we consume and are each essential in varying amounts for healthy growth and body functioning.

A lack of basic nutrition education in primary school all the way through medical school has been a boon for the milk and dairy industries who swooped in to fill the void. These companies have spent large sums to convince people to buy their products. One of the main tactics these industries have used is to create the illusion that their products are healthy. Meat and dairy are associated with the macronutrient "protein" despite the fact that protein comes from plants first and is a macronutrient present, in some amount, in almost all foods. Contrary to the industry's message that meat and dairy are healthy foods, the high levels of protein in animal products have been linked with the development of numerous degenerative diseases and ailments. Doctors and people who have done the research advise people to get their fat and protein from plants. The chart on the following page shows the macronutrient ratio of common foods and demonstrates that, despite common misconceptions, fat and protein are also found in plants.

MACRONUTRIENT RATIO MATTERS

While counting calories or focusing on eliminating certain foods has been the recent craze in managing one's diet, a more effective method would be to pay attention to macronutrients. Paying attention to the big parts of food – the sugar, fat, protein, fiber, and water content – is a more common sense approach to managing health. Consuming foods high in fat over time leads to a buildup of extra fat. Consuming foods high in carbohydrates will reduce the digestive workload and provide the most easily accessible energy for physically and mentally active people. Consuming whole, fresh raw plant foods can help keep your body hydrated. Cooked and processed foods require you to consume more water to not be dehydrated. My own experience with a whole foods, plant-based diet is that I have

1 While fiber is technically a carbohydrate, I find it useful to separate it out since not all carbohydrates are fiber and fiber is an important nutrient many people today are not getting enough of.

Macronutrient Ratio of Common Foods

Food	%Carbs	%Fat	%Protein
Chicken	0%	35%	65%
Beef	0%	41%	59%
Horseradish	46%	18%	36%
Spinach	56%	14%	30%
Cheese	2%	72%	26%
Arugula	53%	22%	25%
Mustard greens	69%	6%	25%
Chard	68%	9%	23%
Black beans	74%	3%	23%
Collards	68%	12%	20%
Broccoli	71%	9%	20%
Cauliflower	78%	3%	19%
Tomatoes	72%	10%	18%
Kale	72%	12%	16%
Wheat Bread	72%	12%	16%
Walnut	6%	80%	14%
Sunflower seed (kernels)	14%	74%	12%
Cabbage	85%	3%	12%
Cucumber	83%	6%	11%
Beet	86%	3%	11%
Almond butter	14%	78%	8%
Peach	87%	5%	8%
Cherries	88%	5%	7%
Watermelon	89%	4%	7%
Donut	51%	43%	6%
Oranges	91%	3%	6%
Potato	94%	0%	6%
Acorn meal	45%	50%	5%
Blueberry muffin	51%	44%	5%
Plum	90%	5%	5%
Carrots	92%	3%	5%
Honeydew melon	92%	3%	5%
Butternut squash	93%	2%	5%
Avocado	19%	77%	4%
Chocolate chip cookie	53%	43%	4%
Blueberries	91%	5%	4%
Banana	93%	3%	4%
Tamarind	94%	2%	4%
Yam	95%	1%	4%
Coconut	18%	79%	3%
Figs	94%	3%	3%
Persimmon	95%	2%	3%
Raisins	96%	1%	3%
Sapodilla	87%	11%	2%
Apples	95%	3%	2%
Dates	98%	0%	2%

never felt the need to count calories, always eat as much as I want when I am hungry, and have maintained a stable healthy weight without getting sick. I focus on the macronutrients – I make sure I get plenty of fresh fruit, raw foods, include a small amount of fat-rich seeds, nuts, and fruits, and minimize any processed foods.

A NEW MACRO VIEW OF FOOD

Paying attention to the macronutrient ratio of food is not necessarily new, but understanding what macronutrients are in foods and how these affect the body is a subject that has been noticeably missing from nutrition education. Many people have no idea that fruit contains protein, for example. Many people also don't know every cell in the brain runs on sugar and that the body has to work extra hard to create energy in the absence of carbohydrates. Also, it's not useful to associate particular foods with one macronutrient. For example, brownies and cakes are generally labeled as "sugar" foods and "junk foods," when most commercially sold baked goods are equally high in fat and a host of other ingredients. Eggs are associated as a "protein" food even though they are high in fat and all foods contain some protein. And while generally brownies and cakes may be classified as "junk" food, a creative and knowledgeable chef can make low-fat cakes from fruit and other whole foods that provide protein, fiber, and many other nutrients, making them a healthy food.

THINKING OUTSIDE THE CEREAL BOX

Food is a centerpiece to the lives of many people and as such it can be hard to imagine different types of diets for some. Many Americans consider "meat and potatoes" a full meal with many not consuming any fresh fruits and vegetables. But, these fatty junk foods cause a buildup of cholesterol and fat in body leading to a host of killer ailments like heart disease, the leading killer of men and women today.

On the flip side, some people consume diets very high in fruits and vegetables. Some people enjoy monomeals, meals comprised of a single food, which are said to be easy on digestion. Even a meal comprised entirely of fruit will contain measurable levels of protein and fat in addition to the sugar, fiber, and water in the fruit.

Just looking up the simple basic nutrition facts, what's in a piece of fruit, can dismantle an entire mythology of food, nutrition, and health. Human beings have ten toes and ten fingers for a reason. We are designed perfectly as tree climbers, fruit pickers, and foragers. Research into diet and disease is helping reveal the hidden secret to human health and thrivation. A diet rich in a variety of plant foods contain all the nutrients necessary for a healthy body.

In school most people learn about the very basics of biology and the food chain by learning to identify carnivores, omnivores, and herbivores. Humans are lumped in the omnivore category along with bears and skunks, who both kill and eat other animals and eat significant amounts of plants as well. Our position as animal-killing and -eating omnivores is further validated by school history classes that paint "prehistoric" humans as primarily hunters who dwelled in caves, carried long spears, and hunted large animals to feed their families. Because of this narrative, many people are under an illusion that human beings are by nature designed to consume the flesh, milk, and other parts of other animals. The truth is, there is another category of eating that humans belong to but many people have never heard of. Humans are biologically frugivores, like all other primates.

MEAT, DAIRY, EGGS, & PROCESSED FOOD MAKES PEOPLE SICK

Study after study has shown a positive correlation between consumption of meat, dairy, and eggs and development of obesity, heart disease cancer, and other disease. While critics will point out that correlation does not equal causation, this correlation is shown over and over, and in people consuming a plant-based diet, we find the reverse. We also see testimony after testimony from people who have reversed their degenerative disease and reclaimed their health with a vegan or raw-food diet.

I have been engaged in researching public health and nutrition, and I have had an interest in creating healthy foods for my family for many years now. In this book I summarize my nutrition science research and present the framework for a diet in line with our human psychology, anatomy, and physiology. This Frugivore Diet stands in direct contrast to the fad diets (Atkins, Paleo, Keto, and the like) and their mythologies that have wrecked the health and caused the premature death of countless millions. The Frugivore Diet is not a fad diet but is a term to describe our natural human diet, the one we are biologically designed to thrive on. The Frugivore Diet may require you to reprogram your habits and attitude around food, but the reward will be increased everyday energy, increased physical and mental capacities, and a key to lifelong wellness.

...The Frugivore Diet's Golden Rule...

ONE SIMPLE RULE: SIMPLY WHOLE PLANTS

There is really just one simple rule to follow if you want to use the Frugivore Diet to lose weight, heal your chronic illness, and regain your health. **The one primary rule is to eat 100% whole-plant foods.** This is your ticket to maximum wellness and healing imbalances caused by poor nutrition. Avoid all processed foods and foods derived from animals—this includes oils!

...Benefits of the Frugivore Diet...

1. PLANTS HAVE ALL THE NUTRIENTS PEOPLE NEED TO THRIVE

A common objection to a plant-based diet is concern over inadequate nutrition, but this concern is not founded in science. Rather, observed nutritional deficiencies in vegetarians and vegans are attributed to diets high in unhealthy processed foods and low in nutrient-rich, whole, fresh plant foods. Still, the food industry, specifically the meat and dairy industries, have worked hard to maintain the myth that meat and dairy are essential for nutrition. They market their products as good for, and even essential for, your health. But simple nutrition facts reveal that plant foods are the most nutrient-rich and healthiest food choices.

I was only very slightly worried that my children might be deficient in vitamin B12 when I took them in to the doctor for a routine physical which included blood work. My children have never tasted animal flesh in their life and have been mostly free of animal products through their entire lives, but strictly vegan for the last five years. As I am a strong believer that whole plant foods contain all the nutrients we need, I have never given them a supplement. They have never had protein powder, protein bars, or a chewable multivitamin. We do however start each day with fresh fruit either on a plate, in a bowl, or blended into a smoothie or other fruity beverage. They eat a variety of plants from the entire rainbow and their blood tests reveal this has given them all the nutrients they require. They were not deficient in any vitamins, minerals, or other nutrients including protein and vitamin B12.[2] All their numbers were well within the healthy range. I already felt they were healthy with no signs of deficiency before their test, but getting the science-backed results certainly helped give me peace of mind. Plants really do have all the nutrients that frugivores like us need to thrive.

Plant foods generally contain all five macronutrients – protein, fat, carbohydrates, water, and fiber in varying amounts. Plant foods also are the most nutrient-dense food choices containing large amounts of vitamins, minerals, and phytochemicals that help protect the body from illness. A common misconception is that animal products are needed to provide adequate nutrition but this is false. Some older people who have practiced a whole-food, plant-based diet for many years are living testimony of the age-defying and health-promoting diet. Some of the world's top performing athletes and body-builders compete and thrive on a vegan diet.

I have not consumed meat in 22 years and have been largely vegan for that time, and strictly vegan for the last five years. I have been through two pregnancies and have two happy healthy children who are thriving on the Frugivore Diet. Like many others practicing this diet, I can say our family doesn't experience sickness like we used to when we included our neighbors' eggs, some dairy, and some processed foods in our diet.

2. A WHOLE-FOOD, PLANT-BASED DIET REDUCES RISK OF DISEASE

A whole-food, plant-based diet is the best health insurance policy known to Man. Science has clearly demonstrated the protective power of eating whole-plant foods. The more energy people consume from whole plants, the more protected they are from heart disease, cancer, diabetes, weight issues, and other disease. Simply eating a diet of whole plants eliminates the great amount of risk that eating animal foods and processed foods pose to your health. Science and basic nutrition facts empower us with the knowledge to chose the right foods for a human, which maintains our health well into old age. Disease is not our destiny, and right nutrition can keep us on a path of wellness and thrivation.

The data supporting the health benefits of a whole-food, plant-based diet can be found at nearly every level and perspective. Vegan diets have been shown to help in maintaining a healthy weight, are linked to healthy cholesterol levels and a healthy blood pressure, produce healthier guts, reduce stress and anxiety, protect against heart disease and cancer, and protect against obesity and type 2 diabetes.

Another way to see the connection between food and disease is to look at the diets and disease rates of large populations for evidence. Countries that consume the greatest percentage of calories from unrefined plant foods also have the lowest rates of heart disease and cancer. The reverse is true: countries who consume the most calories from animal foods and processed foods have the highest rates of chronic disease including obesity, heart disease, diabetes, and cancer. The epidemiologic evidence is further proof that our natural optimal diet is plants.[3]

Besides reducing the risk of disease, a whole plants diet has been shown to reverse and heal numerous ailments. In the Healing With Plants master database are nearly 500 such testimonials of people curing numerous autoimmune disease, various types of cancer, skin conditions, diabetes, obesity, and

2 B12 is a vitamin that many people are deficient in and many people eating a purely plants diet worry about. One reason my children and I may be good with B12 is that we include nutritional yeast in our diet. You will find this ingredient in many of the sauces and soup recipes included in this book. Nutritional yeast contains many B vitamins including B12 and happens to be a tasty addition to whole-plant foods. Besides using nutritional yeast in the sauces and soup recipes in this book, in my family we also often use it as a condiment to sprinkle on plain rice, pasta, or toast. You can find this ingredient in the bulk food section of your local natural food store, or Trader Joe's sells it prepackaged at an affordable price..

3 See *The Frugivore Files, Volume 2*, Epidemiology File for the evidence behind this claim.

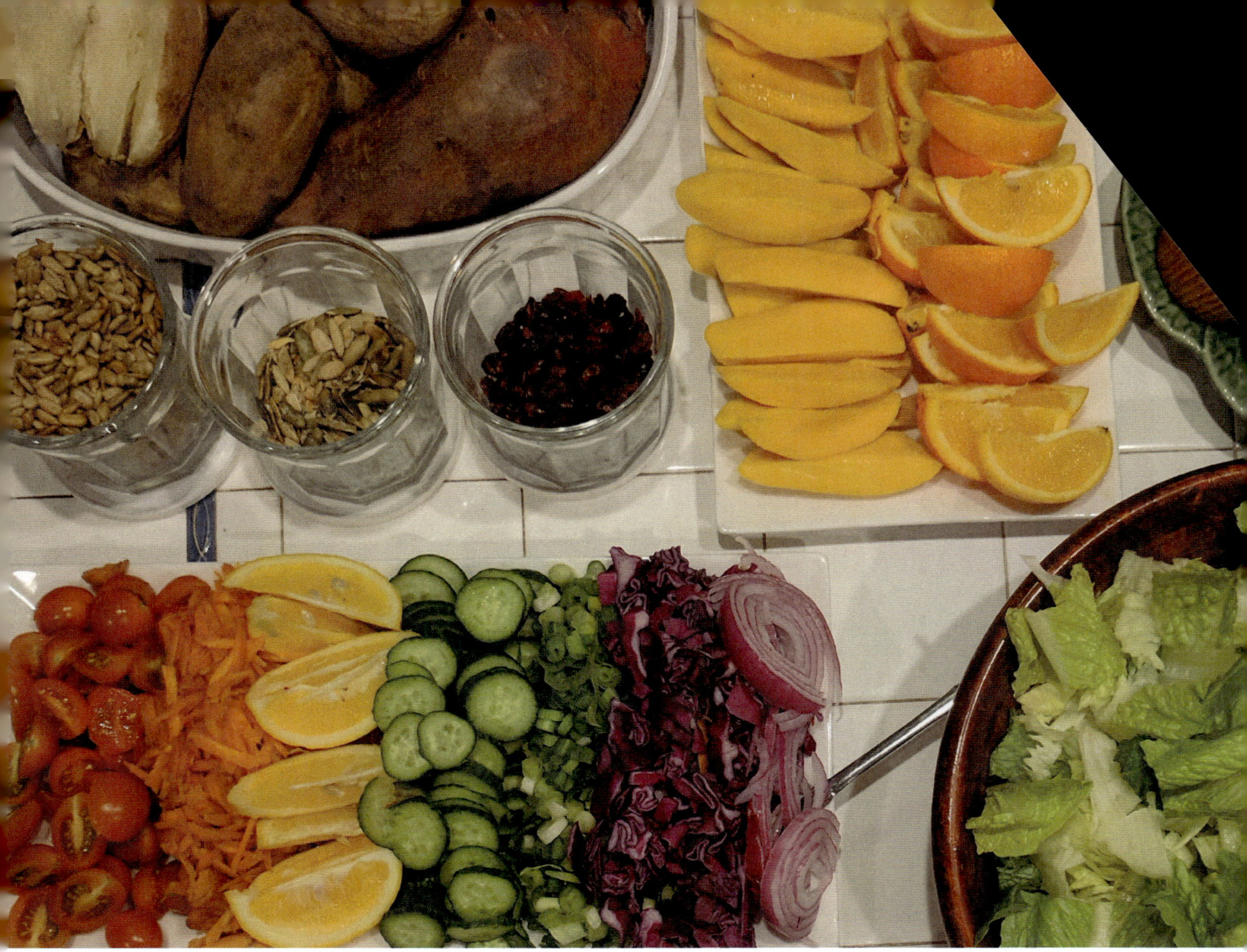

inflammatory conditions simply by eating more fruits and plant foods.

The American Cancer Society acknowledges the role of diet in preventing cancer. In their "Guidelines on Nutrition and Physical Activity for Cancer Prevention" they say:

> *"Evidence suggests that one third of the more than 500,000 cancer deaths that occur in the United States each year can be attributed to diet and physical activity habits, with another third due to cigarette smoking. Although genetic inheritance influences the risk and cancer arises from genetic mutations in cells, most of the variation in cancer risk across populations and among individuals is due to factors that are not inherited."*

Specifically when it comes to eating for cancer prevention they recommend to:

- *"Eat a variety of healthful foods, with an emphasis on plant sources.*
- *Eat five or more servings of a variety of vegetables and fruits each day.*
- *Choose whole grains in preference to processed (refined) grains and sugars.*
- *Limit consumption of red meats, especially those high in fat and processed.*
- *Choose foods that help maintain a healthful weight."*

The American Heart Association's "Dietary Guidelines" also emphasize the importance of a plant-rich diet for preventing heart disease. They say:

A (American Heart Association) strongly endorses the consumption of diets that vide variety of fruits and vegetables throughout the day, both as meals and snacks. vegetables are high in nutrients and fiber and relatively low in calories and hence nutrient density. Dietary patterns characterized by a high intake of fruits and veg- ssociated with a lower risk of developing heart disease, stroke, and hypertension. nsuming a variety of fruits and vegetables (especially those that are dark green, nge, or yellow) helps ensure adequate intakes of micronutrients normally present in this food group."

The AHA acknowledges that excess weight is directly linked to developing heart disease and an important principle of maintaining a healthy weight is to consume enough dietary fiber. Whole-plant foods are rich in dietary fiber and fill up the volume of the stomach triggering a full and satisfied feeling that regulates healthy eating.

3. EATING PLANTS CAN HEAL DISEASES

The most common chronic diseases that plague people today have a simple cure: plants! The Frugivore Diet of 100% whole-plant foods has been known to heal diseases including obesity, overweight, diabetes, heart disease, autoimmune disorders, inflammation, chronic fatigue, psoriasis, arthritis, many cancers, and other conditions. Most of the various diseases known to Man today have their root in the same problem: improper nutrition for the human animal. We wouldn't feed a house cat broccoli and expect it to stay in good health. That's because we know that cats are carnivorous animals. But most people do not extend the same basic logic to themselves. The human animal is a frugivore and if we do not consume our natural diet, we will suffer the consequence of ill health.

4. BRAIN POWER BOOSTED BY PLANTS

The human brain runs on carbohydrates from plants. Although people can survive for a while on a high-fat/low-carb diet, cognitive function will no-doubt suffer. People who follow low-carb diets often report feeling foggy headed. When people switch to a 100% plants diet they often report experiencing a much clearer mind. Science has backed up this phenomenon by showing that eating carbohydrates from plants boost brain function and academic performance.[4] It's no coincidence that many of the leading thinkers and inventors of recent history have practiced a purely or mainly plants diet. In *The Frugivore Files* I present evidence that suggests our large human brain developed over time thanks to our natural affinity for fruit-eating.[5] Our natural frugivore diet is good for our brains.

5. THIS DIET IS BACKED BY PROFESSIONALS

While modern schooling from primary school all the way through medical school contains a noticeable lack of nutrition education, the professionals who have dedicated their careers to the subject are mostly in agreement. The American Dietetic Association states:

> *"It is the position of the American Dietetic Association and Dietitians of Canada that appropriately planned vegetarian diets are healthful, nutritionally adequate, and provide health benefits in the prevention and treatment of certain diseases."*

Even the United States Dietary Guidelines includes this statement supporting a plant based diet as healthy for humans,

> *"Vegetarian diets can be consistent with the Dietary Guidelines for Americans, and meet Recommended Dietary Allowances for nutrients."*

4 See The Frugivore Files V2—The Physiology File for the evidence behind this claim.
5 See The Frugivore Files V1—The Archaeology File for the evidence behind this claim.

The USDA has also come out with a *Healthy Eating for Vegetarians* guide. If only they went a step further with stronger language recommending a plant-based diet and warning against the dangers of meat and dairy consumption. But individual doctors and health practitioners are stepping out of the box more with strong endorsements for a whole-foods, plant-based diet.

Dr. Kim Williams, president of the American College of Cardiology says he became vegan after doing the research. Now a plant-based diet is his number one prescription for reversing and preventing heart disease. In an interview with the *New York Times,* he says after his own experience with diet and throughly reviewing the best science available,

> *"I recommend a plant-based diet because I know it's going to lower their blood pressure, improve their insulin sensitivity and decrease their cholesterol."*

Dr. Michael Greger, MD has dedicated his professional career to staying on top of the latest nutrition research and relating this important information to the public. His perspective as a doctor and nutrition researcher:

> *"The balance of scientific evidence suggests that the healthiest way to eat is a vitamin B12-fortified diet of whole plant foods. For optimum nutrition, we should be sure to include in our daily diet not only an array of whole grains, beans, nuts, seeds, fruit, and as many vegetables as we can eat, but also specifically dark green leafy vegetables, berries, and white (or green) tea."*

While many doctors have not spent time studying nutrition, there is a growing number who have taken up a passion for uncovering the truth in nutrition studies. These doctors, nutritionists, and scientists are helping dismantle food industry propaganda so that the simple truth can reach people – humans are designed to thrive on plants.

6. EASILY MAINTAIN A HEALTHY WEIGHT

With 72% of American adults now clinically overweight, maintaining a healthy weight is a concern facing most of the country. Fortunately the Frugivore Diet, the diet of whole-plant foods that we are biologically designed for, helps regulate weight effortlessly. Whole-plant foods are full of water and fiber that fill up our stomachs, and they are also full of nutrients which help us feel satisfied after eating. These foods are the perfect cocktail of nutrients to give us all we need to thrive and helping us feel satisfied so we don't overeat. When people fill up on processed food lacking fiber, water, and micronutrients, they are left unsatisfied and still hungry. What they are really hungry for is real nutrition, but oftentimes they will eat more junk food which further perpetuates the problem. People who follow a diet of primarily whole-plant foods are able to maintain their ideal weight effortlessly over the years well into old age. It is not our destiny to get fatter and sicker as we age. Maintaining a healthy weight is well within our control if we simply stick to whole plant foods.

7. GIVE YOUR FAMILY THE GIFT OF WELLNESS

Is it not the job of a parent to give their children the best shot at a successful life? A practice of healthy eating, exercise, and mindfulness can be a pathway to a lifetime of wellness. As a mother, I believe that teaching my children how to live healthfully is one of the greatest gifts I can give them for their future happiness and success. If they were to grow up eating nutrient-poor junk foods, it's likely they would be sick often and would be susceptible to numerous diseases. With a healthy body and mind, the possibilities are nearly limitless for what they can do with their lives. Good health makes it possible to walk, run, bike, lift things, make things, have a clear mind to solve problems and develop ideas. As a mother, I have wanted nothing more for my children than to be healthy and happy. Over the years researching, writing about, and practicing a holistic health lifestyle, I have learned just how important good nutrition is to the wellness equation.

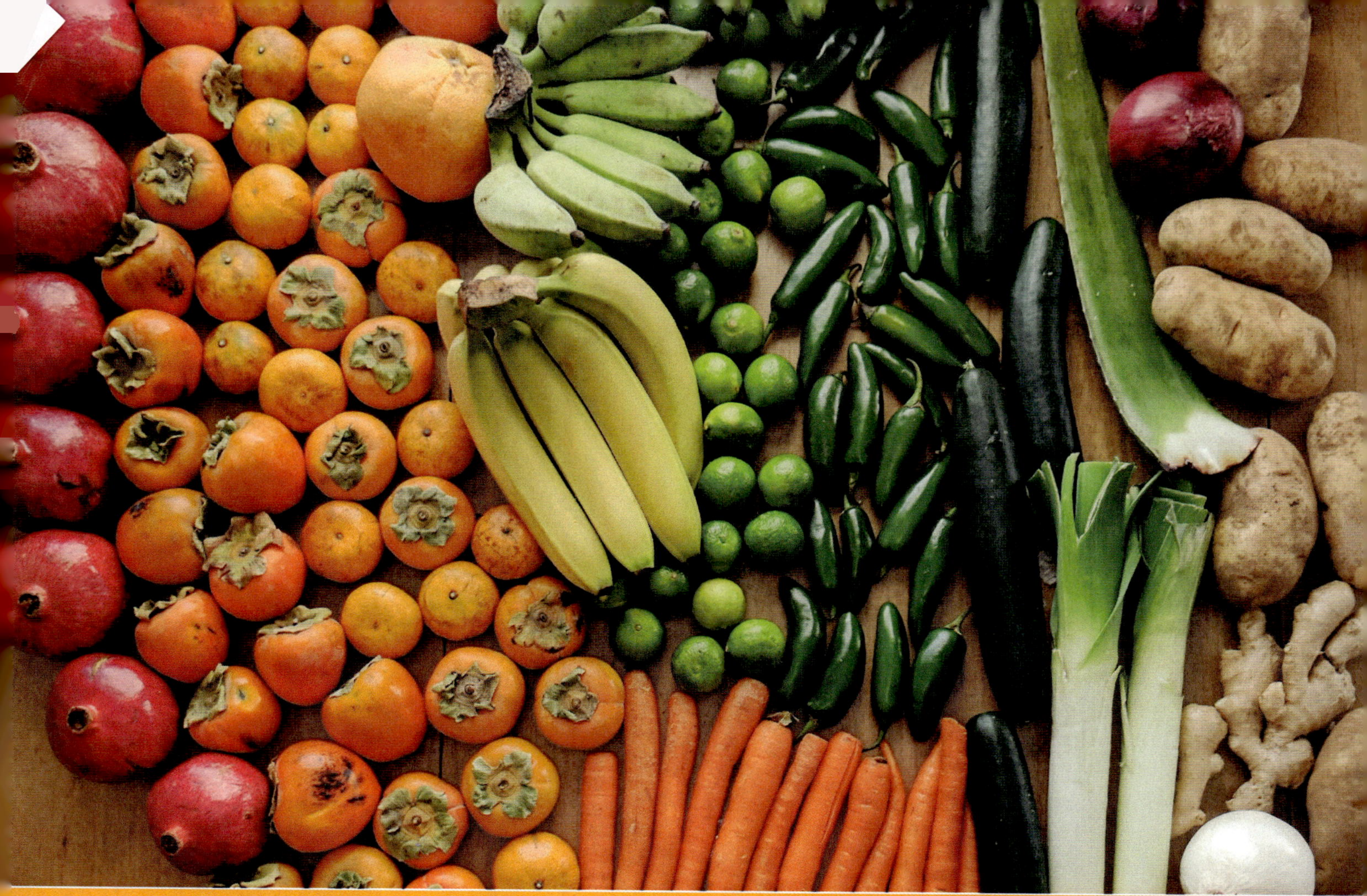

Eating healthy doesn't have to break the bank.
This is a typical grocery haul for the Frugivore Diet, full of affordable produce like whole carrots, potatoes, onions, and bananas. When I shop I load up on ripe seasonal varieties that are on sale—like the persimmons and pomegranates in this photo.

My children are nine and eleven years old and have never tasted animal flesh in their lives. When they were little we still ate cheese, eggs, and dairy, but gave these foods up for a fully, 100% plants diet when my son was six and my daughter was four. My children are very healthy, almost never get sick, are very creative, bright, and are good students. They have always been ahead of their classes in math and reading and test a couple grades above their grade level in standardized tests. What's more, my children love the food I prepare for them and they always have. I have always supplied them with copious amounts of fresh, raw, seasonal fruits. They frequently request the smoothies featured in this book. They are also big fans of the potatoes, beans, and rice dishes that grace these pages. As a mother I am happy to please the palates of my children, but even more happy to know I am giving them the gift of wellness through the food I prepare.

8. THE MOST AFFORDABLE DIET EVER

Many people think that eating healthy means spending a lot of money when this couldn't be further from the truth. While it's true that public policy has favored animal products and processed foods, making them artificially cheap, it's also true that whole-plant foods are still the cheapest way to eat. While it's definitely possible to spend a lot on fancy, rare plant foods, making your grocery bill extra large, it's also possible to focus on foods that are in large supply, seasonal, and very affordable.

Most of the recipes I share in this book are made from ingredients that are very affordable—potatoes, rice, bananas, oranges, apples, and beans are staple foods in our house. These are some of the cheapest foods available. I can buy a large bag of potatoes for $5 that will be the bulk of several meal. A couple bunches of bananas may cost a couple bucks and are packed with delicious energy and loads of nutrients. If you look at the places in the world where people have the least financial wealth, you will find people eating primarily plants. A whole-food, plant-based diet doesn't have to break the bank and is accessible for anyone who shops smart and focuses on seasonal plants and affordable staples.

9. FOOD IS ATTRACTIVE AND TASTY

Is it any surprise that our natural human diet is also the diet that is most naturally attractive to us? There is a reason why fruit bowls are the most common subject of still life paintings throughout history. Fruits are beautiful to us. Whole-plant foods are naturally attractive. Science has shown that people eat with our eyes first, and so filling our plates and bowls with a rainbow of whole fresh plants is not only nutritious and delicious, but also adds beauty to our lives.

10. EXPERIENCE GREATER ENERGY

Anyone I have ever talked to who has switched to a diet of whole-plant foods reports feelings of greater energy. These foods are the easiest for our body to digest and so leave more energy available for our mental and physical functions.

My friend's daughter has become sick with a mysterious illness and couldn't get out of bed. She lacked the energy to get up and go to work and had been unable to support her young son. After I counseled her about nutrition and recommended a whole-food, plant-based diet, it wasn't long before she messaged me that she had so much more energy eating this way. In a short while she was able to get out of bed and got a new job. She lost ten pounds in just a couple weeks and thanked me telling me she was definitely going to stick with it.

A high school wrestler was struggling with extra weight and trying on fad diets had left him feeling foggy and lethargic. After my counsel and switching to a whole-food, plant-based diet he told me he had more energy and was getting better grades at school. I met with his mother to share recipes and their whole family was ready to make a switch. Any person I've ever talked to that has switched to this diet has told me they feel great with an increased energy to move through their day.

...Frugivore Diet's Ten Guidelines...

These ten guidelines will help you to lose weight naturally, heal chronic disease, and thrive on plants!

1. Eat As Many Whole Plants As You Want

The first and most important rule of the Frugivore Diet is simply this: don't skimp on the plants! Eat as many whole-plant foods as you want. By filling up on whole plants, including a variety of leaves, seeds, flowers, fruits, and roots, your stomach will be satisfied by the fullness of the fiber-rich foods. Your stomach will also sense all the nutrition in your meals which will also help you to feel satiated. If you do get hungry suddenly, grab a banana or apple or a healthy, whole-plants snack such as Chocolate Sunflower Balls. On a 100% whole-plant-food diet, there is absolutely no need to restrict your intake. You can eat until you feel satisfied because this is your biologically-specific diet—the one nature intended for you.

2. Avoid All Animal Foods

Rule two follows naturally from the Golden Rule and from rule one—simply avoid all animal foods. Human beings are not to be confused with carnivorous animals who, for the most part, walk on four legs, have razor -harp fangs, have large stomachs and short intestines, have smaller brains, and who usually produce litters of offspring in a relatively short time. Humans are frugivores—we stand upright and have long arms and agile fingers for grasping and plucking ripe fruits and berries. Our teeth are flat and smooth for mashing soft fruits and leaves and the occassional hard seeds. If we want to experience wellness we must consume the food that we are biologically equipped to thrive on.

STOMACH VS STOMACH
~500 Calories of Orange Compared

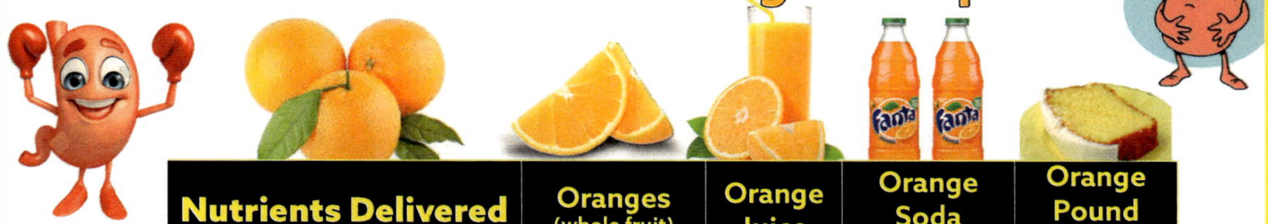

Nutrients Delivered	Oranges (whole fruit)	Orange Juice	Orange Soda (with corn syrup)	Orange Pound Cake
Quantity/Ounces	7 oranges = 35 oz	4 cups = 32 oz	2 cans = 32 oz	1 slice = 4 oz
Calories	480	448	476	490
Macronutrient Content				
Carbohydrates	123 g	103 g	122 g	55 g
Protein	9.1 g	6.8 g	0 g	8 g
Fat	1.4 g	2 g	0 g	27 g
Omega-3 fatty acids	88 mg	109 mg	0 g	~
Omega-6 fatty acids	225 g	288 mg	0 g	~
Fiber	22 g	2 g	0 g	2 g
Water	840 g	876 g	870 g	~
Vitamin Content				
Vitamin A	2,422 U	1,984 IU	0 mg	750 IU
Vitamin B1 (Thiamin)	0.7 mg	0.2 mg	0 mg	~
Vitamin B2(Riboflavin)	0.7 mg	0.4 mg	0 mg	~
Vitamin B3(Niacin)	4 mg	1 mg	0 mg	~
Vitamin B5 (Pantothenic Acid)	3 mg	2 mg	0 mg	~
Vitamin B6	0.7 mg	0.4 mg	0 mg	~
Vitamin B9 (Folate/Folic Acid)	333 mcg	298 mcg	0 mcg	~
Vitamin C (Ascorbic Acid)	580 mg	496 mg	0 mg	1.2 mg
Vitamin E	1.4 mg	0.4 mg	~	~
Vitamin K	0 mg	0.8 mg	~	~
Betaine	0.7 mg	~	0 mg	0 mg
Choline	823 mcg	62 mg	6 mg	0 mg
Mineral Content				
Calcium	421 mg	109 mg	50 mg	150 mg
Copper	0.7 mg	0.4 mg	0.2 mg	0 mg
Iron	1.4 mg	2 mg	0.6 mg	2.7 mg
Magnesium	62 mg	109 mg	10 mg	0 mg
Manganese	~	0 mg	0.2 mg	0 mg
Phosphorus	225 mg	169 mg	10 mg	0 mg
Potassium (K)	1,624 mg	1,984 mg	20 mg	0 mg
Selenium	0 mcg	0.8 mcg	0 mcg	0 mcg
Sodium	10 mg	10 mg	119 mg	380 mg
Zinc	0.7 mg	0.4 mg	1 mg	0 mg

~ = missing value/unknown

Whole plant foods are always nutritionally superior to processed foods

This Stomach vs. Stomach chart that shows nutrients contained in whole oranges, orange juice, orange soda, and orange cake. The more processed food is calorie dense packing a lot of calories into a small package without much nutritional value. In contrast, the whole oranges contain the full spectrum of macronutrients, vitamins, minerals, fiber, and water. Whole foods always win the Stomach vs. Stomach contest!

3. Avoid Processed Oils

The third rule also follows naturally from the Golden Rule and rule one—avoid all processed oils. Processed oils are not much better than animal foods for your health. Oils are an unnatural food because they would never be found growing from the Earth. To make oil, we manipulate natural foods, removing just the fat and leaving behind all the other good stuff, like the protein, carbohydrates, vitamins, minerals, fiber, water, and disease-preventing phytonutrients. Because oil is a very concentrated source of calories from fat, it is very easy to over consume foods with processed oil as they do not trigger the stomach's two satiation sensors: physical fullness and nutrient content.

4. Keep a Well-Stocked Fridge

People eat what's available around them. It's been this way since the beginning of time. People who stock their pantries with processed bars, crackers, and cookies will naturally eat these foods they "harvested" from the store. People who stock their fridges and baskets with fresh fruits and vegetables will naturally eat these foods. Keeping a well-stocked kitchen for success with the Frugivore Diet means harvesting only the foods that are truly good for you because these are the foods that will be available to you when hunger strikes.

- **Eat Your Leaves:** Keep your fridge stocked with multiple varieties of leaves like arugula, lettuce, cabbage, and kale.
- **Add Herbs:** Incorporate fresh herbs from your garden, or start an herb garden in your windowsill or in containers on your front porch.
- **Fill Up On Fruit:** Keep a fruit basket on your kitchen table full of a variety of ripe, seasonal fruits. Bananas are an affordable and nutrient-packed option at any time of year.
- **Stock Up on Seeds:** Seeds are nutrient-packed and add a lot of flavor to the Frugivore Diet. Stock up on seeds like cashews to make Ch-Easy Cashew Sauce or raw sunflower seeds to grind into Chocolate Sunflower Balls. Keep slivered almonds or walnut pieces in your pantry to add a sprinkle of richness to your dinner salad or smoothie.
- **A Steady Supply of Roots:** Roots like potatoes, carrots, and yams are staple foods of the Frugivore Diet. Root vegetables are a tasty dense source of energy and nutrients that are also affordable and easy to store. Practically all of the one-pot meals shared in the recipe section of this book feature wholesome and satisfying roots.
- **Bark, Flowers, Sap, and Stalks:** Keep a variety of whole plant ingredients in your fridge and pantry to make any meal a success. Cinnamon spice—made from ground tree bark—is a nice addition to many breakfast bowls, smoothies, and desserts.

5. Fill Up on Fruit

Fresh, ripe fruit is perhaps the most perfect food known to Man. Ripe fruit entices all our senses from our eyes to our noses to our taste buds. A meal of ripe fruit leaves us feeling hydrated, refreshed, nourished, and energized. We associate an overflowing platter of fruits with royalty for a reason—because this is the fruit we naturally desire. Health is our true wealth and fruit is the natural treasure that becomes our own wellness as we consume it in abundance.

6. Give Digestion a Break

Give your digestive system a break by simply eating foods that don't require it to overwork and use more than its fair share of your body's total energy. Your body benefits when it has enough energy to maintain a state of wellness. Your body is a natural vessel that is always using energy to maintain itself. You use energy to breathe, to sit, to think, and to digest food. If you are continuously devoting energy to eating food, then your body is continuously devoting energy to digesting. This means that less energy is available for other tasks like repairing damaged cells, maintaining a strong immune system, and using your brain to work out complex tasks. Different foods require different amounts of energy to digest. Fruit, not surprisingly, is perhaps the easiest food for a human being to digest. Unlike

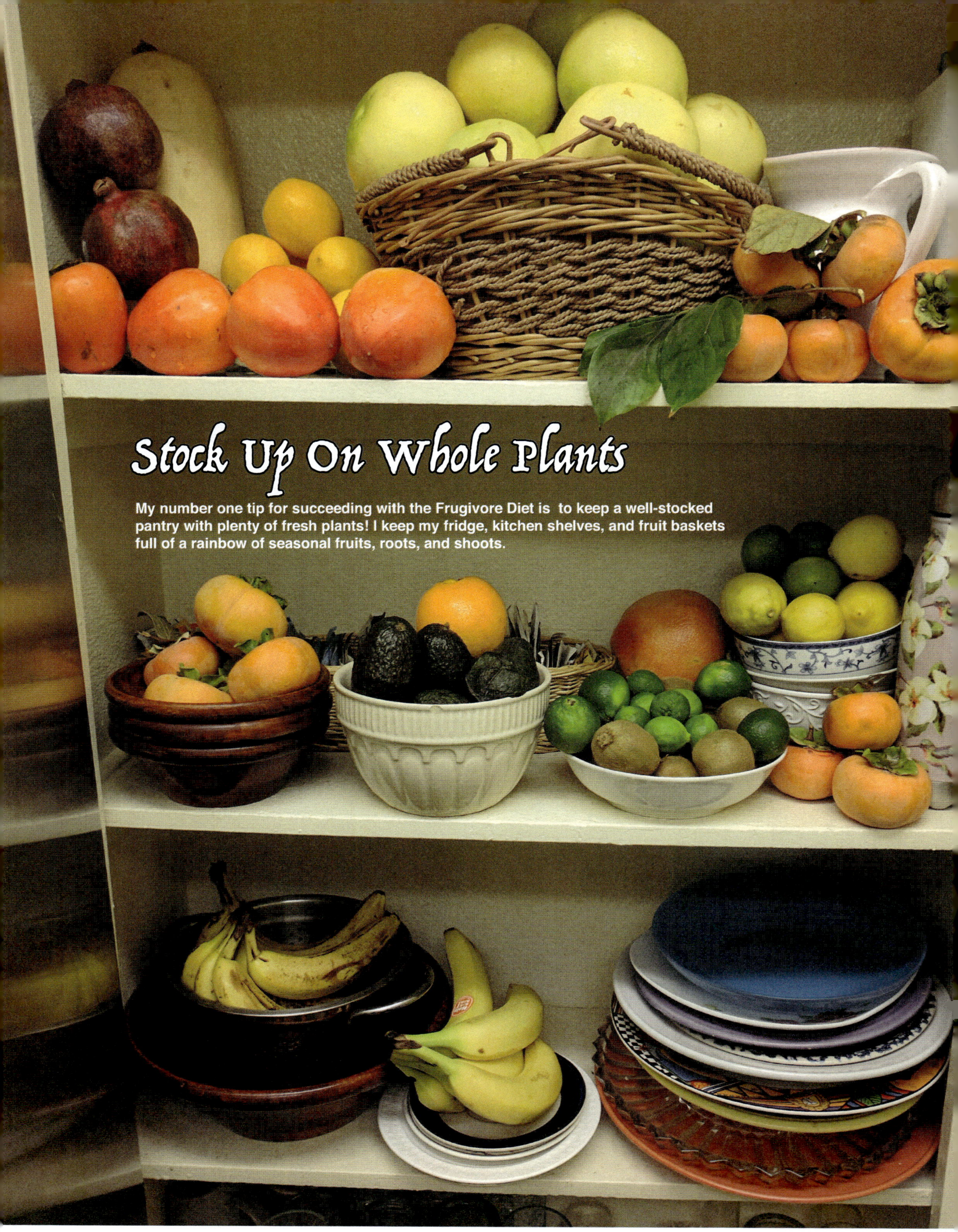

Stock Up On Whole Plants

My number one tip for succeeding with the Frugivore Diet is to keep a well-stocked pantry with plenty of fresh plants! I keep my fridge, kitchen shelves, and fruit baskets full of a rainbow of seasonal fruits, roots, and shoots.

processed sugars which are rapidly released into the bloodstream causing blood sugar spikes, the natural sugars in fruits are released into the blood more slowly because they come with a complete and perfect package of nutrition including a lot of natural fiber, water, vitamins, minerals, and phytonutrients. Eating a meal of fruit will require much less energy to digest than eating a meal of meat or cheese, for example.

7. Limit Salt to Reduce Water Weight

Sodium is a natural mineral found in the earth and that occurs naturally in all plant foods. In it's concentrated form as table salt or sea salt, it can be consumed excessively. Consuming too much salt will lead to your body holding onto water to cope with the internal chemistry created by extra sodium. Your body is essentially trying to dilute the sodium inside itself by holding onto water. To avoid carrying extra water weight and feeling bloated and uncomfortable, limit how much salt you add to your meals. Avoiding processed foods will go a long way towards reducing excess sodium in your diet.

8. Keep Hydrated

Keeping your body hydrated will help avoid you mistaking thirst for hunger, and will help keep you feeling energized and able throughout the day. Lucky for you that keeping hydrated is a no-brainer on the Frugivore Diet. Whole-plant foods are naturally made mostly of water. Most fresh fruits are in the range of 72–93% water. Once you start incorporating an abundance of raw plant foods into your diet you may find your thirst disappears and you have little need to drink water. You will see that recommendations to drink 8–10 glasses of water a day are a response to a culture that was consuming large amounts of over-salted, processed foods. These processed foods lack the natural water content of natural, whole-plant foods.

9. Make Salad Your Supper

Salad is wonderful for supper. Consider making salad a routine part of dinnertime either as the main meal or as a sidekick. Salad is full of raw, living plant nutrition including fiber and water. Salad will fill you up and leave you feeling energized and alert, a sharp contrast to the heavy and tired feelings people experience after a meal of animal products. Hours later you will still feel good and the nutrition releases at a natural pace inside your bloodstream.

While people who are used to meat in the middle of dinner may scoff at the idea of a supper of salad, salad can make a very satisfying meal. The key to a satisfying salad is to combine a complimentary variety of flavors, and to include leaves, roots, fruits, and seeds in the mix. Adding shredded carrots or beets to a salad gives it an attractive color, a slight crunch, and a touch of sweetness. Adding diced cherry tomatoes or dried cranberries contributes fruity goodness and nutrition. Adding a sprinkle of slivered almonds or roasted pumpkin seeds adds a satisfying richness and crunch to your salad. Adding a variety of leaves such as arugula, chopped kale, shredded cabbage, and mustard greens contributes a richness of flavors and nutrients. A salad a day can truly keep the doctor away.

10. Enjoy a Rainbow of Plants

Eating a rainbow of whole-plant food ensures you are giving your body all of the good stuff that keeps you nourished and well. Each color of the plant-food rainbow contributes different phytonutrients, the special disease-protecting nutrients found only in plants. Phytonutrients are most concentrated in the colorful parts of plants. Orange plants are particularly beneficial for healthy eyesight and skin. Red plants are known for fighting and preventing cancer. Blue and purple plants are known for their brain-boosting benefits. The colors of plants are clues to the nutrients they contain, and so in order to get the full array of goodness, aim to eat the rainbow everyday.

...Get Started on The Frugivore Diet...

If your current diet is centered around meat, dairy, eggs, or processed foods, then you might be wondering, *where do I begin?* Old habits, especially ones you've practiced your whole life, can be hard to break. What follows are some tips for getting started with the Frugivore Diet, the diet your human body was designed to thrive on.

THE GREAT PANTRY PURGE

Start with cleaning out your fridge and pantry. Get rid of all animal foods and processed foods. Just throw them in the trash and say goodbye for good. Then say hello to a new, healthy you.

People eat what is available to them so the pantry purge is a key step to clear out the foods that are toxic to your health and set the stage for success with a diet of whole-plant foods. It's also a good excuse to clean your pantry. You'll love the difference you see when you fill your fridge back up with colorful fruits, leaves, roots, and seeds.

FIND A GOOD PRODUCE PLACE

Not all food markets are alike. You may want to spend a little time exploring the markets around you to find the best place to purchase fresh produce. I have a few different markets I like to shop in for different reasons. In one I can get very affordable tropical fruits most any time of the year, in one, I get great sale prices on seasonal fruits and veggies, and the other maintains a consistent and affordable selection of high-quality produce. Getting to know the produce markets near you will help you succeed on your path to everyday wellness.

KITCHEN EQUIPMENT

You don't need a lot of fancy kitchen equipment to succeed on this diet, but it helps to have a few tools.

Cutting tools: The most basic tools you need are a good cutting board and a good fruit knife. I also use kitchen scissors frequently for cutting green onions and herbs. You can find a decent pair at the dollar store for $1.

Measuring tools: After that it helps to have a measuring cup and measuring spoons for making many of these recipes.

Blending tools: Next on the list would be getting a good high speed blender. While you don't need to purchase the most expensive blender out there, you won't want to purchase the cheapest variety either. Go for a high-powered motor and a good quality brand that will make smoothies with ease and puree soups to creamy perfection. I previously had purchased multiple cheap blenders only to have them fail to perform and end up in the trash. I have had a Ninja blender for the last five years which has served me well for making the smoothies and sauces in this book. For blending thicker nice-creams and making energy balls and raw pie crusts, I use a food processor. This handy machine works wonders and can help you achieve some really nice desserts, but it is the priciest kitchen tool I own. A good-sized one like I use will cost you at least $150, but there are smaller-capacity ones on the market for as little as $40.

Juicing tool: Another tool which is very handy is a citrus juicer. You can find hand-held lemon squeezers at the dollar store for $1 which work at a basic level to squeeze the juice from lemons and limes while preventing their seeds from entering the mix. These are low-quality, however, and I have had a few of them break. It's worth it to spend $8–10 on a hand-held juicer made of metal that will extract citrus juice effortlessly and will last you for many years.

Eat Your Fruits

FILL UP ON FRUITS

Whole fruits are loaded with nutrients that frugivores like us need. Counter to decades of anti-carb and anti-sugar propaganda, which has often lumped fruit in with other processed sugar foods and scared well-intentioned people away from fruit, science says whole fruits are a healthy choice any time of day. You truly cannot eat too much fruit! Eating a meal of just fruit is a way to keep meal prep simple while loading up on dietary fiber, essential macronutrients, and healthy carbohydrate energy, all while hydrating your body with the purest water on the planet, filtered through fruits! Most primates in nature eat over 50% of their calories from fresh, ripe fruits, and studies show they are not starving for variety. Many primates have been observed eating over 100 types of fruits, while most people today eat considerably less variety. Consider becoming a fruit explorer and venture to try new varieties when they come to market. There is so much goodness to enjoy in the rainbow of fruits available to us, and I hope this book gives you some ideas for incorporating more fruit into your life.

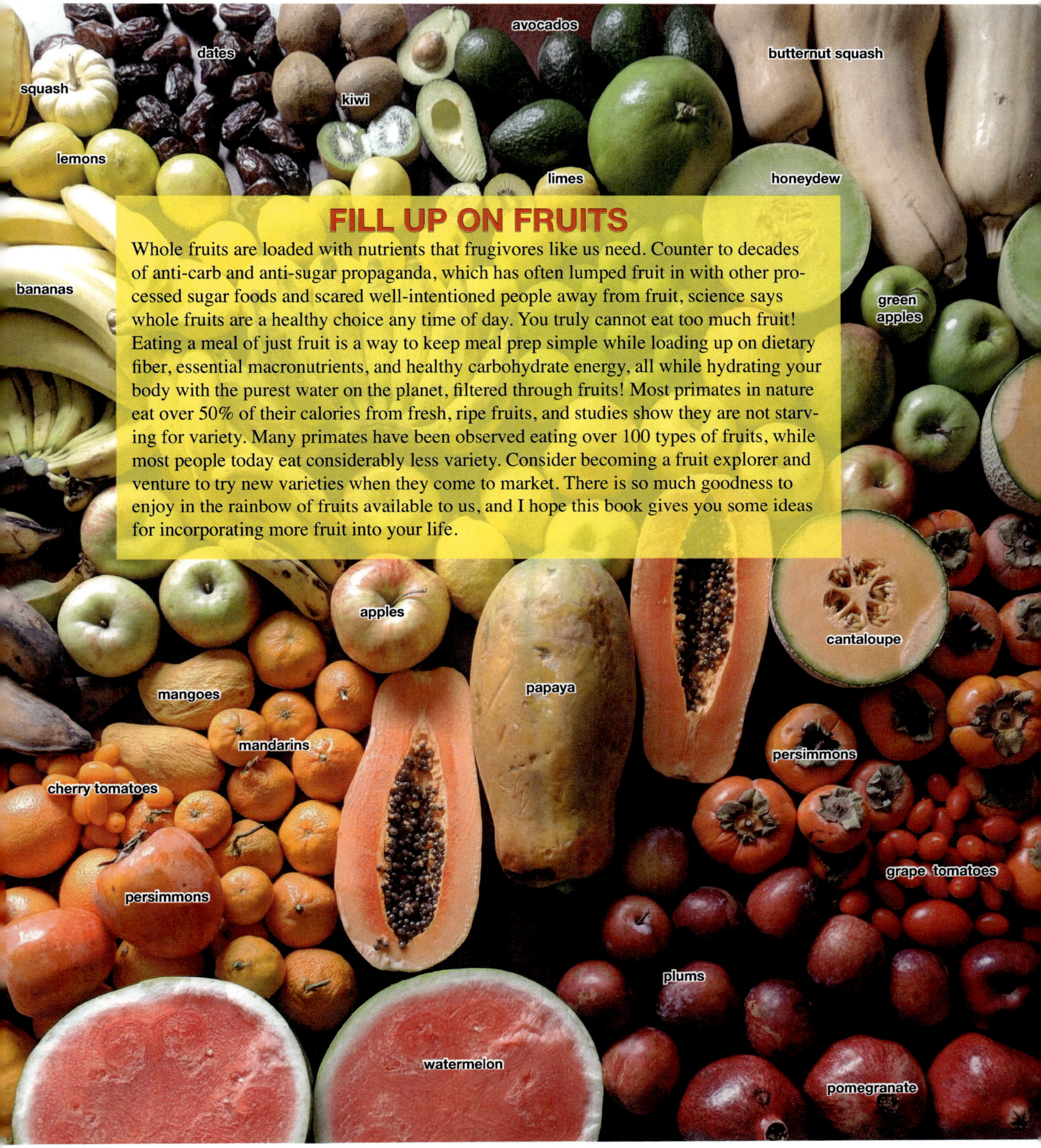

Fill Up On Fruits

ONE-INGREDIENT MONO MEALS

When people realize the nutritional superiority of whole fruits and other plant foods, it is easy to imagine more people experimenting with fruit mono-meals. Again to bust the myth that someone would have to consume an excessive amount of fruit to get by, the chart below proves this isn't so. It is fairly easy to reach 1,000 calories with one fruit alone. If whole fruit numbers seem intimidating, remember it's also possible to consume fruit as juice or blended into a smoothie which many raw foodists say can make consuming large amounts of raw plant foods easier to adjust to. Incorporating juice and smoothies into the diet can also add variety while delivering loads of nutrition. Fresh fruits have been made into a "junk" food by industry-backed junk science and mis-educated health professionals, but the stories people tell about food are changing as real nutrition facts are exposed and shared.

How many fruits make a 500 calorie mono-meal?

Fruit	Calories per piece of fruit	Quantity
Cantaloupe	200	2.5
Avocado	150	3.5
Apple	130	4
Grapefruit	120	4
Banana	110	4.5
Pear	100	5
Orange	80	6.5
Date	67	7
Tangerine	64	8
Nectarine	60	8.5
Peach	60	8..5
Kiwi	50	10
Fig	40	12.5
Plum	35	14.5
Cherries	4.8	104

Notes: Apple and tangerine values are for large fruits. All other values are for medium fruits. Date values are for Medjool dates. Cherry values are for sweet cherries. Nutrient data source: USDA SR-21.

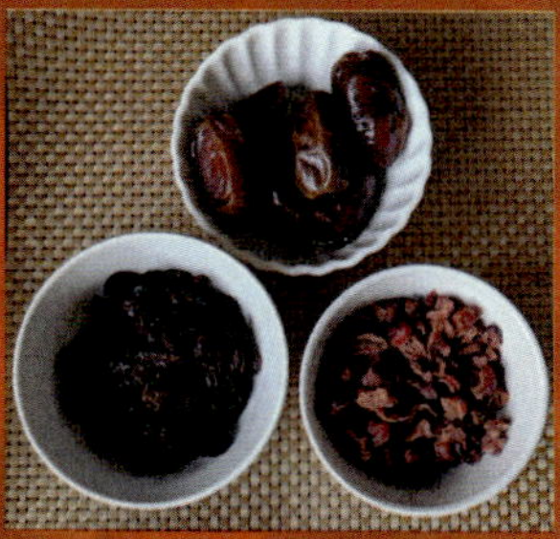

MONO MEALS

While it's essential to get variety in your diet, there is absolutely nothing wrong with enjoying an all-fruit meal or monomeals of a single fruit or other plant. Some people have found healing through eating meals of just potatoes or bananas. Focusing in keeping it simple and enjoying one food at a time can help you tune back into your body's natural hunger and satiation mechanisms.

Purely Fruit Meals

500-Calorie Fruit MonoMeals: NUTRITION FACTS

Nutrients Delivered	Banana	Mango	Kiwi	Strawberries
~500 Calorie Serving Size	5 fruit	4 fruit	9 fruit	86 berries
Calories (exact)	525	540	499	498
Macronutrients				
Carbs	135 g	140.8 g	135 g	120.4 g
Protein	6.5 g	4.4 g	0 g	8.6 g
Fat	2 g	2.4 g	0 g	8.6 g
Fiber	15.5 g	14.8 g	0 g	34.4 g
Water	442 g	676 g	1,163 g	1,410.4 g
Mirconutrients: **Vitamins**				
Vitamin A	377.5 IU	6,336 IU	712.8 IU	189.2 IU
Vitamin B1 (Thiamin)	0.15 mg	0.4 mg	0 mg	0 mg
Vitamin B2 (Riboflavin)	0.5 mg	0.4 mg	0 mg	0 mg
Vitamin B3 (Niacin)	4 mg	4.8 mg	2.7 mg	8.6
Vitamin B5 (Pantothenic Acid)	2 mg	1.2 mg	1.8 mg	0 mg
Vitamin B6	2 mg	1.2 mg	0.9 mg	0 mg
Vitamin B9 (Folate/Folic Acid)	118 mcg	116 mcg	204.3 mcg	369.8 mcg
Vitamin C (Ascorbic Acid)	51.5 mg	229.2	759.6	911.6
Vitamin E	0.5 mg	9.2 mg	11.7 mg	8.6 mg
Vitamin K	3 mcg	34.8 mcg	330.3 mcg	34.4 mcg
Mirconutrients: **Minerals**				
Calcium	29.5 0 mg	82.8 mg	278.1 mg	249.4 mg
Copper	0 0 mg	0.8 mg	0.9 mg	0 mg
Iron	1.5 0 mg	1.2 mg	2.7 mg	8.6 mg
Magnesium	159.5 0 mg	74.4 mg	139.5 mg	197.8 mg
Manganese	1.5 0 mg	0.4 mg	0.9 mg	8.6 mg
Phosphorus	130 0 mg	91.2 mg	278.1 mg	369.8 mg
Potassium (K)	2,110 0 mg	1,292 mg	2,556 mg	2,365 mg
Selenium	6 0 mcg	4.8 mcg	1.8 mcg	8.6 mcg
Sodium	6 0 mg	16.4 mg	24.3 mg	17.2 mg
Zinc	1 0 mg	0.4 mg	0.9 mg	0 mg

POST-PANTRY PURGE: Your New Healthy Pantry Awaits

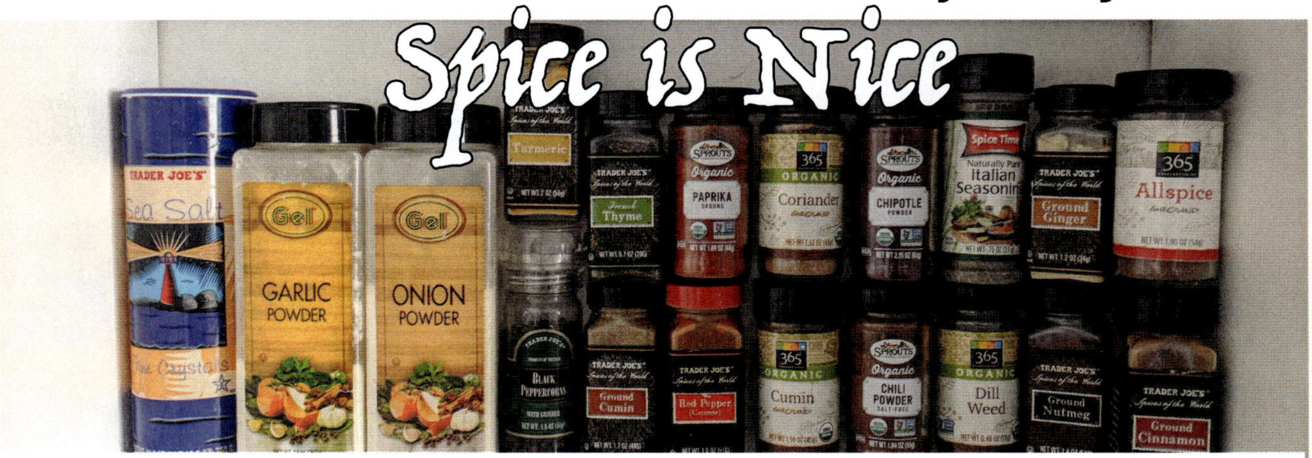
Spice is Nice
Sea Salt
GARLIC POWDER
ONION POWDER
Turmeric
Thyme
PAPRIKA
Coriander
CHIPOTLE
Italian Seasoning
Ground Ginger
Allspice
Black Peppercorns
Ground Cumin
Red Pepper
Cumin
CHILI POWDER
Dill Weed
Ground Nutmeg
Ground Cinnamon

These are the dried spices I keep handy in my pantry and which are used to make the recipes included in this book.

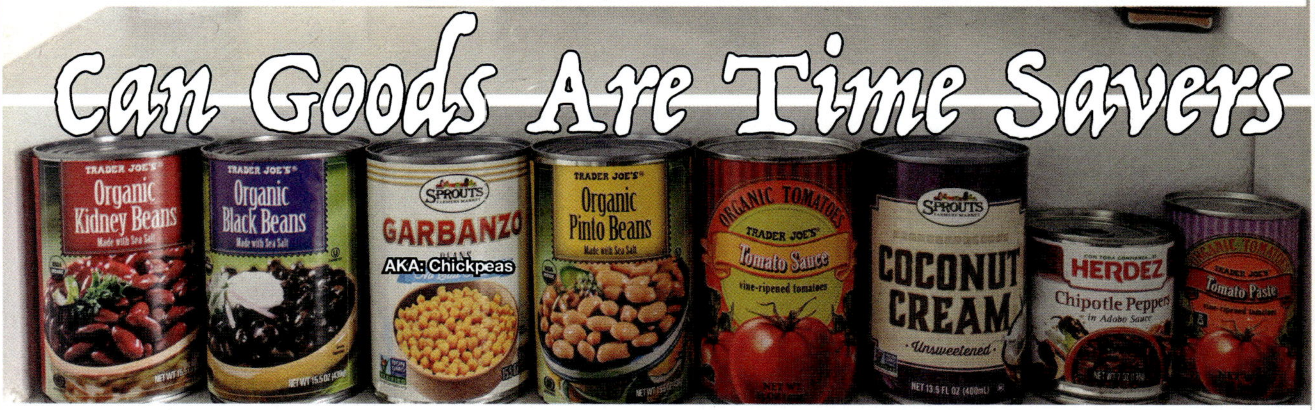
Can Goods Are Time Savers
Organic Kidney Beans
Organic Black Beans
GARBANZO
AKA: Chickpeas
Organic Pinto Beans
Tomato Sauce
COCONUT CREAM
Unsweetened
HERDEZ
Chipotle Peppers in Adobo Sauce
Tomato Paste

If you have these ingredients in your pantry you will be able to make most of the recipes included in this book. While the Frugivore Diet prioritizes whole plant foods, canned goods can be an affordable time-saver that adds ease to your food preparation. Many recipes include just one can of beans or coconut cream for ease. Some recipes call for using a portion of a can of coconut cream or chipotle peppers and you can store the remainders in the fridge for use later.

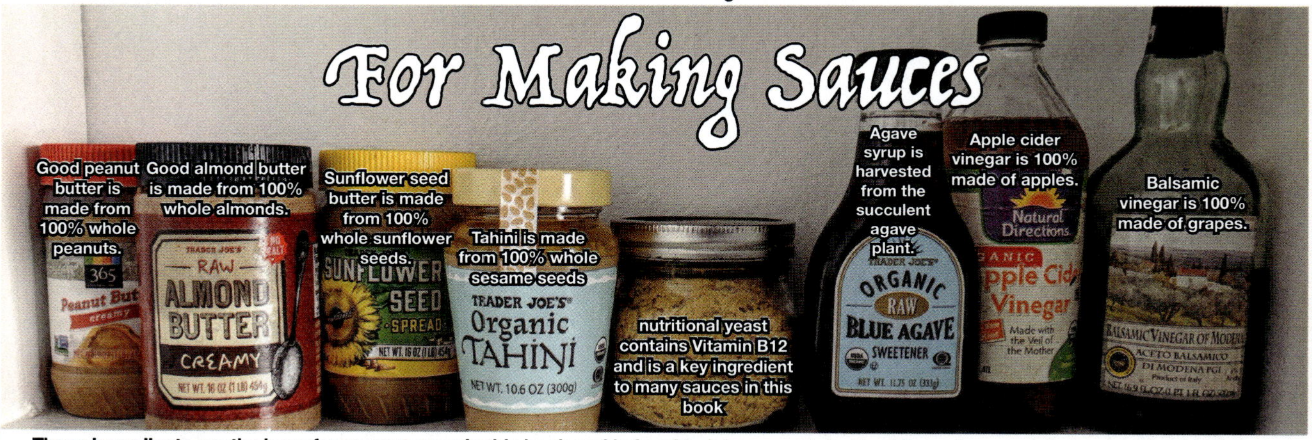
For Making Sauces
Good peanut butter is made from 100% whole peanuts.
Good almond butter is made from 100% whole almonds.
Sunflower seed butter is made from 100% whole sunflower seeds.
Tahini is made from 100% whole sesame seeds
nutritional yeast contains Vitamin B12 and is a key ingredient to many sauces in this book
Agave syrup is harvested from the succulent agave plant.
Apple cider vinegar is 100% made of apples.
Balsamic vinegar is 100% made of grapes.
ALMOND BUTTER
CREAMY
SUNFLOWER SEED SPREAD
Organic TAHINI
ORGANIC RAW BLUE AGAVE SWEETENER
Apple Cider Vinegar
BALSAMIC VINEGAR OF MODENA

These ingredients are the base for many sauces in this book and help add richness and depth of flavor to many whole plant food dishes.

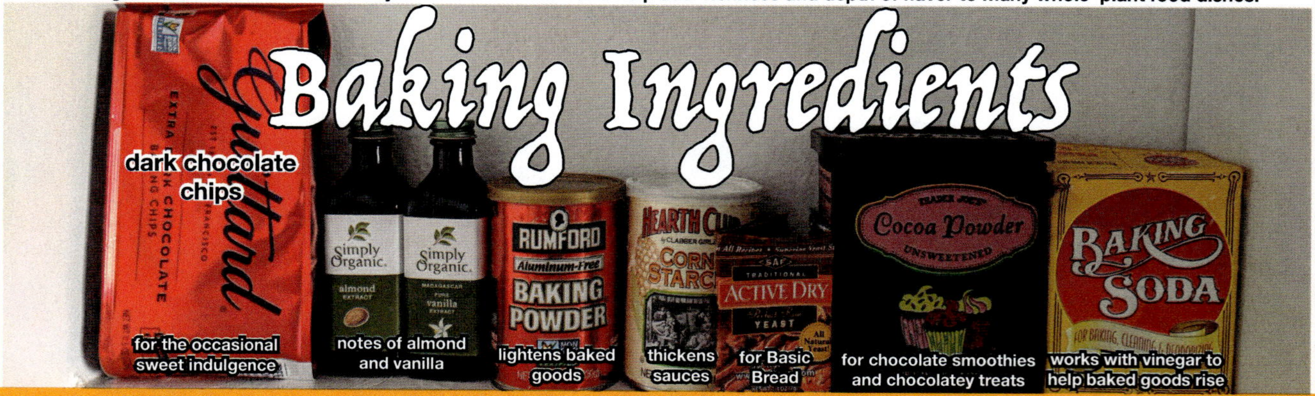
Baking Ingredients
dark chocolate chips
for the occasional sweet indulgence
notes of almond and vanilla
RUMFORD
BAKING POWDER
lightens baked goods
CORN STARCH
thickens sauces
ACTIVE DRY YEAST
for Basic Bread
Cocoa Powder
UNSWEETENED
for chocolate smoothies and chocolatey treats
BAKING SODA
works with vinegar to help baked goods rise

Cooking Vessels: To make the One-Pot Wonders and many of the Savory Sidekicks and Bountiful Bowls in the recipe section of this book, you will need at least one good pot for the stovetop. I recommend investing in a crockpot or slow cooker because of how easy it makes this diet. Most of the One-Pot Wonders can be prepared in a crockpot. Simply chop and combine the ingredients in your crockpot in the morning and go about your day. When you return home later, your home will smell like someone's been hard at work in the kitchen and you will have a warm meal ready and waiting for you.

While some people have a variety of cooking vessels: multiple size pots, rice cooker, slow cooker, steamer, special tea pots, etc., these are not essential. Use what works for you, but don't be discouraged if all you have is a single pot with a lid. There is so much you can do by just starting with that. If you want to do baking, it can help to have a baking sheet, though simple baked potatoes and squash can cook perfectly fine simply placed on the metal bars of your oven's rack. I make frequent use of my glass baking pans for roasted potatoes, baked ch-easy mac, and other whole-plant delights.

TIPS WHEN ON A TIGHT BUDGET

If you're on a budget, here are a few tips to help you succeed:

1. ***Find a good place to shop:*** As already discussed, the best tip to help with your budget is to identify an affordable produce spot. You might have a few stores that you end up frequenting. I go between 99 Cent Only stores for great deals on some basic staples, Trader Joe's or Sprouts for a consistent variety of good quality produce, and a local Hispanic market that has great deals on some of the tropical fruits we love.
2. ***Focus on the most affordable plants:*** Whole-plant staples such as bananas, potatoes, apples, oranges, rice, and beans are almost always affordable options. My local 99 Cents Only stores carry these staples regularly. A bag of rice or a pound of dried beans costs 99 cents. A bag of organic apples or a bag of baking potatoes can be purchased for $2. Meals built around these ingredients can be made very cheaply.
3. ***Don't be afraid to substitute:*** If you don't have one ingredient on hand, feel free to substitute. Black beans are almost always a good substitute for kidney beans and vice versa. Dried herbs can substitute for fresh. Substitute seasonal fruits for more pricey fruits that aren't in season near you.
4. ***Plan for your budget:*** If you are cooking just for yourself it can be easy to make a pot of soup stretch for dinners for the entire week. You can always stretch a pot of soup by including baked potatoes with your soup meals. Bake enough potatoes to last the week and they will be quick and easy to warm up at suppertime. If you are feeding a family, you might need to plan a bit more carefully. Many meals in this book, including the One-Pot Wonders and Bountiful Bowls, are made from the same basic ingredients. If you get a good deal on bananas you can make banana bowls for breakfast and smoothies for after school. If you cook up a large pot of beans you could make a salad with beans for supper one night, a Bountiful Bowl of beans and rice the next night, and baked Taquitos the next.

INVITING PLANTS INTO YOUR LIFE

Once you get going with the Frugivore Diet, you may want to invite plants into your life in more ways than on your fork and spoon. If you have the space, time, and interest, consider starting a garden. Besides growing your own plant foods that will be fresher and tastier than store-bought varieties, you will also benefit in other ways from the practice of gardening. Science has proven there are numeous measurable mental health benefits to gardening, being outside, and simply being around plants.[6] If you are currently land-challenged, like me, there are still ways to invite gardening into your life. I currently am growing baby avocado trees and green onions indoors in my kitchen. Right outside my apartment door I have aloe plants and a large pot containing mint, basil, green onions,

6 For the evidence behind this claim see The Frugivore Files V1—The Psychology File.

tree collards, and a few baby fruit trees I started from seeds. I have also started fruit trees that I have passed onto friends which is fun and rewarding. My dearest friend adopted a few of the avocado trees I started from seed and after just purchasing her first home, is getting ready to plant one in her new back yard.

If you don't have the land for a garden of your own and don't have room inside for many plants there is also the option of adopting a vacant parklet to start a garden in, renting a vacant back-yard space from somebody, or renting a spot in a community garden. At different places in my life I have had the fortune to have a front porch sunny enough for a container garden, land to plant a large kitchen garden, and land to cultivate perennial plants. When I haven't had land of my own, I have found other ways to engage in gardening. I have personally planted gardens in public parklets, rented a vacant backyard where I started a garden, helped start a garden in a friends backyard, and have enjoyed watching the plants growing in the community garden where I teach. I have started papaya trees and date trees in ziploc bags on top of my fridge and avocado trees in pots on the kitchen windowsill. Where there's a will, there's a way, and growing plants is a great way to relax, learn more about plants, and grow skills you might need for a healthy and self-reliant future.

GROWING A HEALTHY FUTURE

If you have the space available, consider planting a fruit tree or two, or several. Fruit trees generally are easy to grow once established and produce an abundance of delicious and nutritious fruits for decades to come. According to my calculation, using typical fruit-tree productivity data, just eight fruit trees could feed you delicious nutrient-rich hydrating food, supplying most of your calorie needs year-round. This is of course a rough estimate. The productivity of your edible forest garden will depend on the type of tree, age of the tree, climate, rainfall or watering, and numerous other factors such as soil type, presence or absence of pests, location of plant relative to the sun, and more. The most repeated wisdom about fruit trees is that the best time to plant a fruit tree was ten years ago. Still, the second best time to plant a fruit tree is today. Fruit trees take time to grow, but once they do, most are prolific producers.

...More Recipes, Nutrition Info, Resources...

On the following pages you will find a suggested meal plan and shopping list including the most common ingredients needed to make the recipes in this book. Once you clean out your pantry and fill your fridge and fruit basket with healthy, whole plants, you will be ready to rock and roll on the way to a healthier you. With the new energy you receive from your natural diet, you may want to explore even more nutrition science, whole-plant recipes, and resources to help you on your way. Visit my website at www.HealingWithPlants.us for more resources to help you thrive on the Frugivore Diet. There I include recipes, healing stories, and nutrition science articles with links to numerous scientific studies which I purposefully have left out of this book so as not to bog you down. If you want to explore the science and evidence backing this diet in greater depth, you will want to check out *The Frugivore Files* where I make the bullet-proof case that our natural diet is a fruit-rich rainbow of whole-plant foods.

Finally, I wish you the best transitioning to your natural diet, the *Frugivore Diet* your human body is designed to thrive on.

Eat Your Shoots

EXPLORE FRESH HERBS

While dried herbs are great because they are cheap, readily available, and store on the shelf with ease, fresh herbs can add another level of flavor to the meals you create. If you aren't used to using fresh herbs, I suggest experimenting with one at a time. Fresh garlic and ginger are great places to start. Fresh parsley, basil, and cilantro add tantalizing flavor to many dishes. I like to keep fresh herbs in my fridge at all times and I prefer fresh if I have them available, though I also frequently use dried herbs. On page 20 you can see the dried herbs I keep in my pantry and use to create the recipes in this book. Below, I photographed the fresh green herbs I use in these recipes (I also love using fresh ginger and garlic). Feel free to convert dried to fresh or fresh to dried in the recipes depending on what you have available. To help, here's basic conversion rates for the most common herbs.

Fresh Herbs Add Flavor

Fresh to Dry Herb Conversation Rate

Herb	Fresh	Dry
Basil	2 tbsp.	1 tbsp.
Cilantro	1 tbsp.	2 tbsp.
Dill	1 tbsp.	1 tsp.
Garlic	1 clove	1/2 tsp.
Ginger	1 tbsp.	1/4 tsp.
Parsley	1 tbsp.	1 tsp.
Rosemary	1 tbsp.	1 tsp.
Sage	1 tbsp.	1 tsp.
Thyme	1 tbsp.	3/4 tsp.

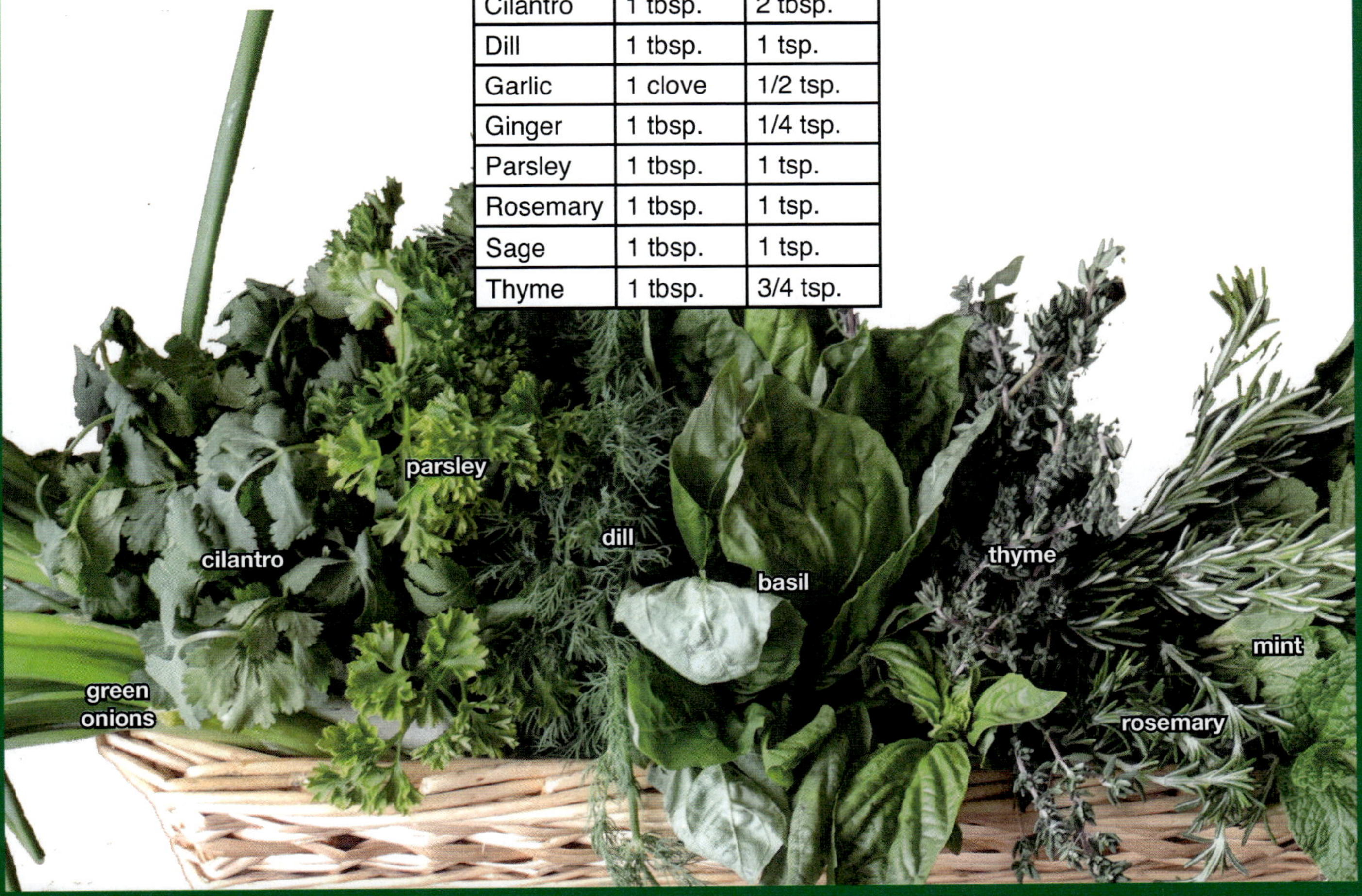

Eat Your Roots

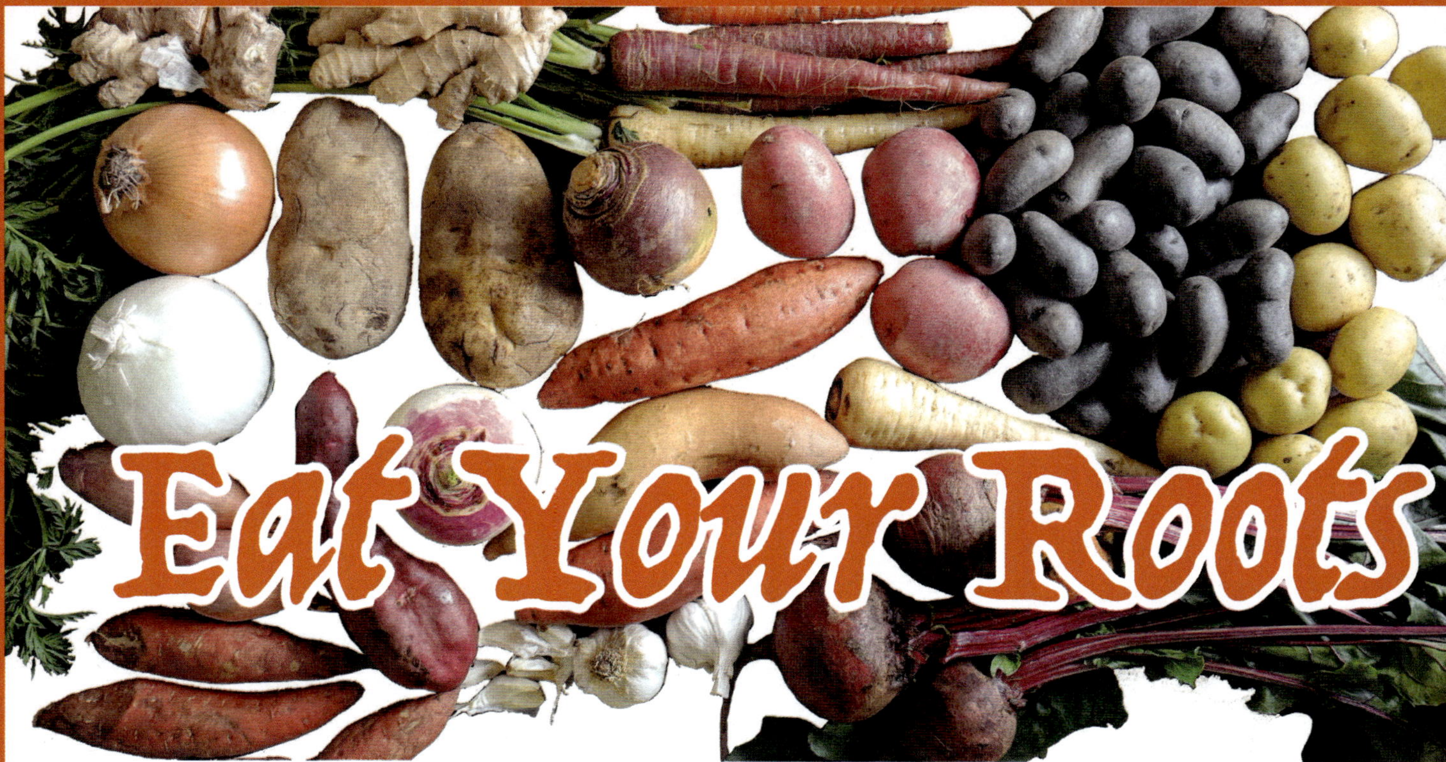

DIG INTO ROOTS

Potatoes, yams, sweet potatoes, parsnips, beets, turnips, rutabagas, carrots, onions, ginger, garlic, turmeric, horseradish, jicama, Jerusalem artichokes, and radishes are all roots that are central to the diets of people around the world. While some of the foods in this group—such as potatoes, yams, and sweet potatoes—are technically tubers (the elongated stems and storage organs of these plants) and others like onions and garlic are technically bulbs (another type of elongated stem that's also a storage organ for these plants) most people classify these foods as roots simply because they grow underground. Edible roots are the delicious and nutritious plant parts that we can't see before we dig them up. When we do, they reward us with a nutritious source of energy that's delicious baked, steamed, or boiled. Roots such as potatoes and yams can easily be the staple food of a healthy diet and there are endless ways to prepare them into tasty meals. Other roots such as onions, garlic, turmeric, and ginger are powerful spices and medicinal plant parts that confer many health benefits. Just consider all the nutrition in one large Russet potato baked (299 g):

NUTRITION IN 1 BAKED POTATO

- Calories: 290 g

MACRONUTRIENTS:

- Carbohydrates: 64.1 g
- Protein: 7.9 g
- Fat: 0.4 g
- Omega-3 fatty acids: 29.9 mg
- Omega-6 fatty acids: 95.7 mg
- Fiber: 6.9 g
- Water: 223 g

VITAMINS:

- Vitamin A: 29.9 IU, 1%
- Vitamin C: 38.6 mg, 64%
- Vitamin E: 0.1 mg, 1%
- Vitamin K: 6.0, mcg, 7%
- Thiamin: 0.2 mg, 13%
- Riboflavin: 0.1 mg, 8%
- Niacin: 4.0 mg, 25%
- Vitamin B6: 1.1 mg, 53%
- Folate: 77.7 mcg, 19%
- Pantothenic Acid: 1.1 mg, 11%
- Choline: 44.8 mg
- Betaine: 0.6 mg

MINERALS:

- Calcium: 53.8 mg, 5%
- Iron: 3.2 mg, 18%
- Magnesium: 89.7 mg 22%
- Phosphorus: 212 mg, 21%
- Potassium: 1645 mg, 47%
- Sodium: 41.9 mg, 2%
- Zinc: 1.0 mg, 7%
- Copper: 0.3 mg, 16%
- Manganese: 0.7 mg, 34%
- Selenium: 1.5 mcg, 2%

How many roots make a 500 calorie mono-meal?

ROOT	Calories per root	Quantity
Potato, baked (medium)	161	3
Sweet potato, baked (medium)	103	5
Yam, 1 cup boiled	158	3
Carrot (large, 72g)	30	17

Eat Your Seeds

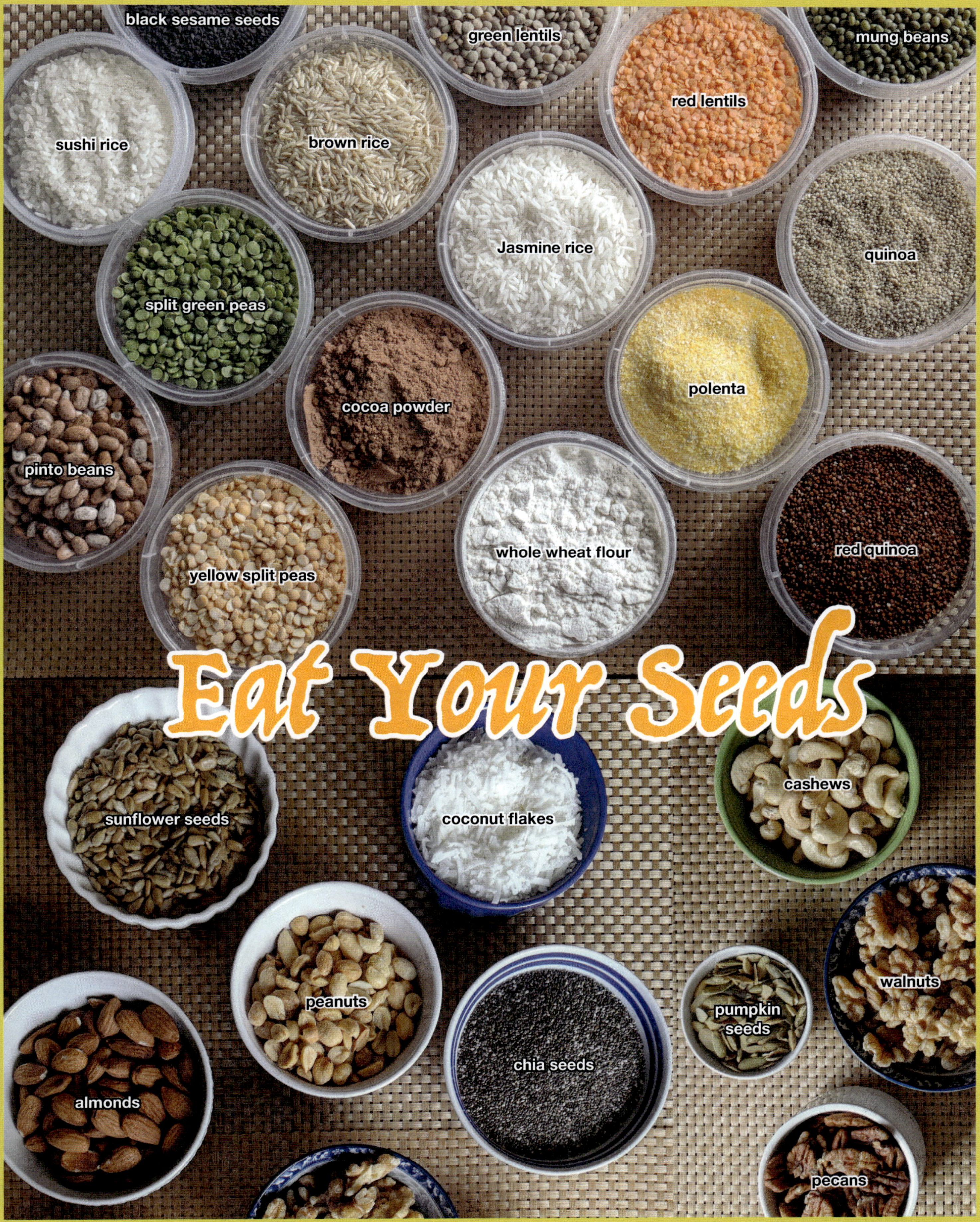

The 28-Day Life Changer

4-WEEK FRUGIVORE DIET MEAL PLAN

Use the meal plan below as a rough guide to help you organize your transition to a diet of health and wellness. Since how much food you make depends on how many people you are serving and how active you and your family are, it is impossible for me to create a plan here that will work for everyone.

WEEK 1: If you are cooking for just you, then it's likely you can make one recipe stretch over more than one meal, potentially over two or three days. A big pot of soup could last a single person the entire week or could be gobbled up by a large family in a single meal. So feel free to modify this to work for you based on your family size, budget, and what foods are in season and available to you.

MEALS	MON	TUES	WED	THURS	FRI	SAT	SUN
BREAKFAST	Simply Mangoes Platter	Mango Banana Bowl	Fruit Flowers + Cucumber Avocado Toast	Citrus Platter	Banana Plate	Persimmon Smoothie Bowl	I am Royalty Fruit Platter
LUNCH	Seven Greens Salad	Open Face Pizza Sandwich	Marinated Cucumbers and Heavenly Hummus Sandwich	Rainbow Sticks N' Hummus	Seedy Slaw	Garden Sushi Cups	Chickpea Tacos
DINNER	Lentil Lover Soup	Vegetable Curry Soup	Red Rice n Beans Bowl	Roasted Potato Bowl	Chickpeas N' Rice Bowl	Green Power Soup	Mashed Potatoes and Gravy
SNACK/ DESSERT	Chocolate Shake	Pineapple Lime Crush	Peppermint Smoothie	Peppermint Smoothie	Peanut Butter Balls	Peanut Butter Balls	Peanut Butter Balls

WEEK 2: Also remember that a simple baked potato or butternut squash can make a meal on its own and simply adding some fresh greens and one of the sauces here can make it a tasty and satisfying meal.

MEALS	MON	TUES	WED	THURS	FRI	SAT	SUN
BREAKFAST	Citrus Platter	Tri-Fruita Bowls	Bananas for Bananas	Blueberry Banana Chia Pudding	Simply Strawberries	Strawberry Banana Bowl	Fruit Balls Salad
LUNCH	Cucumber Salad	Chickpea of the Sea Salad with greens	Rainbow Salad	Pinto Beans N' Rice Bowl	Taquito	Fresh Spring Rolls	Peanut Butter Tofu Salad
DINNER	Irish Garden Stew	Ch-Easy Mac	Rainbow Rice N' Tofu Bowl	Vegetable Soup	Red Pepper & Corn Chowder	Red Pepper & Corn Chowder	Curry Cabbage
SNACK/ DESSERT	Mango Smoothie	Raspberry Nice-cream	Fresh Mint Lemonade	Fresh Mint Lemonade	Chocolate Sunflower Balls	Chocolate Sunflower Balls	Chocolate Sunflower Balls

WEEK 3: I have gone weeks of eating banana bowls for breakfast every morning.

MEALS	MON	TUES	WED	THURS	FRI	SAT	SUN
BREAKFAST	Simple Mandarins Bowl	Apple Salad	Fruit Flowers + Cucumber Avocado Toast	Purely Pineapple	Papaya Boats	Trinity Greens Fruit Salad	Scrambled Tofu, Almond Milk Biscuit, and Breakfast Gravy
LUNCH	Pear Mandarin Green Salad	King Kale Salad	Peas and Carrots and Brown Rice	Baked Sweet Potato and Yellow Rice	Carrot Salad	Basic Baked Tofu and Mushroom Risotto	Garden Sushi Salad
DINNER	Roots Stew	Squash on Squash	Split Pea Soup	Vegetable Curry Bowl	Tortilla Soup	Yam Curry Soup	Green Potato Soup
SNACK/ DESSERT	Watermelon Icee	Blueberry Nice-cream	Cinnamon Banini Shake	Piña Colada Smoothie	Mango Nice-cream	Mint Tea	Mint Tea

WEEK 4: Do what works for you in your budget. Enjoy, and cheers to your health!

MEALS	MON	TUES	WED	THURS	FRI	SAT	SUN
BREAKFAST	Kiwi Mandala Plate	Tri-Fruita Bowls	The Real Grape Nuts	Overnight Mango Chia Pudding	Citrus Platter	Melon Bowls	I am Royalty Fruit Platter
LUNCH	Green Potato Salad	Rainbow Salad	Go Garbanzo Bowl	3 Sisters Salad	Caribbean Rice N' Beans	Caribbean Rice N' Beans	Rainbow Raw Tacos
DINNER	Broccoli Bowl	Vegetable Curry Bowl	Mushroom Barley Soup	Steamed Broccoli Baked Potato and	3 Bean Chili	Red Lentil Coconut Curry	Potato Chowder
SNACK/ DESSERT	Blueberry Blissard	Mango Lime Crush	Grape Icee	Ginger Tea	Ginger Tea	Mom's Hot Cocoa	Mom's Hot Cocoa

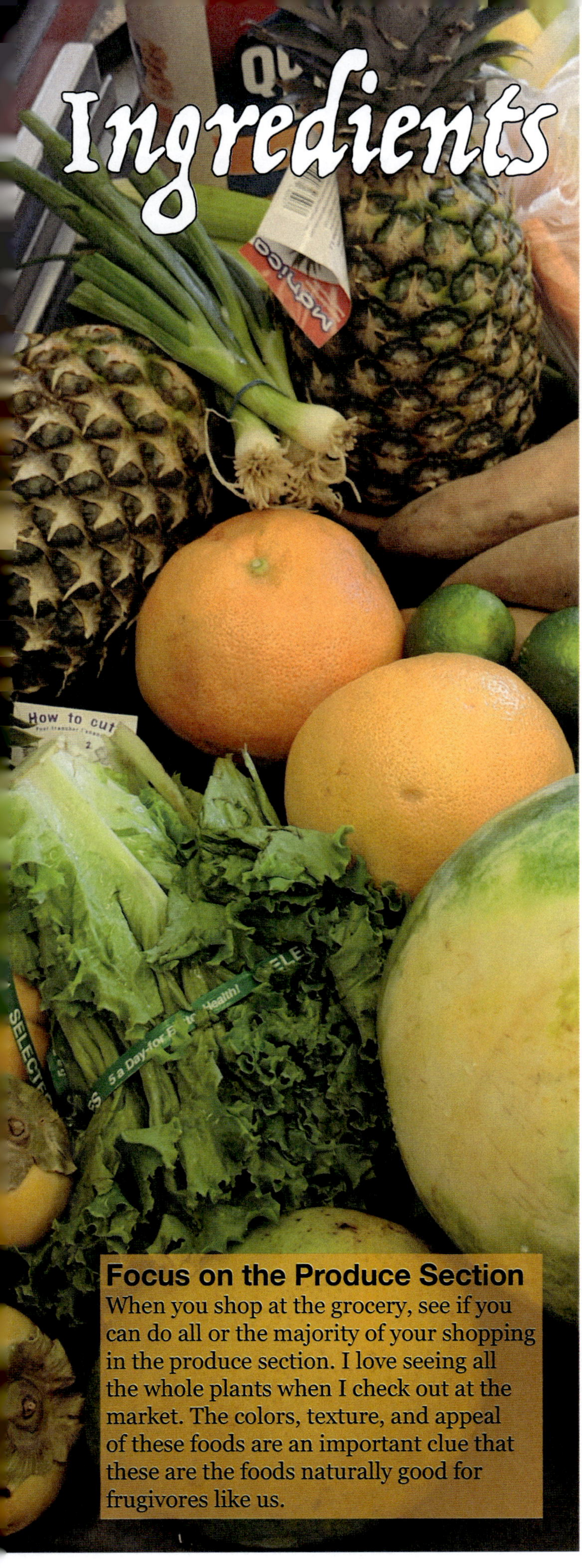

Ingredients

Focus on the Produce Section

When you shop at the grocery, see if you can do all or the majority of your shopping in the produce section. I love seeing all the whole plants when I check out at the market. The colors, texture, and appeal of these foods are an important clue that these are the foods naturally good for frugivores like us.

FRUGIVORE DIET SHOPPING LIST

Flowers

- ❍ artichoke hearts
- ❍ broccoli
- ❍ cauliflower

Fruits

- ❍ apples: fresh & cider vinegar
- ❍ apricots
- ❍ avocados
- ❍ bananas: fresh & frozen
- ❍ bell pepper: red, green, yellow
- ❍ blackberries
- ❍ black pepper: dried & ground
- ❍ blueberries: fresh & frozen
- ❍ butternut squash
- ❍ cantaloupe
- ❍ cayenne pepper: dried & ground
- ❍ cranberries: dried
- ❍ chili peppers: fresh, dried, ground
- ❍ cucumbers
- ❍ dates
- ❍ delicatta squash
- ❍ grapes: fresh
- ❍ grapes: dried—raisins
- ❍ grapefruits
- ❍ honeydew melon
- ❍ kiwis
- ❍ lemons
- ❍ limes
- ❍ mangoes: fresh & frozen
- ❍ oranges
- ❍ papaya
- ❍ peaches
- ❍ pear
- ❍ persimmons
- ❍ pineapple: fresh & frozen
- ❍ plums
- ❍ pomegranate
- ❍ pummelo
- ❍ pumpkin
- ❍ raspberries: fresh & frozen
- ❍ spaghetti squash
- ❍ strawberries: fresh & frozen
- ❍ tangerines
- ❍ tomato: fresh, cherry, red, yellow, paste, sauce
- ❍ tomatillos
- ❍ watermelon
- ❍ zucchini squash

Roots

- ❍ beets
- ❍ carrots
- ❍ garlic: fresh and dried
- ❍ ginger: fresh and dried
- ❍ onion: red, white, yellow, green, fresh and dried
- ❍ parsnip
- ❍ potatoes: Russet, white, red
- ❍ radish
- ❍ rutabaga
- ❍ shallots
- ❍ sweet potato
- ❍ turmeric: fresh and dried
- ❍ turnip
- ❍ yams

Shoots

SALAD GREENS

- ❍ arugula
- ❍ butter lettuce
- ❍ cabbage, green and red
- ❍ celery
- ❍ collards
- ❍ endive
- ❍ green lettuce
- ❍ green onions
- ❍ horseradish
- ❍ kale
- ❍ mustard greens
- ❍ red lettuce
- ❍ romaine lettuce
- ❍ spinach

HERBS FOR FLAVOR

- ❍ basil
- ❍ cilantro
- ❍ dill
- ❍ lemongrass
- ❍ mint
- ❍ parsley
- ❍ rosemary
- ❍ sage
- ❍ thyme

Seeds

BEANS & LEGUMES

- ❍ black beans
- ❍ chickpeas
- ❍ edamame, fresh
- ❍ green beans
- ❍ kidney beans
- ❍ lentils, brown
- ❍ lentils, red
- ❍ mung beans
- ❍ navy beans
- ❍ peas, fresh green
- ❍ peas: split green
- ❍ peas: split yellow
- ❍ pinto beans
- ❍ soy sauce
- ❍ tempeh (soy bean and grains)
- ❍ tofu (soy bean)

GRAINS

- ❍ barley
- ❍ brown rice
- ❍ corn: fresh
- ❍ corn meal
- ❍ Jasmine rice
- ❍ polenta (coarsely ground cornmeal)
- ❍ sushi rice
- ❍ wheat flour

NUTS & OTHER SEEDS

- ❍ almonds: whole, ground, & milk
- ❍ cacao: powder, dark chocolate chips
- ❍ cashews
- ❍ chia seeds
- ❍ coconut: flakes, cream, milk
- ❍ peanuts: whole & ground
- ❍ pecans
- ❍ pumpkin seeds
- ❍ sesame: whole & ground, tahini
- ❍ sunflower seeds: whole & ground
- ❍ walnuts

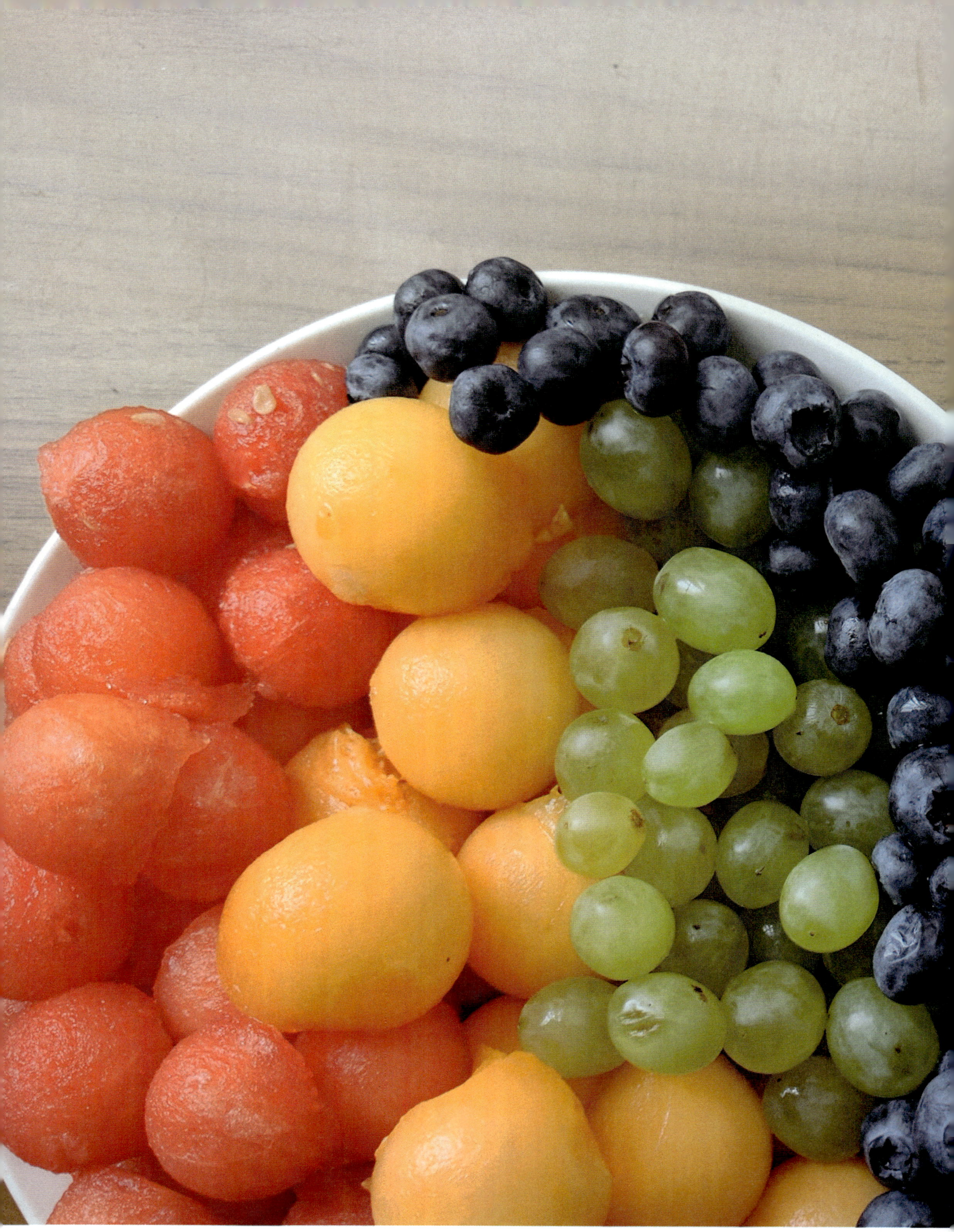

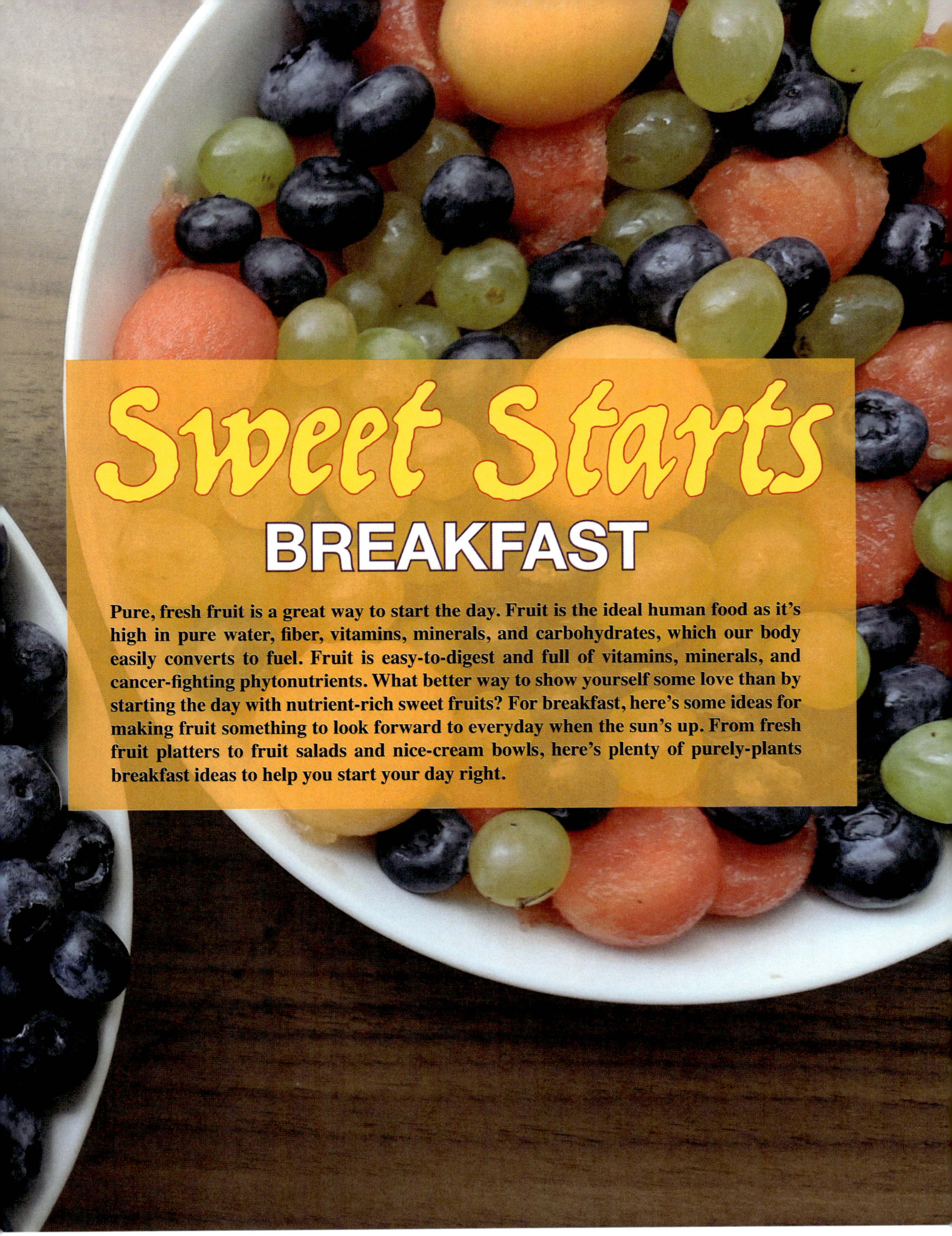

Sweet Starts

BREAKFAST

Pure, fresh fruit is a great way to start the day. Fruit is the ideal human food as it's high in pure water, fiber, vitamins, minerals, and carbohydrates, which our body easily converts to fuel. Fruit is easy-to-digest and full of vitamins, minerals, and cancer-fighting phytonutrients. What better way to show yourself some love than by starting the day with nutrient-rich sweet fruits? For breakfast, here's some ideas for making fruit something to look forward to everyday when the sun's up. From fresh fruit platters to fruit salads and nice-cream bowls, here's plenty of purely-plants breakfast ideas to help you start your day right.

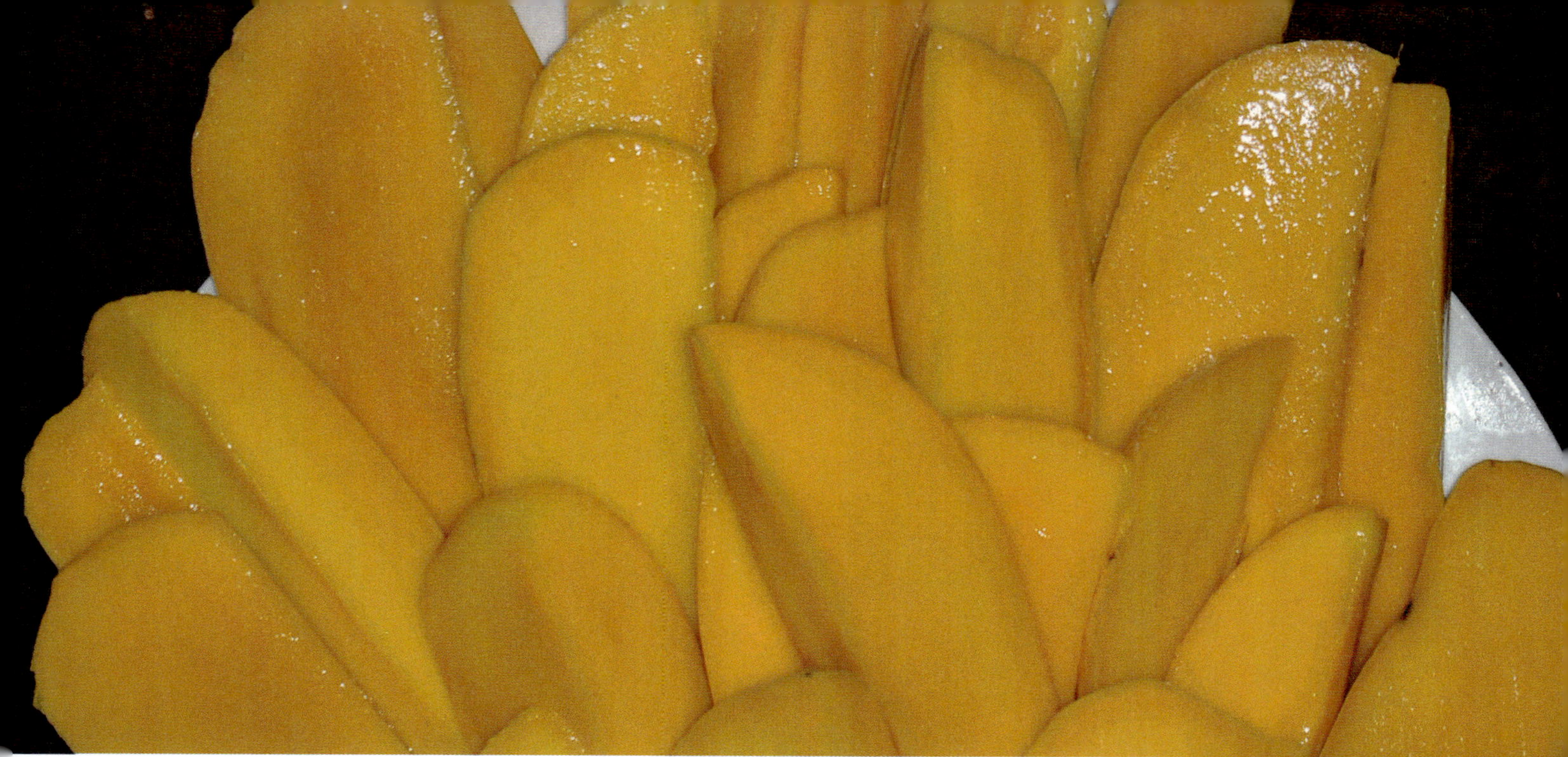

SIMPLY MANGOES

Just mangoes to make your mouth water.

Mango Nutrition Facts

Nutrients Delivered	1 Mango
Calories	135
Macronutrients	
Carbs	35.2 g
Protein	1.1 g
Fat	0.6 g
Fiber	3.7 g
Water	169 g
Mirconutrients: Vitamins	
Vitamin A	1584 IU
Vitamin B1 (Thiamin)	0.1 mg
Vitamin B2 (Riboflavin)	0.1 mg
Vitamin B3 (Niacin)	1.2 mg
Vitamin B5 (Pantothenic Acid)	0.3 mg
Vitamin B6	0.3 mg
Vitamin B9 (Folate/Folic Acid)	29 mg
Vitamin C (Ascorbic Acid)	57.3 mg
Vitamin E	2.3 mg
Vitamin K	8.7 mcg
Mirconutrients: Minerals	
Calcium	20.7 mg
Copper	0.2 mg
Iron	0.3 mg
Magnesium	18.6 mg
Manganese	0.1 mg
Phosphorus	22.8 mg
Potassium (K)	323 mg
Selenium	1.2 mcg
Sodium	4.1 mg
Zinc	0.1 mg

INGREDIENT:

- 4 mangoes

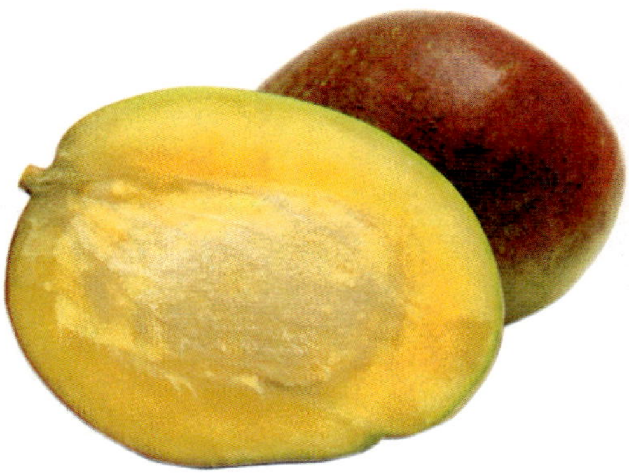

STEPS:

1. Slice mangoes and remove any bad spots with a knife.
2. Arrange mango slices onto plate.
3. Enjoy!

DELICIOUS WITH:

- Almond milk
- Orange juice
- Banana slices
- Lime squeeze
- Sprinkle of shredded coconut

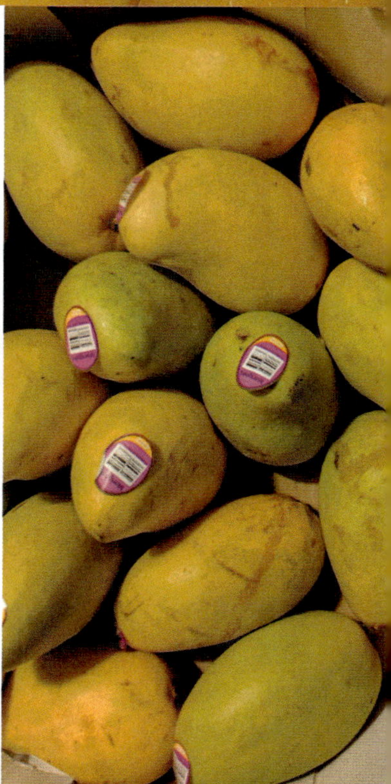

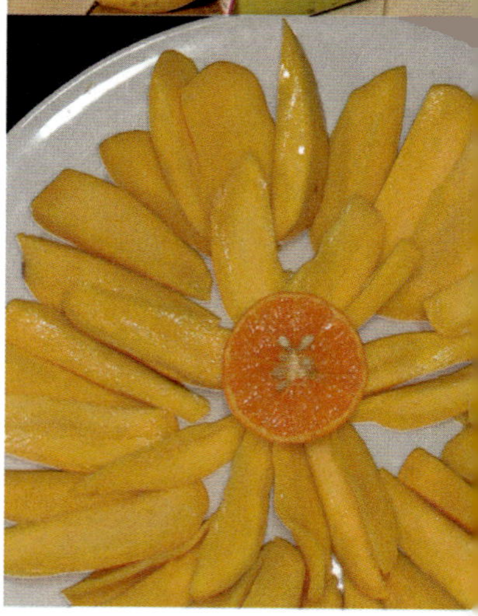

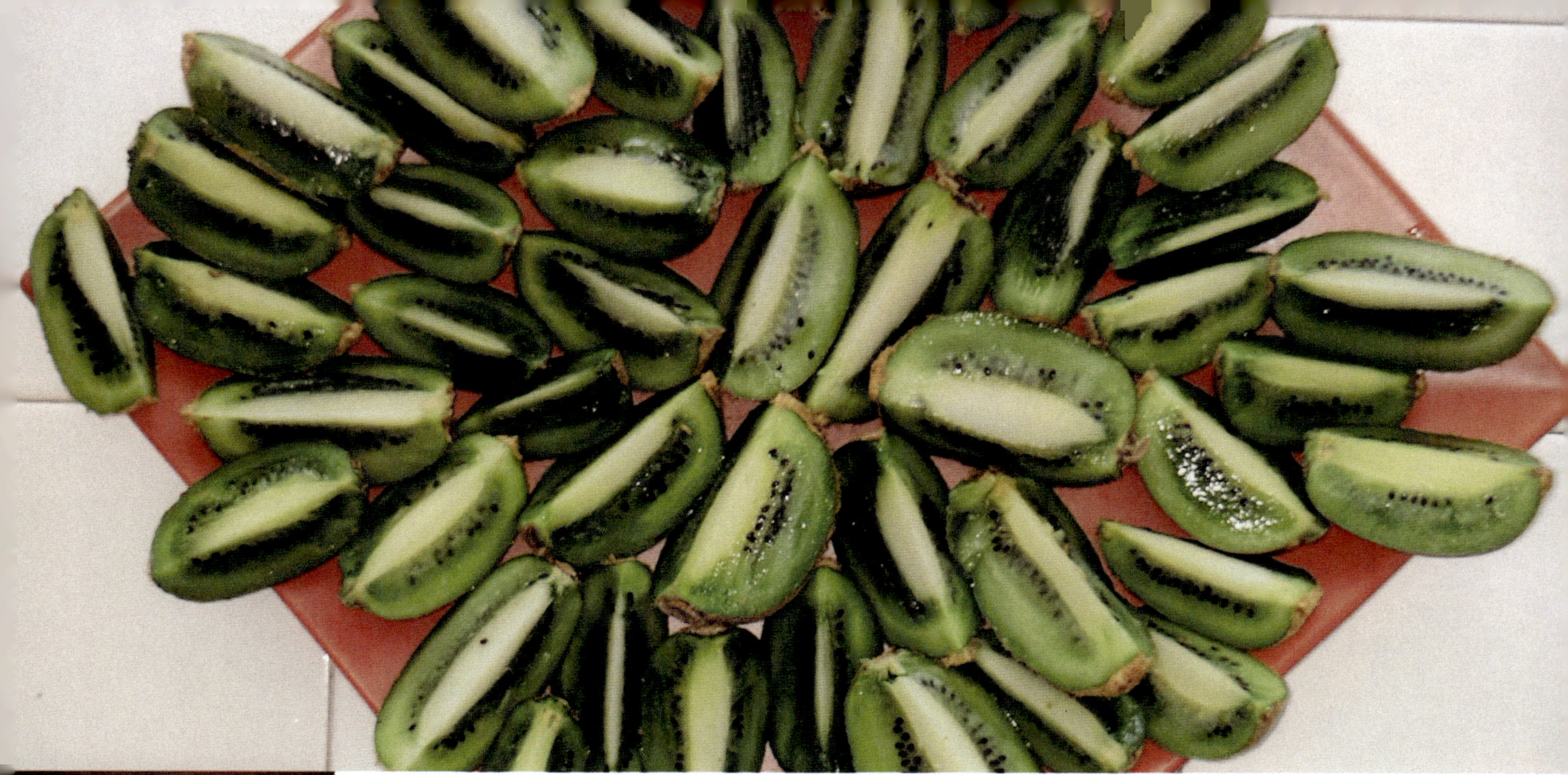

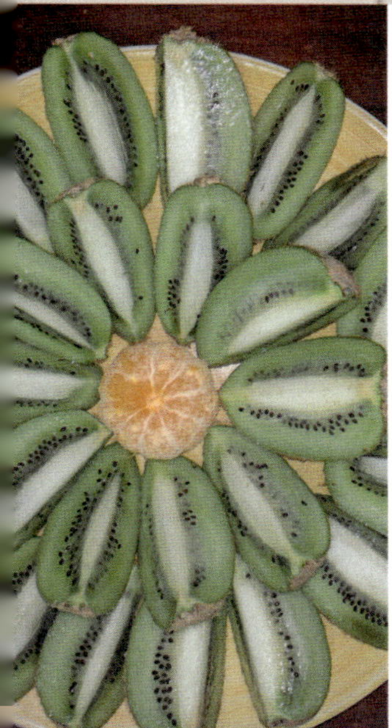

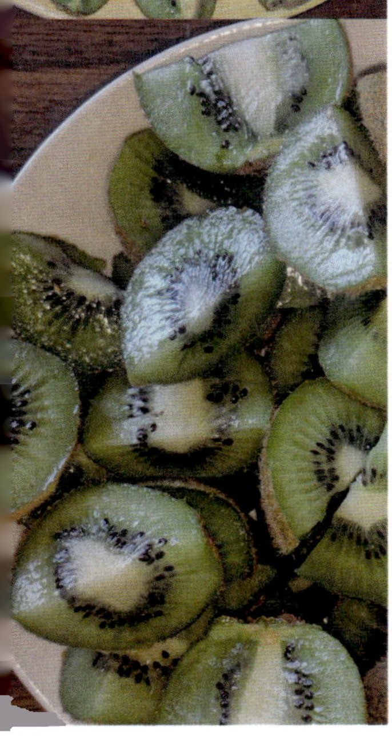

KIWI MANDALA PLATE

A copious plate of kiwis fit for a king.

INGREDIENT:

- 6–10 kiwis

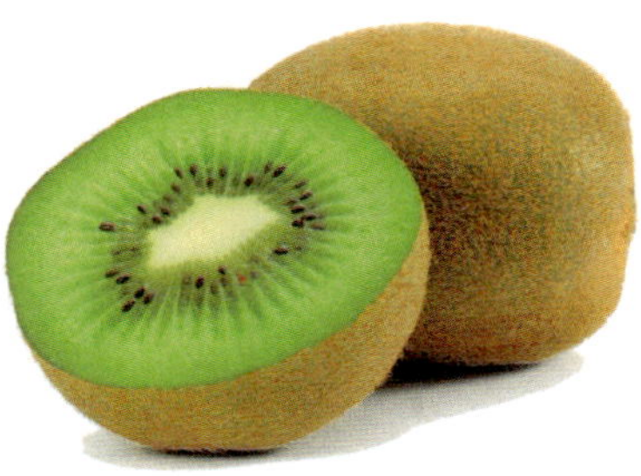

STEPS:

1. Slice kiwi into wedges or into round slices that are halved.
2. Arrange kiwi slices onto plate in a circular fashion.
3. Enjoy!

Kiwi Nutrition Facts

Nutrients Delivered	1 Kiwi
Calories	55.5
Macronutrients	
Carbs	13.3 g
Protein	1 g
Fat	0.5 g
Fiber	2.7 g
Water	75.6 g
Mirconutrients: Vitamins	
Vitamin A	79.2 IU
Vitamin B1 (Thiamin)	0 mg
Vitamin B2 (Riboflavin)	0 mg
Vitamin B3 (Niacin)	0.3 mg
Vitamin B5 (Pantothenic Acid)	0.2 mg
Vitamin B6	0.1 mg
Vitamin B9 (Folate/Folic Acid)	22.7 mg
Vitamin C (Ascorbic Acid)	84.4 mg
Vitamin E	1.3 mg
Vitamin K	36.7 mcg
Mirconutrients: Minerals	
Calcium	30.9 mg
Copper	0.1 mg
Iron	0.3 mg
Magnesium	15.5 mg
Manganese	0.1 mg
Phosphorus	30.9 mg
Potassium (K)	284 mg
Selenium	0.2 mcg
Sodium	2.7 mg
Zinc	0.1 mg

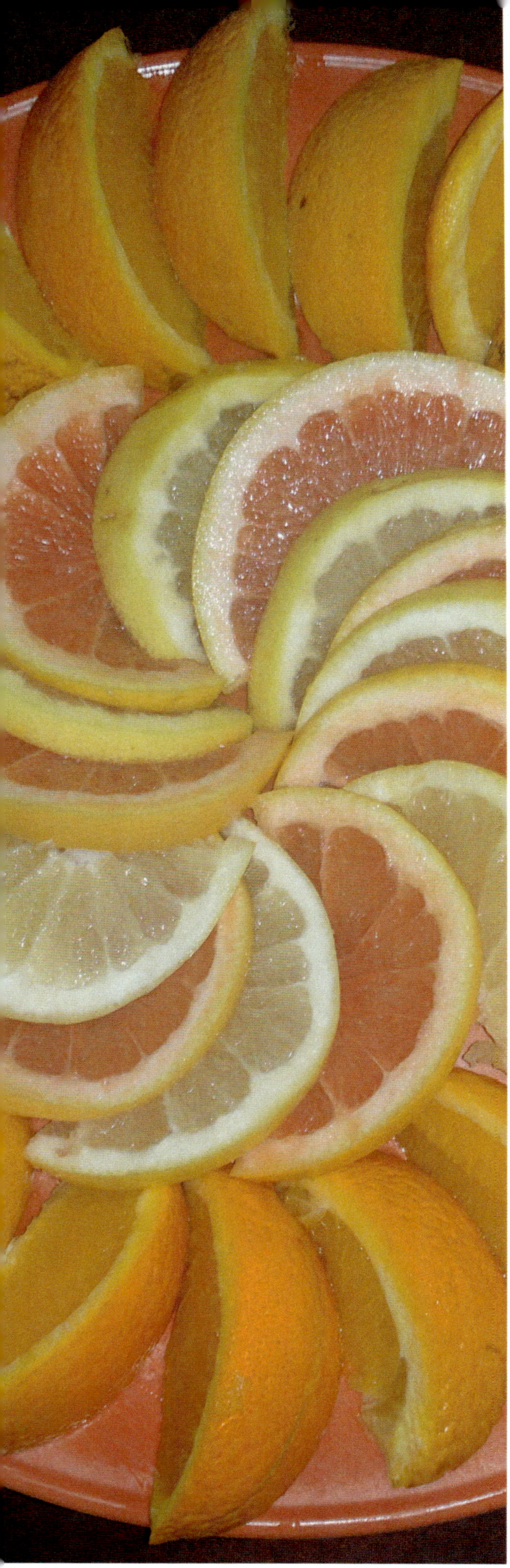

CITRUS MANDALA PLATE

Sweet, sun-fired, citrus shapes to tantalize the taste buds.

INGREDIENT:

- 5–8 citrus fruits

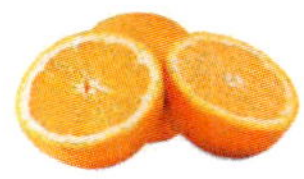

STEPS:

1. Slice citrus into wedges or into round slices that are halved.
2. Arrange citrus slices onto plate in a circular fashion.
3. Voilà, enjoy!

Orange Nutrition Facts

Nutrients Delivered	1 Orange
Calories	68.6
Macronutrients	
Carbs	17.6 g
Protein	1.3 g
Fat	0.2 g
Fiber	3.1 g
Water	120 g
Mirconutrients: Vitamins	
Vitamin A	346 IU
Vitamin B1 (Thiamin)	0.1 mg
Vitamin B2 (Riboflavin)	0.1 mg
Vitamin B3 (Niacin)	0.6 mg
Vitamin B5 (Pantothenic Acid)	0.4 mg
Vitamin B6	0.1 mg
Vitamin B9 (Folate/Folic Acid)	47.6 mg
Vitamin C (Ascorbic Acid)	82.8 mg
Vitamin E	0.2 mg
Mirconutrients: Minerals	
Calcium	60.2 mg
Copper	0.1 mg
Iron	0.2 mg
Magnesium	15.4 mg
Phosphorus	32.2 mg
Potassium (K)	232 mg
Selenium	0 mcg
Sodium	1.4 mg
Zinc	0.1 mg

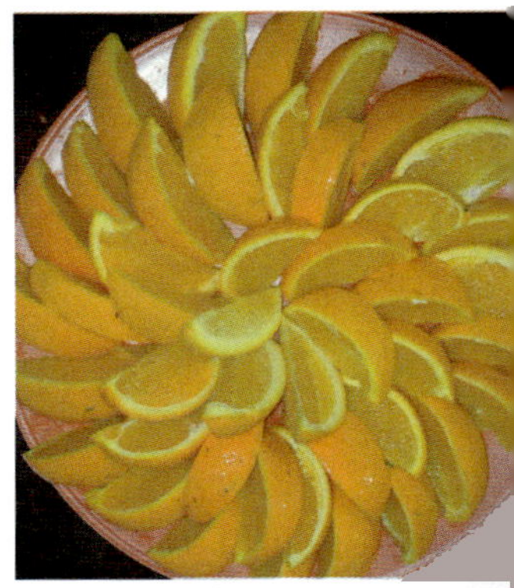

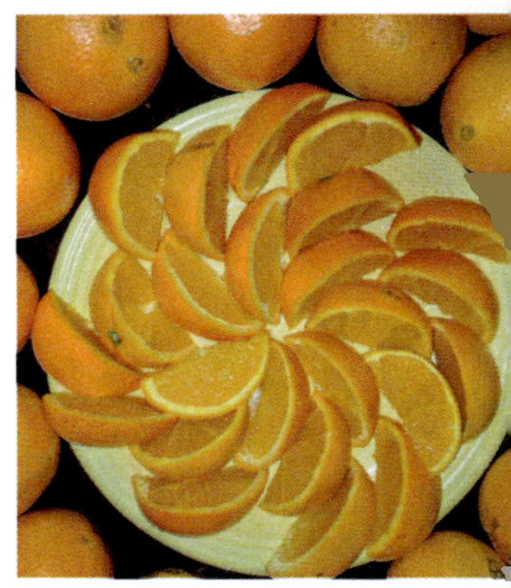

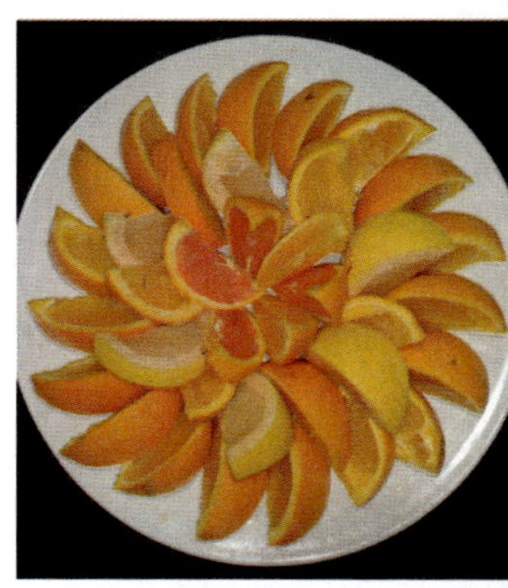

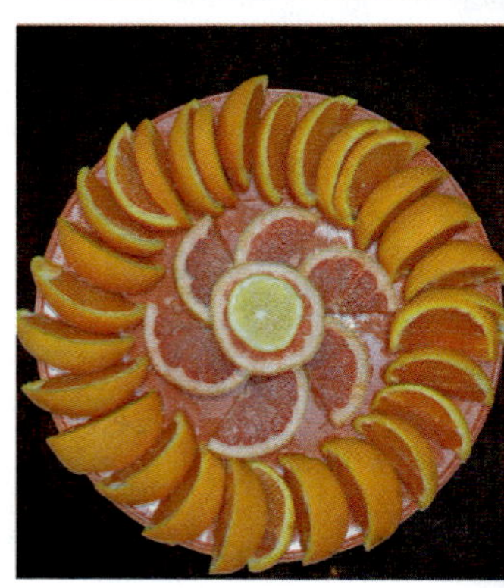

MANDARINS FOR MY MEAL

When a bowl of sweet clementines is all you need.

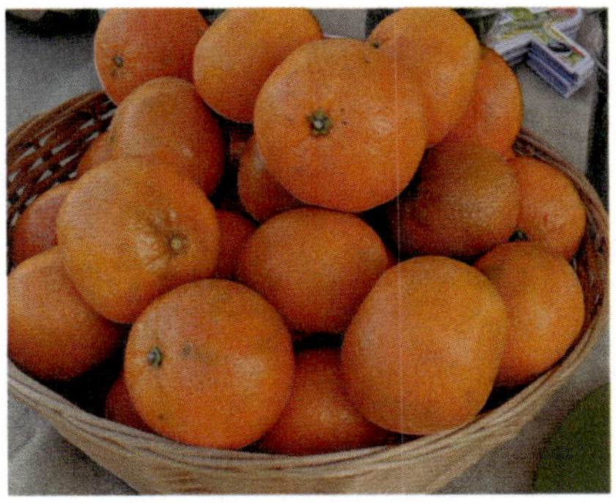

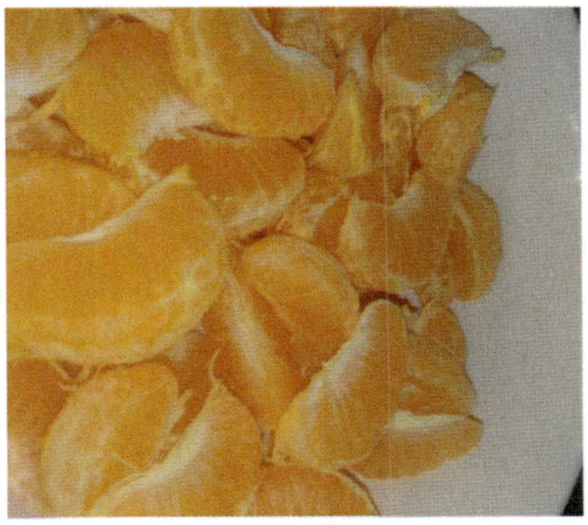

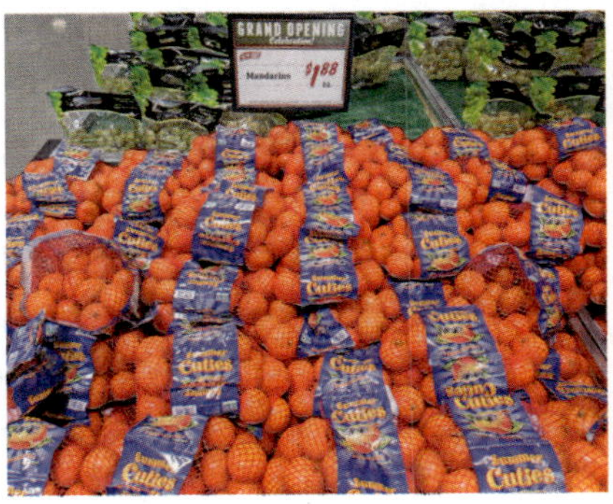

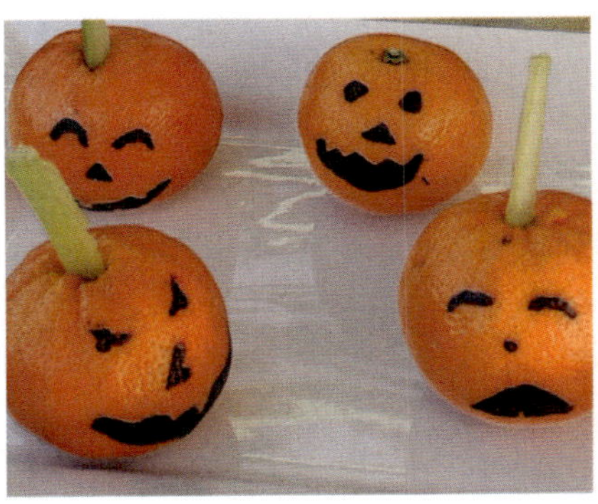

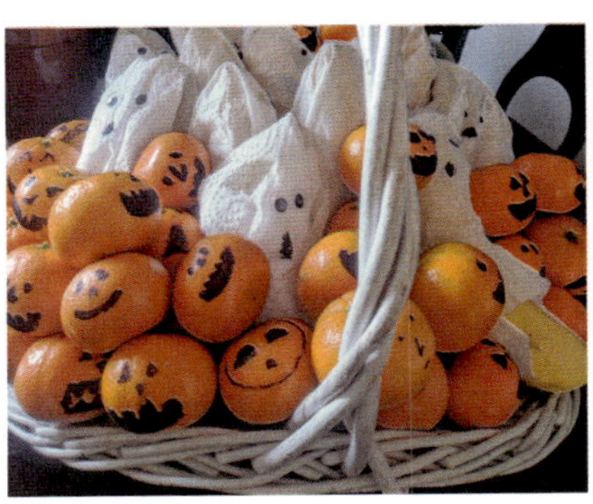

INGREDIENT:

- 8–15 mandarins, clementines

STEPS:

1. Peel mandarins.
2. Divide mandarins slices into a bowl.
3. Enjoy!

DELICIOUS WITH:

- Dried cranberries
- Dried raisins
- Fresh grapes
- Lime squeeze

Mandarin Nutrition Facts

Nutrients Delivered	1 Mandarin
Calories	34.8
Macronutrients	
Carbs	8.9 g
Protein	0.6 g
Fat	0.1 g
Fiber	1.3 g
Water	64.1 g
Mirconutrients: Vitamins	
Vitamin A	0 mg
Vitamin B1 (Thiamin)	0.1 mg
Vitamin B2 (Riboflavin)	0 mg
Vitamin B3 (Niacin)	0.5 mg
Vitamin B5 (Pantothenic Acid)	0.1 mg
Vitamin B6	0.1 mg
Vitamin B9 (Folate/Folic Acid)	17.8 mg
Vitamin C (Ascorbic Acid)	36.1 mg
Vitamin E	0.1 mg
Mirconutrients: Minerals	
Calcium	22.2 mg
Copper	0 mg
Iron	0.1 mg
Magnesium	7.4 mg
Manganese	0 mg
Phosphorus	15.5 mg
Potassium (K)	131 mg
Selenium	0.1 mcg
Sodium	0.7 mg
Zinc	0 mg

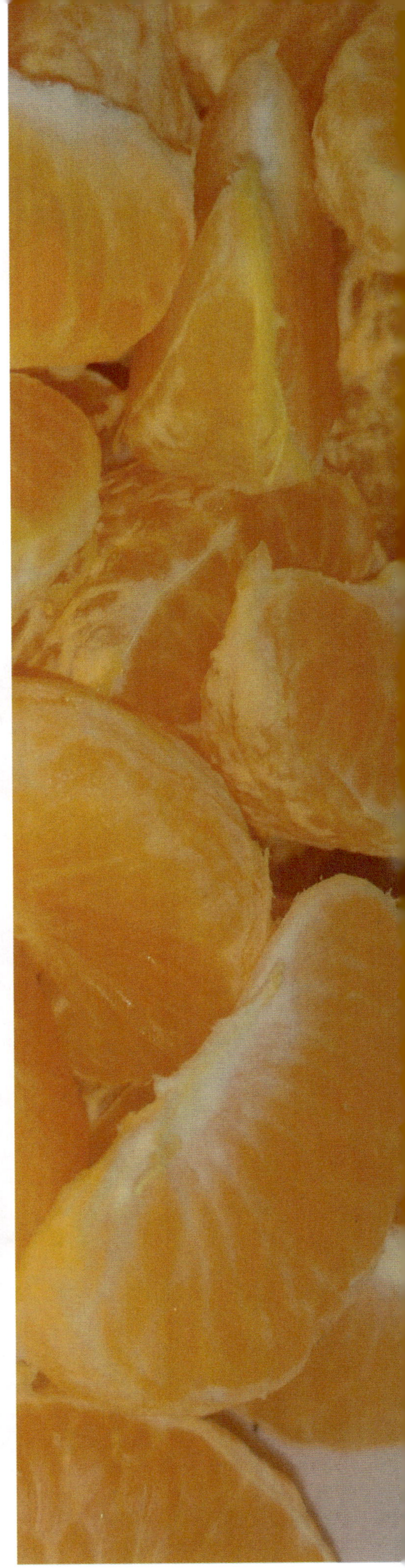

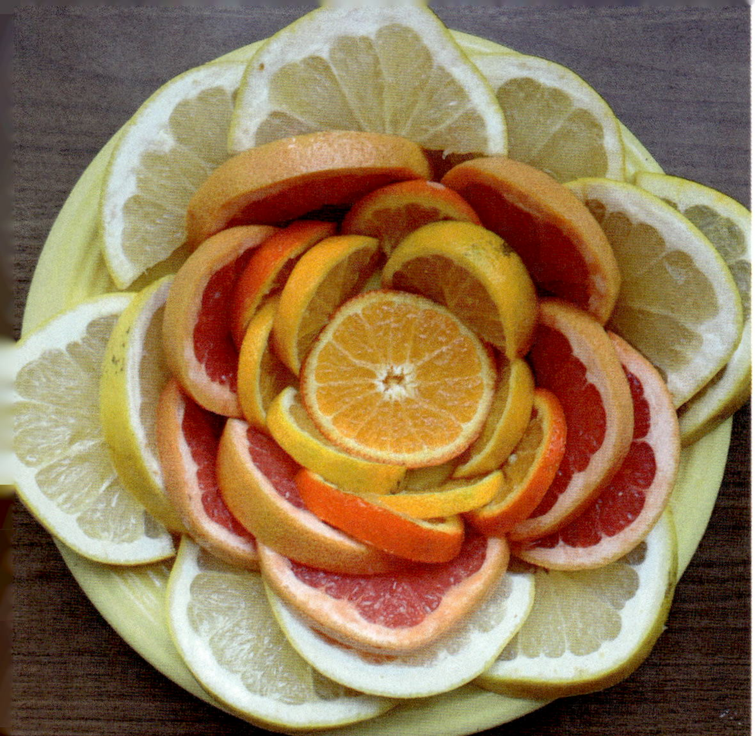

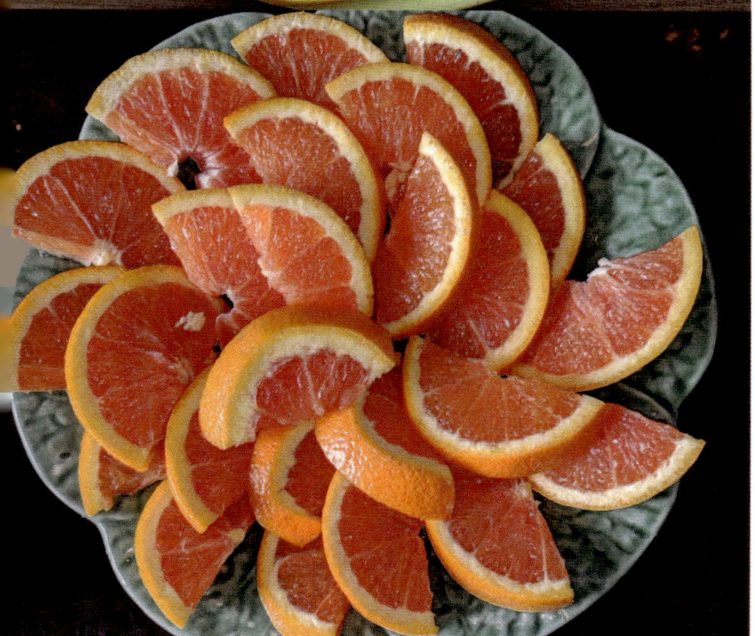

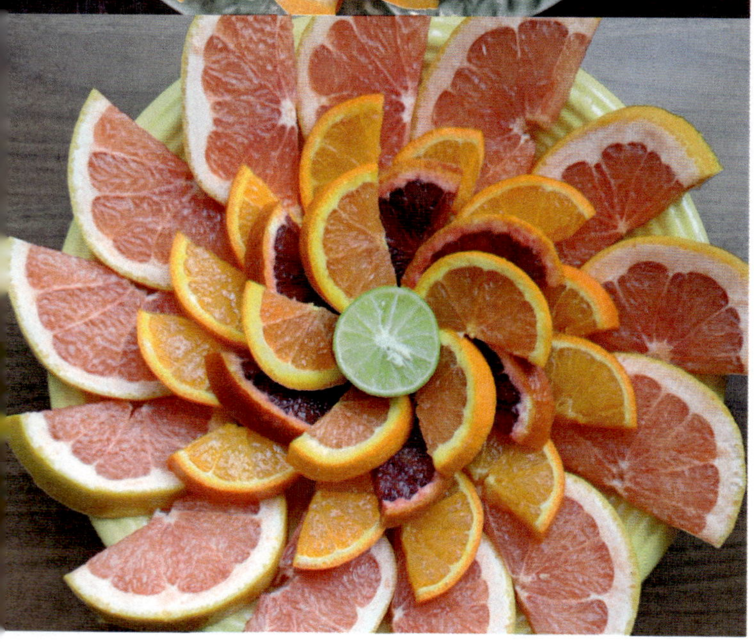

GRAPEFRUIT MANDALA

A gratifying plate of grapefruits.

INGREDIENT:

- ~6 grapefruits

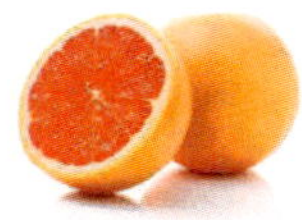

STEPS:

1. Slice citrus into wedges or into round slices that are halved.
2. Arrange citrus slices onto plate in a circular fashion.
3. Voilà, enjoy!

DELICIOUS WITH:

- Dried cranberries
- Lime squeeze

Grapefruit Nutrition Facts

Nutrients Delivered	1 Grapefruit
Calories	51.7
Macronutrients	
Carbs	13.1 g
Protein	0.9 g
Fat	1.4 g
Fiber	2 g
Water	108 g
Mirconutrients: Vitamins	
Vitamin A	1415 IU
Vitamin B1 (Thiamin)	0.1 mg
Vitamin B2 (Riboflavin)	0 mg
Vitamin B3 (Niacin)	0.3 mg
Vitamin B5 (Pantothenic Acid)	0.3 mg
Vitamin B6	0.1 mg
Vitamin B9 (Folate/Folic Acid)	16 mg
Vitamin C (Ascorbic Acid)	38.4 mg
Vitamin E	0.2 mg
Vitamin K	0 mcg
Mirconutrients: Minerals	
Calcium	27.1 mg
Copper	0 mg
Iron	0.1 mg
Magnesium	11.1 mg
Manganese	0 mg
Phosphorus	22.1 mg
Potassium (K)	166 mg
Selenium	0.1 mcg
Sodium	0 mg
Zinc	0.1 mg

Grapefruits Make Us Smile 😊

There's so much goodness inside this juicy fruit we can't help but smile!

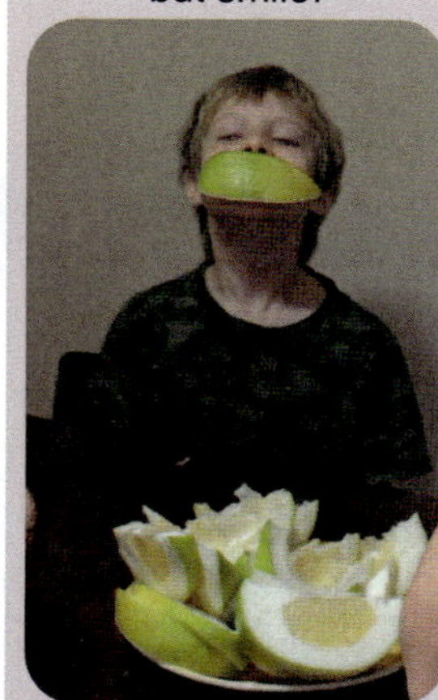

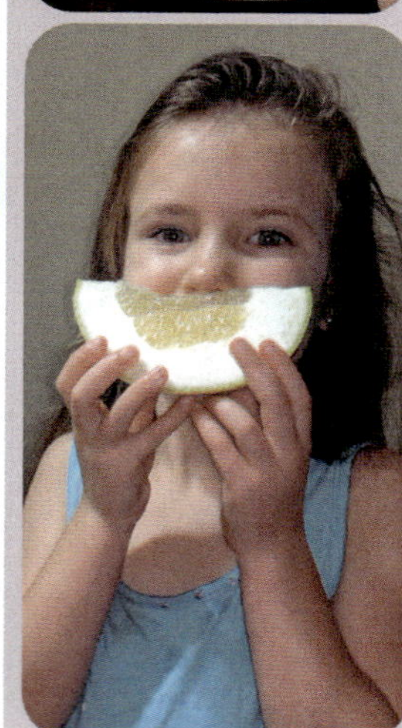

PURELY PINEAPPLE

A sweet and tangy pineapple to nourish the body and pleasure the palate.

INGREDIENT:

- 1 pineapple

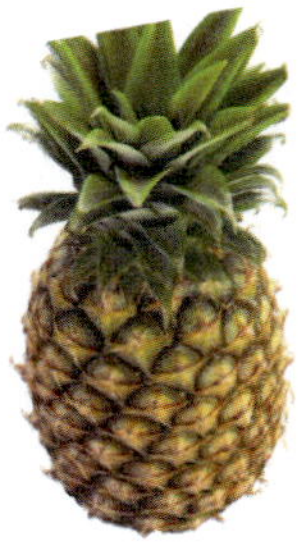

STEPS:

1. With a sharp knife slice off pineapple top and remove hard outer pineapple skin.
2. Cut four sides of pineapple away from central hard core.
3. Chop pineapple into chunky pieces and serve.
4. Enjoy!

Pineapple Nutrition Facts

Nutrients Delivered	1 Pineapple
Calories	452
Macronutrients	
Carbs	119 g
Protein	4.9 g
Fat	1.1 g
Fiber	12.7 g
Water	778 g
Mirconutrients: Vitamins	
Vitamin A	525 IU
Vitamin B1 (Thiamin)	0.7 mg
Vitamin B2 (Riboflavin)	0.3 mg
Vitamin B3 (Niacin)	4.5 mg
Vitamin B5 (Pantothenic Acid)	1.9 mg
Vitamin B6	1.0 mg
Vitamin B9 (Folate/Folic Acid)	163 mg
Choline	49.8 mg
Vitamin C (Ascorbic Acid)	433 mg
Betaine	0.9 mg
Vitamin E	0.2 mg
Vitamin K	6.3 mcg
Mirconutrients: Minerals	
Calcium	118 mg
Copper	1.0 mg
Iron	2.6 mg
Magnesium	109 mg
Manganese	8.4 mg
Phosphorus	72.4 mg
Potassium (K)	986 mg
Selenium	0.9 mcg
Sodium	9.1 mg
Zinc	1.1 mg

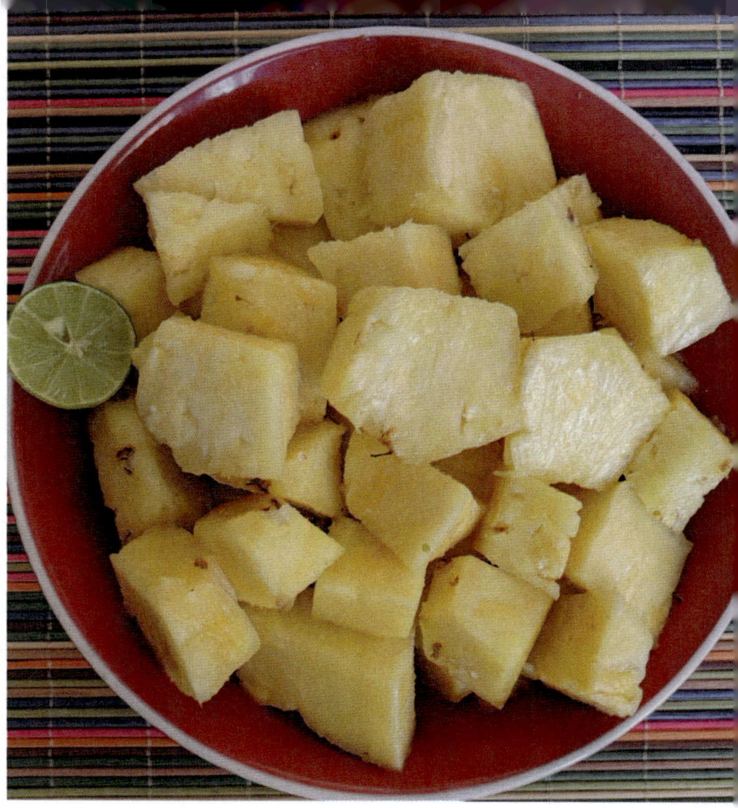

DELICIOUS WITH:

- Lime squeeze
- Strawberries
- Coconut flakes
- Banana slices
- Blueberries

Eating The Whole Pineapple

I wasn't a big fan of pineapple growing up since I wasn't really exposed to fresh pineapple. Canned pineapple chunks in syrup didn't appeal to me. When I grew up and finally tasted fresh pineapple I found a new love. I still wouldn't have thought of eating a whole pineapple by myself until I was pregnant with my son.

I craved pineapple and ate it frequently throughout my pregnancy. The day before my daughter Ayla was born, I ate my first whole pineapple all by myself. When I told people about my fruit-eating feat they were shocked, but it really shouldn't be too shocking, for one pineapple contains the enzyme bromelain, which helps soften the cervix and prepare a woman's body for labor. I had read that it would be a good way to get labor moving on time around my due date, and for me it seemed to work. I started having contractions at midnight that night and Ayla was born at 5 am after a fairly uncomplicated labor.

There are less than 500 calories in a single pineapple, and it's packed with hydration and nutrition. If you're a pineapple fan, why not eat the whole thing? No one says you have to share!

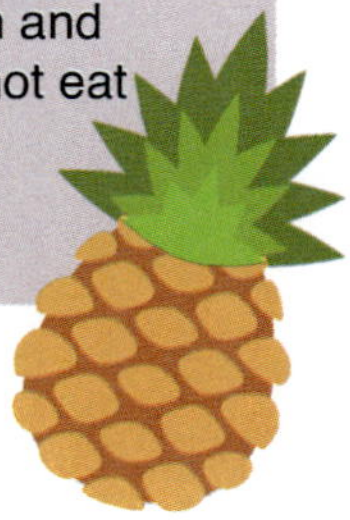

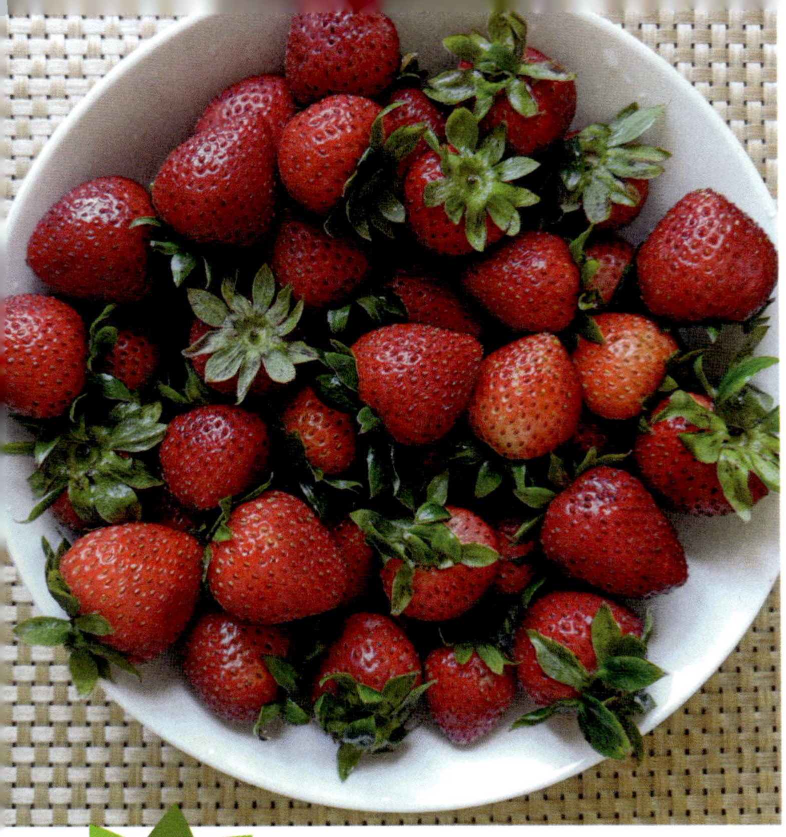

SIMPLY STRAWBERRIES

Berry goodness.

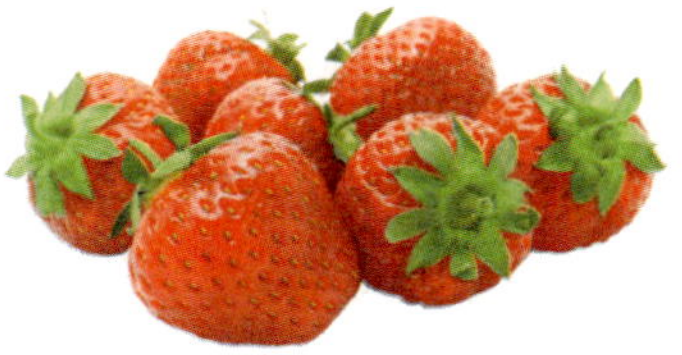

INGREDIENT:

- strawberries

STEPS:

1. Wash fresh fruits and remove any bad spots with a knife.
2. Chop strawberry tops off if you like, or simply bite into the whole fruits.
3. Enjoy!

TIP: 1 quart of strawberries contains approximately 50 medium-size berries and weighs approx. 2 lbs. 50 medium strawberries provide 190 calories of energy. 50 large strawberries provide 290 calories of energy.

Red Defends You

Red foods have a reputation for the protective powers they pass on to us when we eat them. Studies have shown that consuming red foods high in the phytonutrient lycopene greatly reduce the risk of heart disease, cancer, and other ailments.

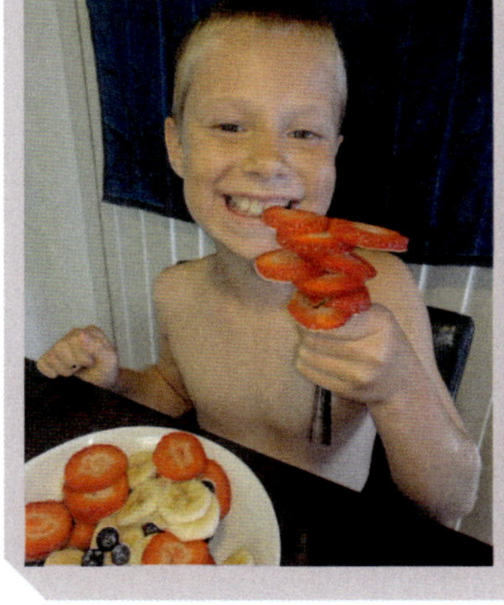

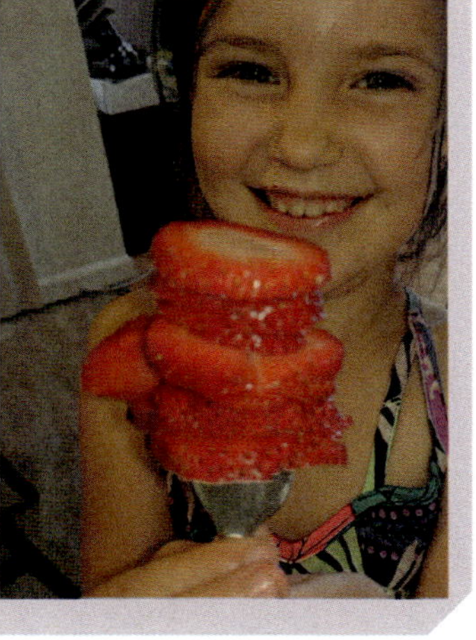

Strawberry Nutrition Facts

Nutrients Delivered	1 LG Strawberry
Calories	5.8
Macronutrients	
Carbs	1.4
Protein	0.1
Fat	0.1
Fiber	0.4
Water	16.4
Mirconutrients: Vitamins	
Vitamin A	2.2 mg
Vitamin B1 (Thiamin)	0 mg
Vitamin B2 (Riboflavin)	0 mg
Vitamin B3 (Niacin)	0.1 mg
Vitamin B5 (Pantothenic Acid)	0 mg
Vitamin B6	0 mg
Vitamin B9 (Folate/Folic Acid)	4.3 mg
Vitamin C (Ascorbic Acid)	10.6 mg
Vitamin E	0.1 mg
Vitamin K	0.4 mcg
Mirconutrients: Minerals	
Calcium	2.9 mg
Copper	0 mg
Iron	0.1 mg
Magnesium	2.3 mg
Manganese	0.1 mg
Phosphorus	4.3 mg
Potassium (K)	27.5 mg
Selenium	0.1 mg
Sodium	0.2 mg
Zinc	0 mg

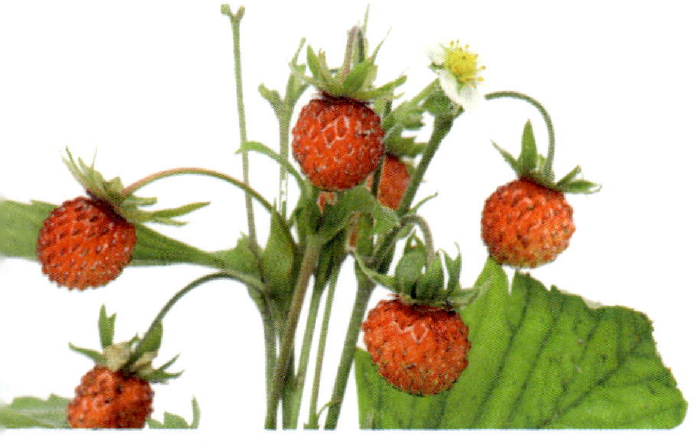

BANANA LOVE PLATE

Simply the most perfect food known to Man.

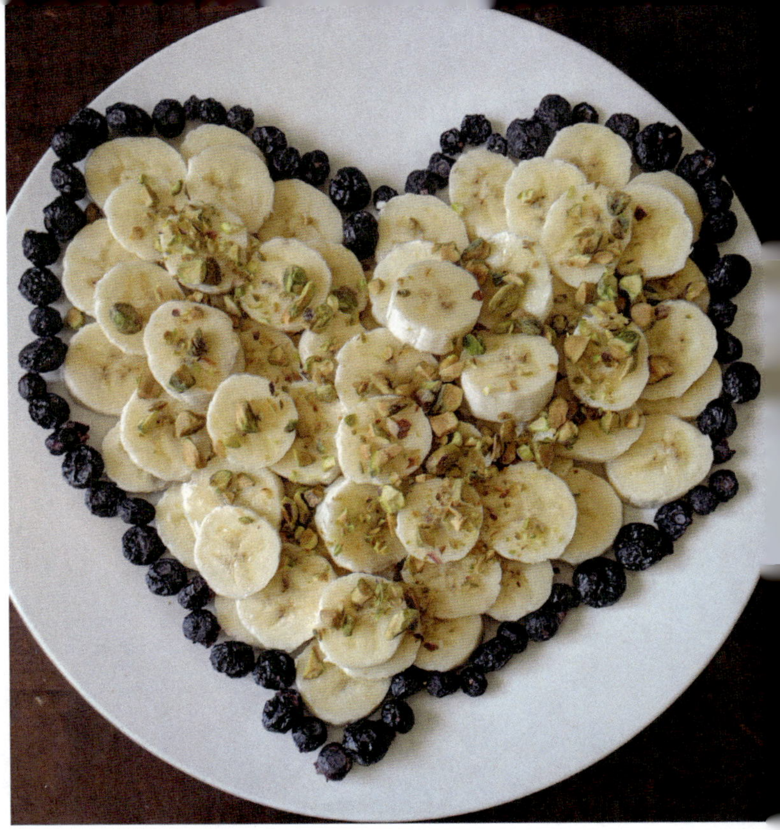

INGREDIENT:

- 3–5 bananas

STEPS:

1. Peel bananas and remove any bad spots with a knife.
2. Slice bananas into thin rounds.
3. Arrange bananas onto plate in the shape of a giant heart.
4. Top bananas with your desired toppings. Enjoy!

DELICIOUS WITH: Shredded, dried coconut, fresh or dried blueberries, raisins, cinnamon spice, ginger spice, peanut butter or almond butter drizzle, slivered almond sprinkle, crushed walnuts, choppe pistachios, sprinkle of sesame seeds.

Banana Nutrition Facts

Nutrients Delivered	1 Banana
Calories	105
Macronutrients	
Carbs	27 g
Protein	1.3 g
Fat	0.4 g
Fiber	3.1 g
Water	88.4 g
Mirconutrients: Vitamins	
Vitamin A	75.5 IU
Vitamin B1 (Thiamin)	0.03 mg
Vitamin B2 (Riboflavin)	0.1 mg
Vitamin B3 (Niacin)	0.8 mg
Vitamin B5 (Pantothenic Acid)	0.4 mg
Vitamin B6	0.4 mg
Vitamin B9 (Folate/Folic Acid)	23.6 mg
Vitamin C (Ascorbic Acid)	10.3 mg
Vitamin E	0.1 mg
Vitamin K	0.6 mcg
Mirconutrients: Minerals	
Calcium	5.9 mg
Copper	0.1 mg
Iron	0.3 mg
Magnesium	31.9 mg
Manganese	0.3 mg
Phosphorus	26 mg
Potassium (K)	422 mg
Selenium	1.2 mcg
Sodium	1.2 mg
Zinc	0.2 mg

Benefits of Bananas

The fruit of banana plants are more than just tasty, they have many medicinal uses as well.

- TREAT DEPRESSION: Bananas are useful for those suffering depression because they contain serotonin, a "happy hormone", which produces glad feelings.
- CURE ANEMIA: Bananas are good for anemia because they are high in iron, which supports the production of hemoglobin.
- HEALTHY DIGESTION: Bananas are effective at regulating the bowels and are used to treat both diarrhea and constipation. Eat a banana after a meal to improve digestion.
- FIGHT ULCERS: Eat bananas to heal intestinal disorders such as ulcers. Bananas are one of the few fruits that ulcer patients can safely consume. The chemical composition of the fruit helps neutralize internal acidity and relieve pain caused by ulcers.
- HANGOVER MEDICINE: Bananas are effective to counteract a hangover due to their high sugar and water content.
- POTASSIUM POWERHOUSE: Bananas are rich in potassium which helps us to be alert.
- PROMOTES HEALTHY INTERNAL PH: Bananas neutralize acidity in the body and are good for stomach ulcers and heart-burn.
- GOOD FOR PREGNANT WOMEN: Bananas are effective at relieving symptoms of morning sickness.
- ANTACID: Skip the Tums, eat a banana! Bananas are a natural antacid. Eat the creamy fruit to treat and prevent acid reflux and heartburn.
- PROMOTES HEALTHY WEIGHT LOSS: Bananas have long been regarded as a super food for those seeking to lose excess weight. Bananas are low in fat and high in fiber and water so they are a great food for regulating the appetite.

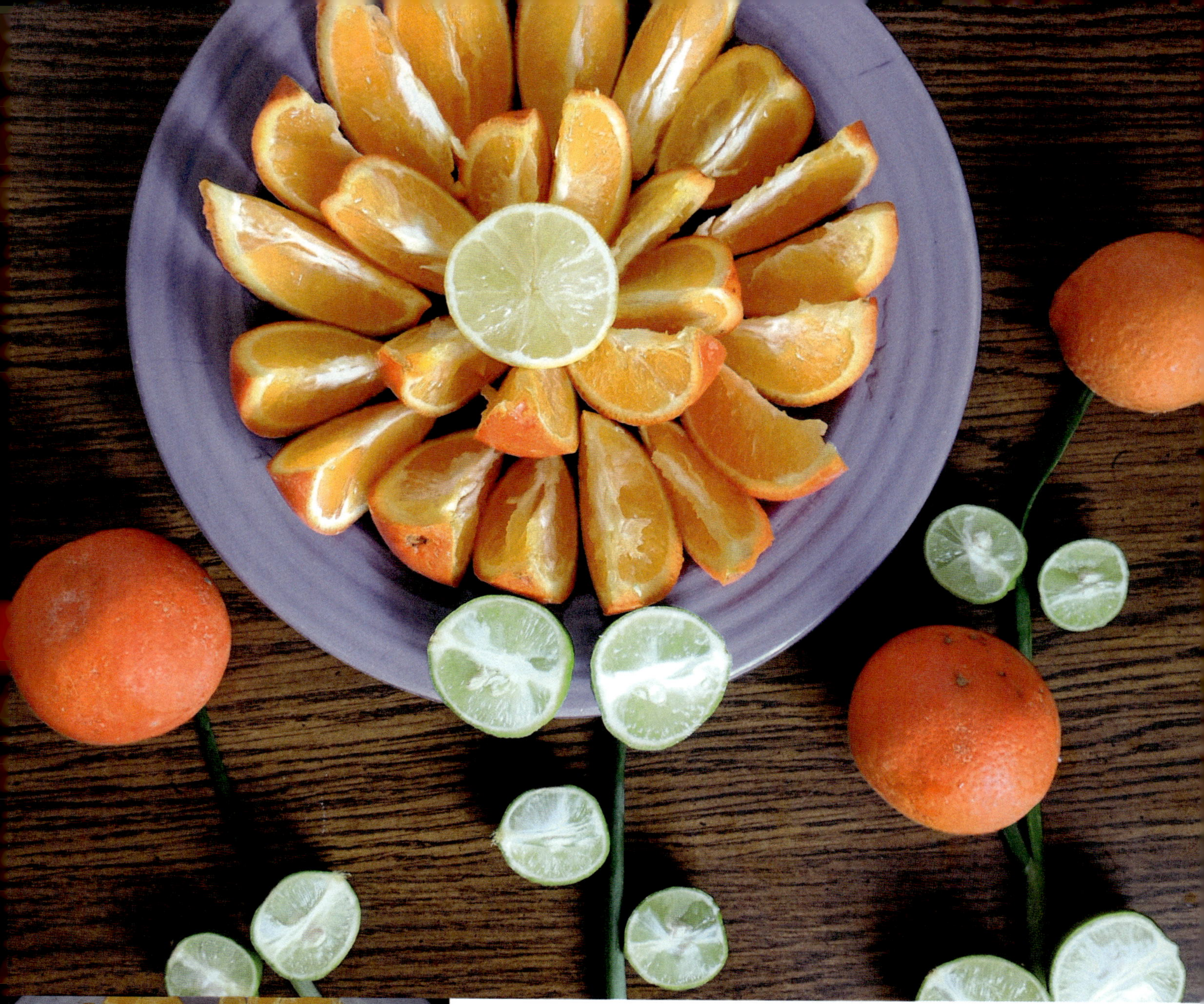

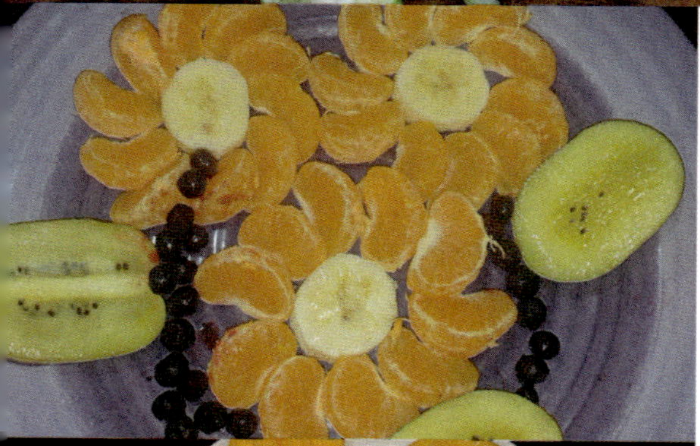

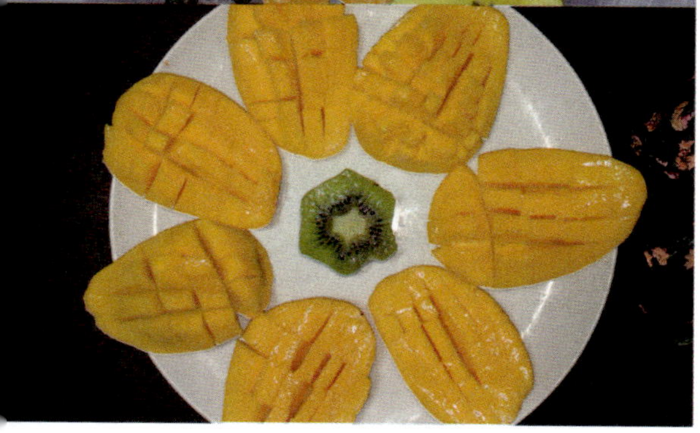

☀FRUIT FLOWERS☀

Make fruit more fun with the shape of flowers.

INGREDIENTS:

- 4 oranges, mandarins, or mangoes for petals
- 1 banana, kiwi, or lemon for center of flower
- kiwi, blueberries, or limes for stem and leafs

STEPS:

1. Wash fresh fruits and remove any bad spots with a knife.
2. Chop fresh fruits into desired flower-shaped parts.
3. Arrange fruit in the shape of one or more flowers.
4. Share with friends or family, enjoy!

SUBSTITUTE: Swap other seasonal ripe fruits to make your own version of fruit flowers.

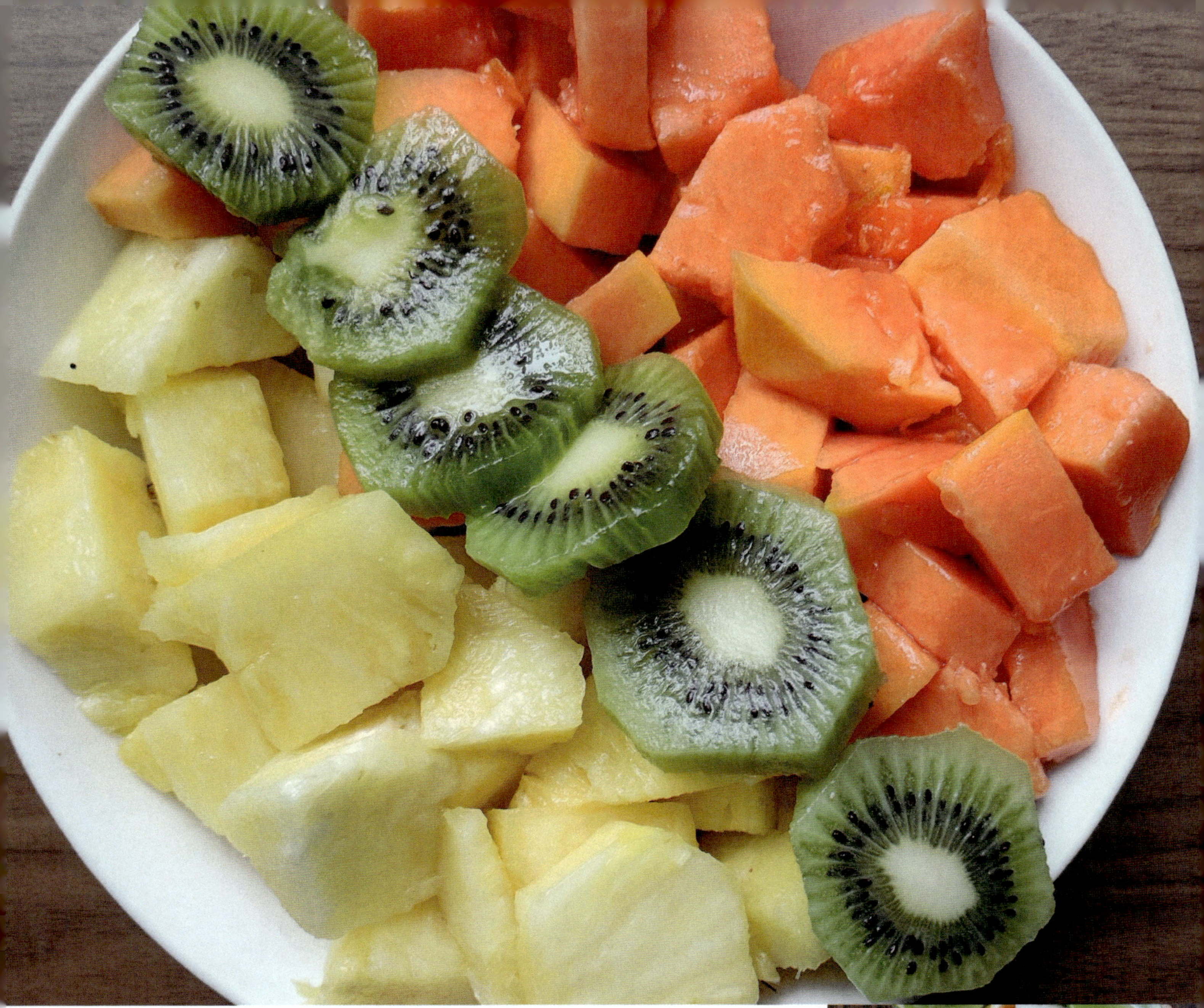

TRI-FRUITA SALAD

Infinite flavors combinations await in this three-fruit salad.

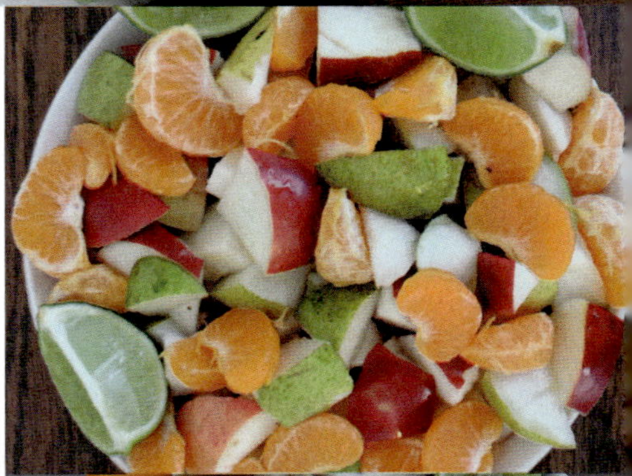

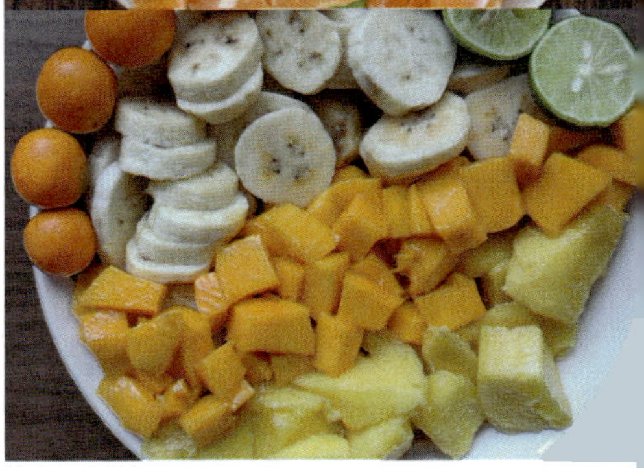

INGREDIENTS:

- 3 types of fruits (enough to fill a bowl for a 300–500 calorie meal)
- Try: pineapple, papaya, and kiwi
- Try: cantaloupe, strawberry, and banana
- Try: mandarin, kiwi, and banana
- Try: banana, blueberries, and strawberries

STEPS:

1. Wash fresh fruits and remove any bad spots with a knife.
2. Chop fresh fruits into bite-size pieces.
3. Combine fruit in bowl.
4. Enjoy!

TIPS:

- Experiment with different combinations of fruit.
- Use seasonal fresh fruits for maximum flavor and affordability.
- Add a handful of chopped nuts, seeds, or dried fruit to your salad.
- Try it with a cinnamon sprinkle.

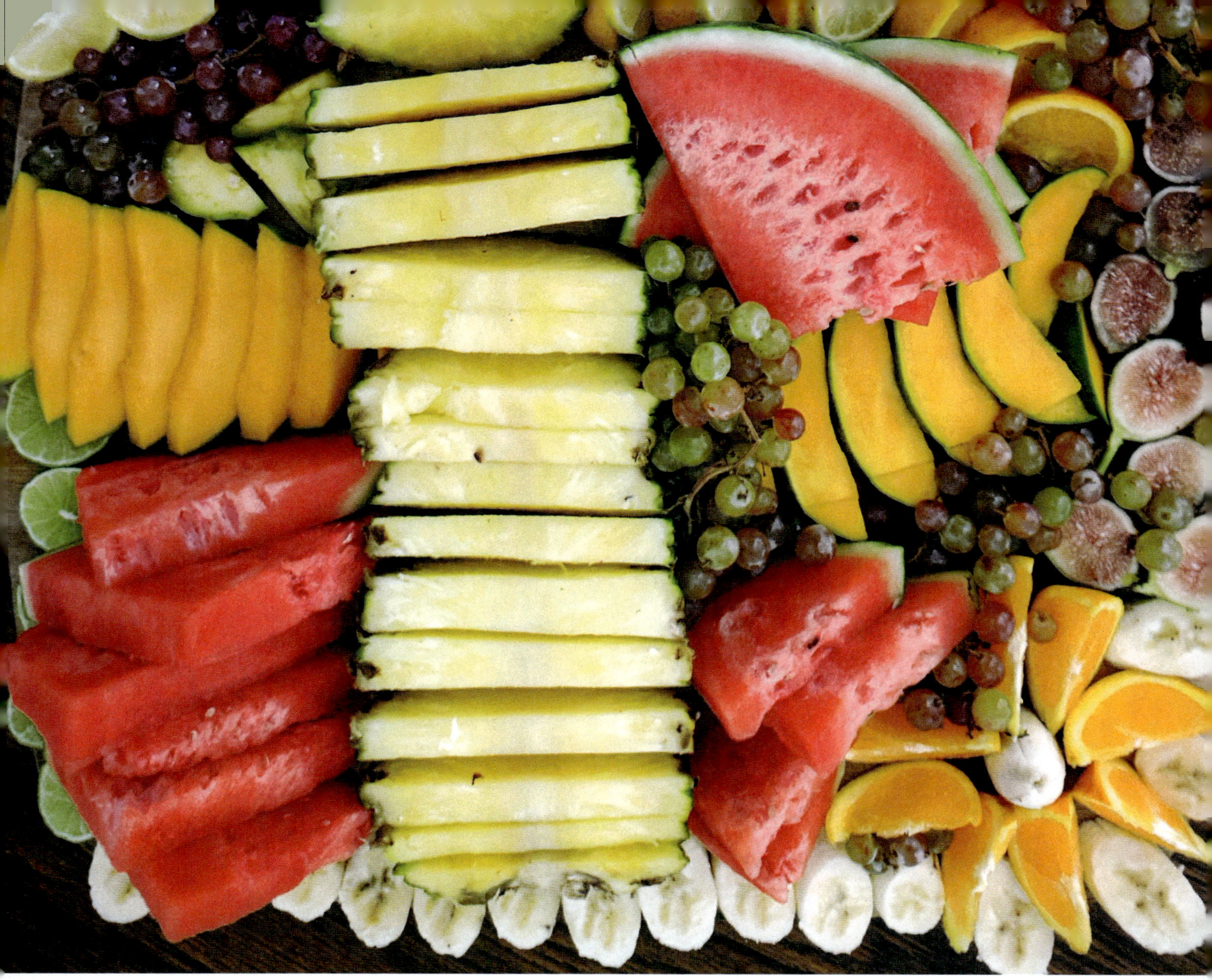

I AM ROYALTY FRUIT PLATTER

A fruit platter that makes you feel as rich as royalty.

INGREDIENTS:

- 1 small watermelon
- 1 pineapple
- 1 bunch grapes
- 3–4 citrus fruits
- 1–3 mangoes
- 2 bananas
- 6 figs
- any fresh seasonal fruit can substitute for the any of the fruits above.

STEPS:

1. Wash fresh fruits and remove any bad spots with a knife.
2. Chop fresh fruits into attractive slices.
3. Arrange fruit slices onto large platter or cutting board.
4. Share with friends, enjoy!

DELICIOUS WITH:

- Apples
- Apricots
- Blackberries
- Blueberries
- Cantaloupe
- Cherries
- Cranberries
- Currants
- Dates
- Gooseberries
- Grapefruit
- Honeydew
- Kiwi
- Kiwi berries
- Lime wedges
- Nectarines
- Papaya
- Passionfruit
- Peaches
- Pears
- Persimmon
- Plums
- Raspberries
- Star fruit
- Strawberries

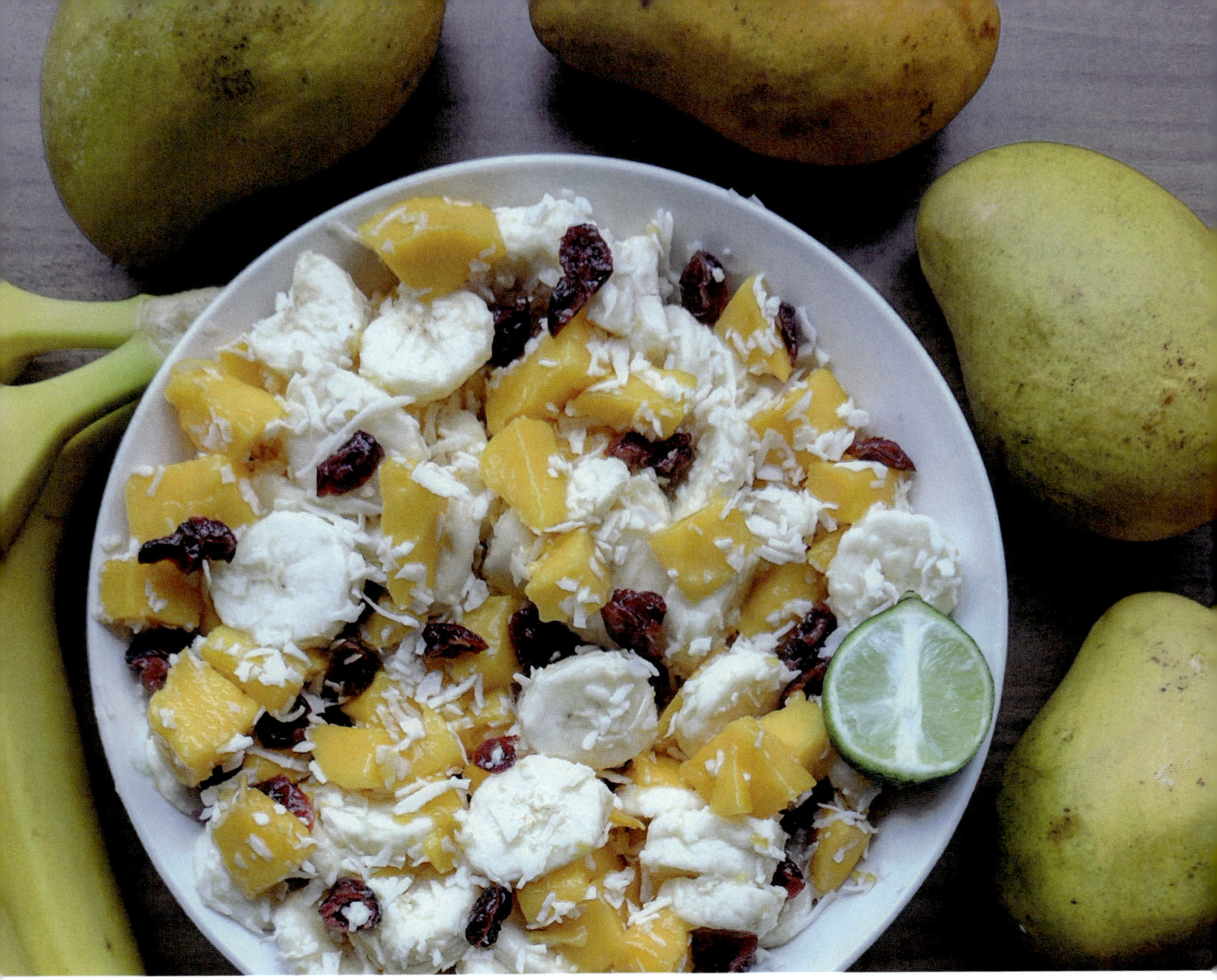

MANGO BANANA BOWL

Mangoes and bananas make a delectable duo in this simple two-fruit salad.

Serves: 1

INGREDIENTS:

- 2 bananas
- 2 mangoes

STEPS:

1. Peel bananas and slice into rounds.
2. Remove skin from mangoes and dice fruit into bite-sized pieces.
3. Combine fruit in bowl.
4. Stir until well combined.
5. Enjoy!

DELICIOUS WITH: Dried cranberries, raisins, strawberries, shredded coconut flakes, chopped pecans, walnuts, or hazelnuts. Experiment with adding your favorite dried fruits, nuts, or seeds on top. This dish is excellent with a lime wedge squeeze.

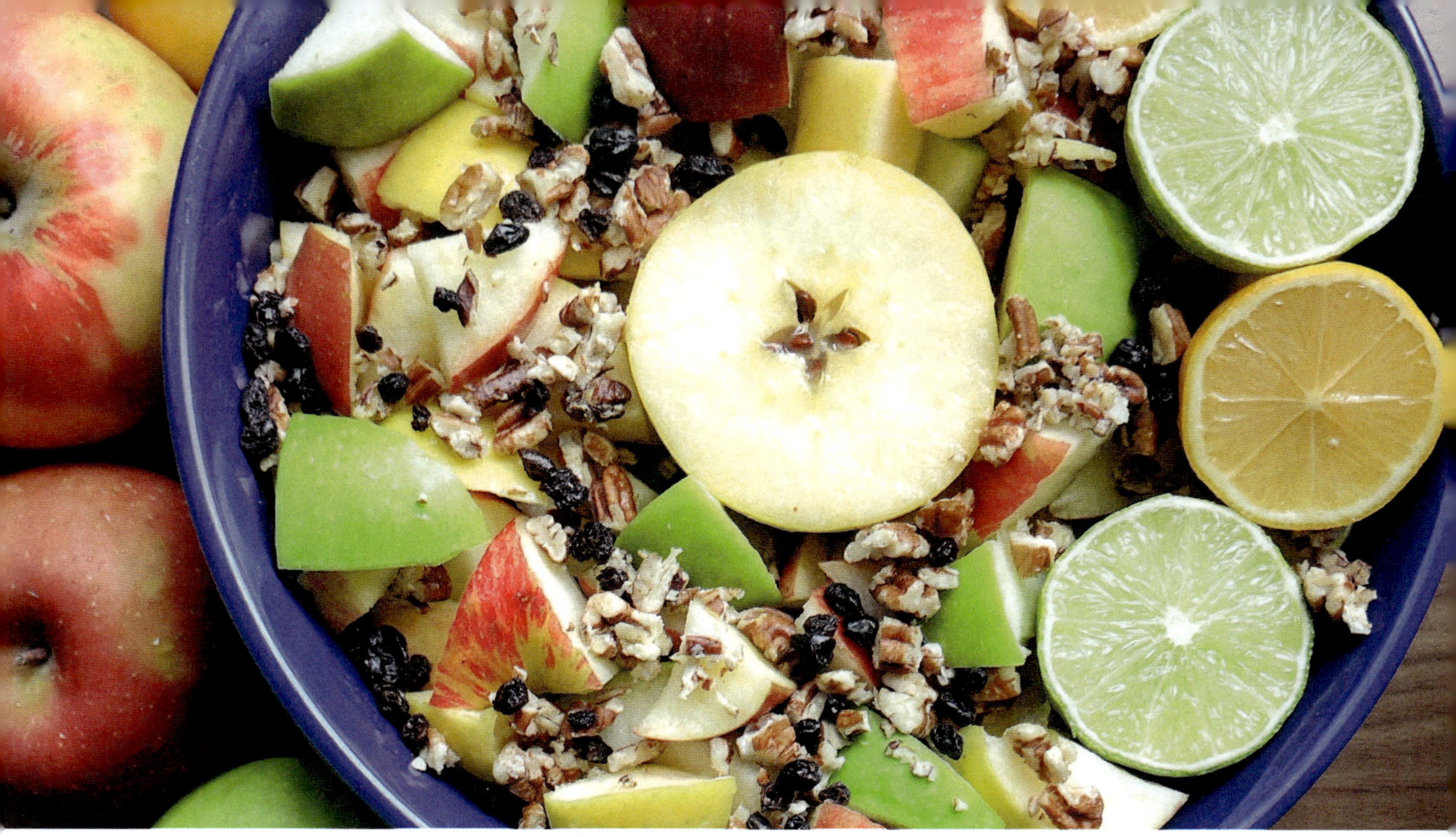

APPLE SALAD

An array of apples combine to ignite your appetite and satisfy your frugivorous senses.

INGREDIENTS:

- 6–9 apples, different varieties (aim to include red, green, and yellow apples)
- 1 lime
- 1 lemon
- 1/2 cup pecans, chopped
- 1/2 cup dried currants

STEPS:

1. Wash fresh fruits and remove any bad spots with a knife.
2. Chop apples into bite-sized pieces, leaving peel on.
3. Add chopped apples to large bowl and squeeze a large lemon on top.
4. Stir apples to coat with lemon juice. The acid in the citrus will help prevent the apples from turning brown.
5. Add chopped pecans, currants, and remaining citrus to top of apples.
6. Share with friends, enjoy!

An Apple A Day

Apples have long been hailed through folk wisdom as having the power to protect our health. Recently modern science has shown apples help defend our bodies against cancer. Illustrating this cancer-fighting power of apples are several studies where scientists introduced ground up apple peels to various cancer cell cultures. In every such study, researchers have found that apple peels, or extracts of, either kill cancer cells or inhibit their growth.

DELICIOUS WITH:

- Walnuts, or another chopped nut can substitute for pecans.
- Dried raisins or cranberries can substitute for currants.
- Fresh grapes add more texture and flavor to this salad.
- Try it with a cinnamon sprinkle.
- Try serving with a drizzle of almond butter or peanut butter.

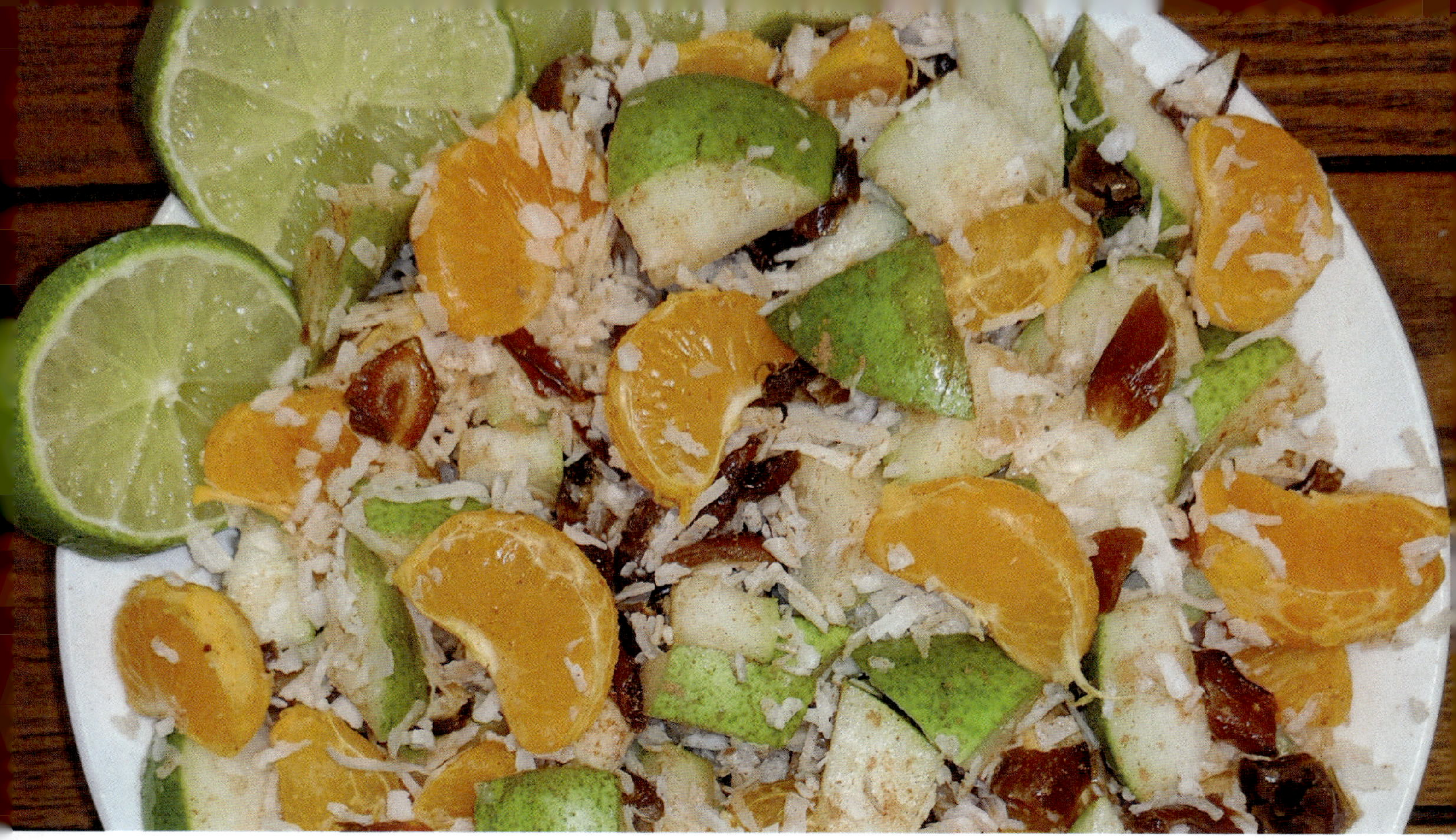

SEVEN TREES FRUIT SALAD

A delicious way to enjoy nutrient-rich, fiber-full, hydrating tree fruits.

Serves: 1

INGREDIENTS:

- 1 lime, cut in half and squeezed
- 1 mandarin, peeled and divided
- 1 pear, washed and diced in cubes
- 4 dates, pitted and diced small
- 1/4 cup shredded coconut
- 1/2 tbsp. maple syrup
- 1/2 tsp. cinnamon sprinkled

DELICIOUS WITH:

- Use cranberries or raisins instead of dates.
- Drizzle a spoonful of peanut butter or almond butter on top.
- Use crisp apples or persimmons instead of pears.
- Add a sprinkle of ginger powder.
- Use more than one type of crisp fruits.
- Try chopped walnuts, pecans, hazelnuts, or almonds in place of coconut.
- Enjoy this salad on top of banana nice-cream: just blend frozen bananas with almond milk for a smooth creamy treat.

STEPS:

1. Wash fresh fruits and remove any bad spots with a knife.
2. Chop fresh whole fruit into small bite-sized pieces.
3. Add fruit to a bowl and squeeze lime juice on top to cover fruit in the juice.
4. Remove pits from dates and chop into small pea-sized pieces. *(Save the date pits for planting. Each date pit is a potential future date tree!)*
5. Combine fruit in bowl with coconut, cinnamon, and maple syrup.
6. Stir until well combined.
7. Share with friends, enjoy!

Tree Food

All seven ingredients in this salad grow on trees. Trees are not only beautiful, they provide shade, clean groundwater, clean the air we breathe, provide animal habitat, and can produce an abundance of nutritious and delicious food that frugivores like us enjoy and thrive on!

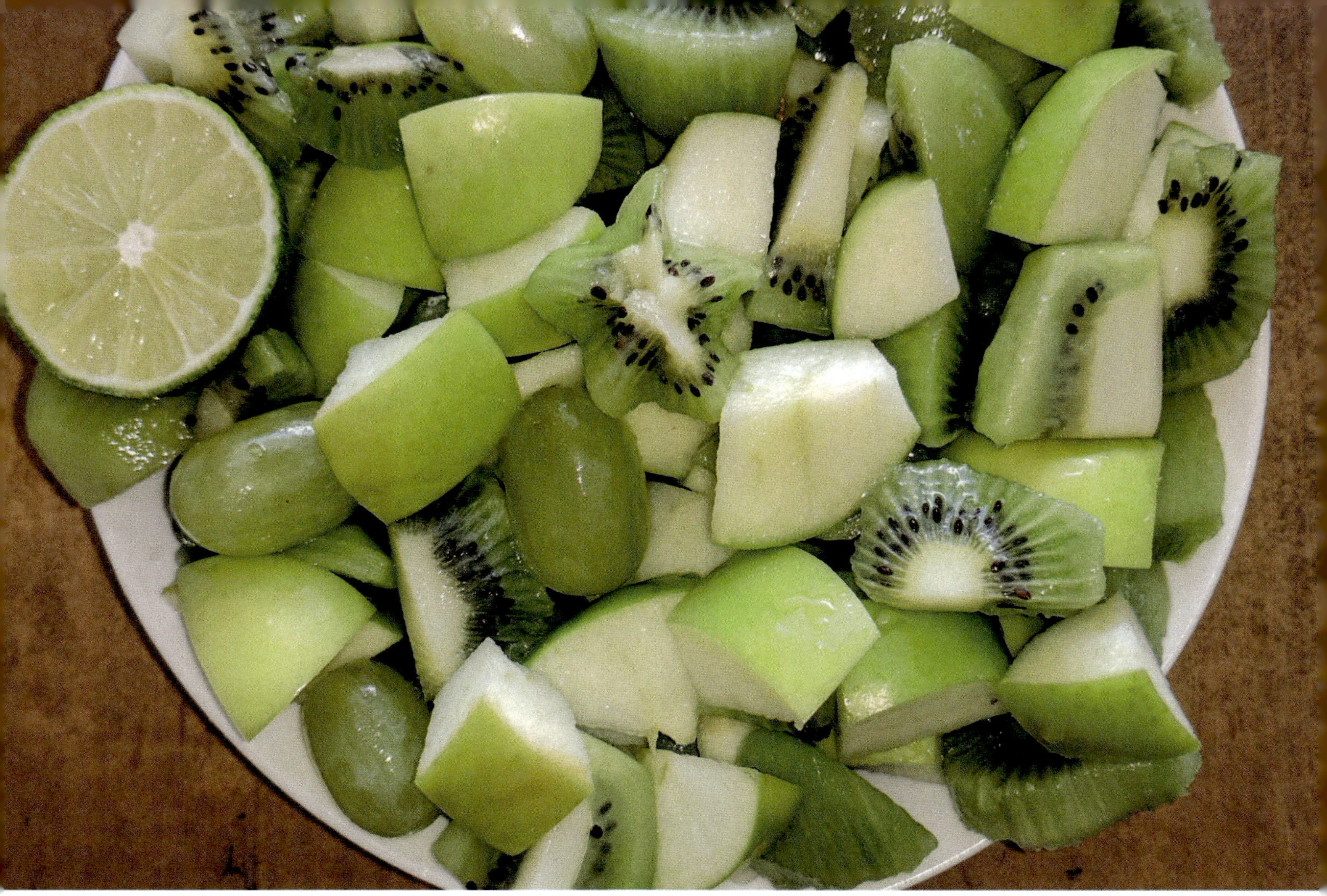

TRINITY GREENS FRUIT SALAD

Three green fruits combine for a tart, tasty, and hydrating meal.

Serves: 1

INGREDIENTS:

- 3 kiwis
- 2 green apples
- handful of green grapes

STEPS:

1. Wash fresh fruits and remove any bad spots with a knife.
2. Chop fresh apples into bite-sized pieces.
3. Peel kiwis and chop into bite-sized pieces.
4. Remove grapes from stems.
5. Combine fruits in bowl.
6. Enjoy!

DELICIOUS WITH:

- Garnish with a lime wedge or a kiwi star.
- Squeeze a lime or lemon on top of salad to prevent apples from browning.
- Green honeydew melon can substitute for one of the green fruits here.

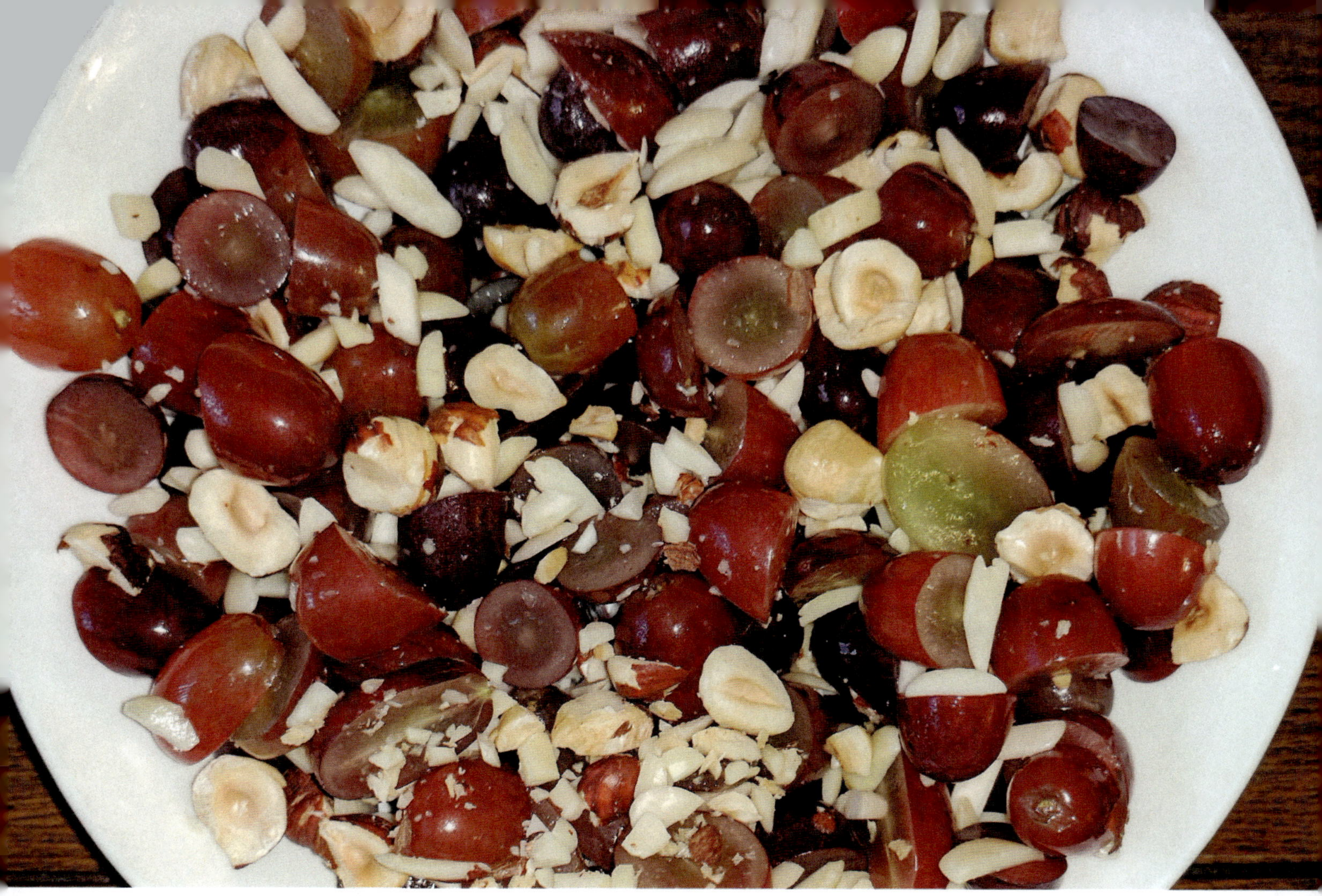

THE REAL GRAPE NUTS

Purely fruits and nuts in this hydrating and nutrient-packed bowl.

Serves: 1

INGREDIENTS:

- 2 cups fresh grapes
- 1/4 cup nuts, chopped any variety

STEPS:

1. Wash fresh grapes and slice in half.
2. Chop nuts.
3. Combine grapes and nuts in a bowl and stir.
4. Enjoy!

DELICIOUS WITH: Vanilla almond milk or add a splash of granola to the bowl.

Bunches of Reasons to Go for Grapes

Grapes are the perfect bite-sized packages of pure water, fiber, sugar, nutrients and antioxidants that frugivores like us just can't seem to get enough of. Grapes have long been praised not just for their sweet taste, but also for their impressive health benefits.

- **Antioxidants:** These juicy fruits pack a whopping punch of antioxidant power. The antioxidants in grapes interact with free radicals in the body to reduce oxidative stress, helping to prevent some of today's leading diseases from developing.
- **Heart Health:** Studies published in peer-reviewed scientific journals have shown that eating grapes can help promote a healthy heart by reducing the risk of atherosclerosis and decreasing inflammation. This may explain what's known as the "French-Paradox" where French people who drink a good amount of wine appear to live long and healthy lives despite also being in the habit of smoking and eating foods high in saturated fats.
- **Strong Bones:** Just one cup of grapes provides 25% of your daily vitamin K needs. Vitamin K has been associated with preventing breaks and fractures according to multiple scientific studies.
- **Prevent Diabetes:** A 2013 study followed a large group of women for nearly 2 decades and found those who ate more whole fruits, especially grapes, blueberries, and apples, had significantly lower risk of type 2 diabetes.
- **Don't' skip the peels!** The flesh contains just 5% of the antioxidants found in the skin and seeds.

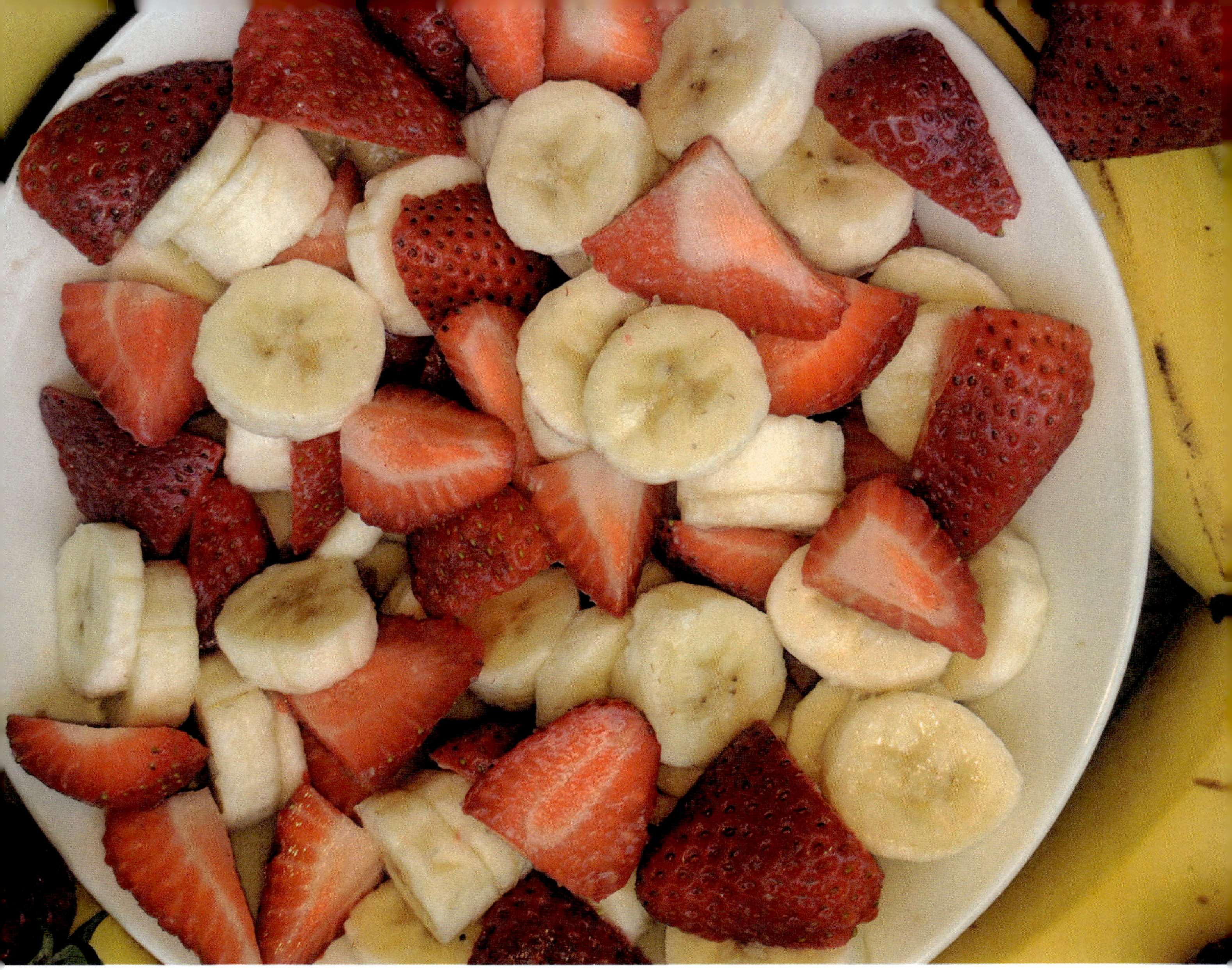

BERRY BANANA BOWL

Just strawberries and bananas make a delectable breakfast duo.

Serves: 1

INGREDIENTS:

- 2 bananas
- 10–30 strawberries

STEPS:

1. Wash strawberries and remove any bad spots with a knife.
2. Remove tops of strawberries with a sharp knife and chop strawberries into quarters.
3. Peel bananas and slice into thin rounds.
4. Combine fruit in bowl.
5. Enjoy!

DELICIOUS WITH:

- Blueberries, blackberries, or raspberries can substitute for strawberries in this bowl.
- Add a lime wedge to squeeze on top.
- Diced mango makes a great addition to strawberries and bananas.
- Sprinkle a handful of shredded coconut on top.
- Dust with cocoa powder.
- Enjoy with a glass of fresh almond or coconut milk.
- Goes well with a cup of orange juice.

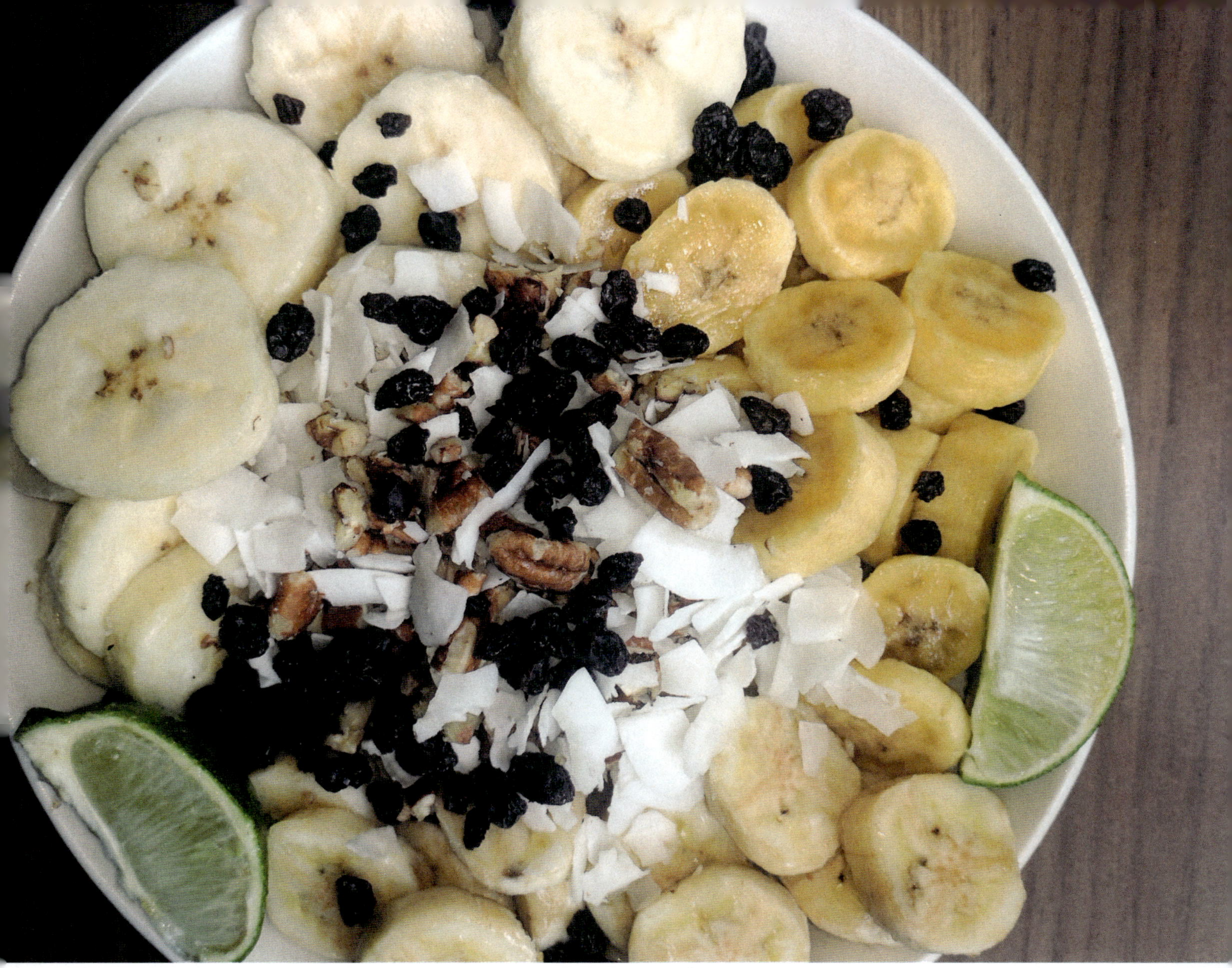

BANANAS FOR BANANAS BOWL

Fill up with fruit, get hydrated, and start the day right with this creamy, sweet breakfast bowl.

Serves: 1

INGREDIENTS:

- 2–5 bananas, chopped, 1–3 varieties
- sprinkle of shredded coconut
- sprinkle of dried currants

STEPS:

1. Slice bananas into a bowl.
2. Add desired toppings.
3. Enjoy!

DELICIOUS WITH: Garnish with shredded coconut, dried raisins, cranberries, currants, and a lime wedge. Enjoy with fresh, creamy almond or coconut milk, or a cup of herbal tea.

Bioactive Bananas

Bananas aren't the only plant foods that contain a large symphony of essential & beneficial nutrients, but they are a great example! Not only do bananas contain all the macronutrients: protein, carbohydrates, fat, fiber, & water (a banana is 72% water on average, same as a newborn human). Bananas also contain dozens of vitamins and minerals. And, so you can appreciate your next banana snack a little bit more... Bananas also contain the following bioactive compounds:

Tannic acid · Catechin · Gallic ad · Cinnamic acid · p-Coumaric acid · Gallocatechin · Quercetin · Ferulic acid · Trans-α carotene · Trans-β carotene · Violaxanthin · Cryptoxanthin · Serotonin · Dopamine · Catecholamines · β-Sitosterol · Campesterol and stigmasterol

..........Wow, bananas!!!! Go, go bananas!

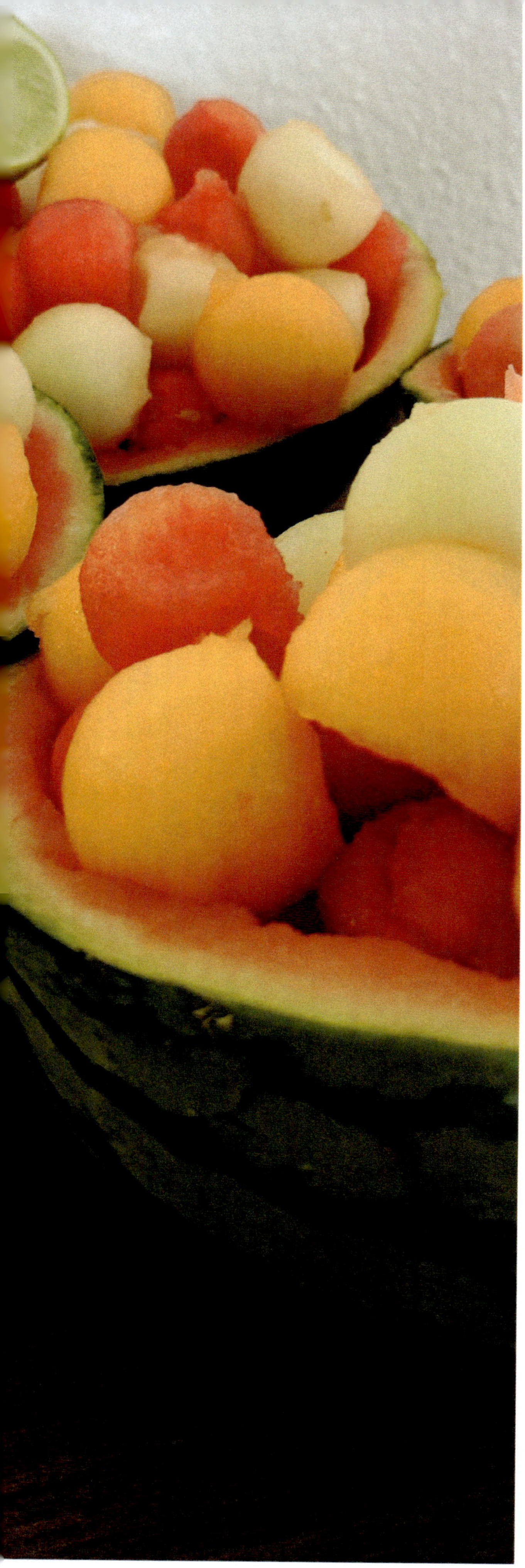

FRUITY MELON BOWLS

Fruit salad becomes more festive in natural melon bowls.

Serves: 2

INGREDIENTS:

- 1 watermelon, baby
- 1 cantaloupe, small
- 1 honeydew melon, small
- 1 mango
- 2 bananas
- 1 lime

TIP: Any type of melon can work as a melon bowl to make a fruity meal more fun.

STEPS:

1. Slice baby watermelon in half.
2. Scoop out watermelon fruit using a melon baller. If you don't have a melon baller, simply dice into bite-sized chunks.
3. Slice cantaloupe and honeydew melons in half and remove seeds with a large spoon.
4. Scoop out melon fruit with a melon baller.
5. Dice mango into bite-sized chunks, removing the skin.
6. Combine fruits into empty melon bowls and use a regular kitchen bowl to store any of the remaining fruit that doesn't' fit.
7. Serve soon. This fruit salad is best fresh.
8. Enjoy!
9. Store leftovers in the fridge and enjoy later.

DELICIOUS WITH:

- Try using a melon baller to make beautiful fruit balls from bananas, papaya, and any type of melon.
- Swap any of the fruits in this simple fruit salad with your favorite seasonal fruit varieties.
- Excellent fruit salad breakfast for two.
- Use a large watermelon and adapt recipe to make an attractive fruit salad for sharing at family gatherings, parties, and potlucks.

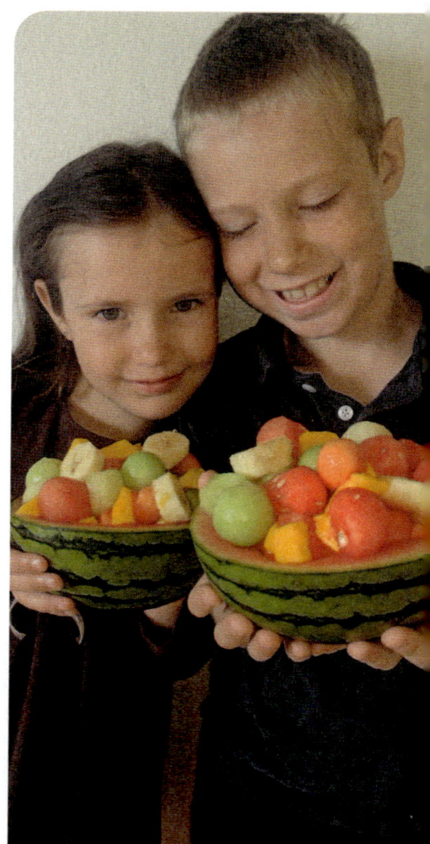

FRUIT BALLS SALAD

Taste the raw fruit rainbow with this sweet bowl.

Serves: 2

INGREDIENTS:

- 1 small watermelon
- 1 small cantaloupe
- 2 pints of blueberries
- 4 cups green grapes

STEPS:

1. Wash fresh fruits.
2. Cut melons in half and remove seeds from cantaloupe.
3. Use melon ball scooper to scoop balls from watermelon and cataloupe.
4. Remove stems from grapes and blueberries.
5. Combine fruits in serving bowls.
6. Enjoy soon after making.

DELICIOUS WITH:

- If you are feeling adventurous, try scooping balls out of bananas.
- Honeydew and other melon varieties also work great in this salad.
- Try red or black grapes instead of green.
- Add a lime squeeze for an extra flavorful burst of tart.

Essential Tool

To create the recipes on these two pages you will need a melon baller. While this tool isn't essential to a healthy diet, it is essential for creating perfect spheres of fruit to make fruit salads and fruit kabobs even more magnificent. Many grocers and stores selling kitchen tools will have this item, but sometimes it can be hard to find. For your fruit-balling convenience I have included a melon baller just like this in the Frugivore Diet store found at https://healingwithplants.us/store/kitchen-tools/ for just $9.99.

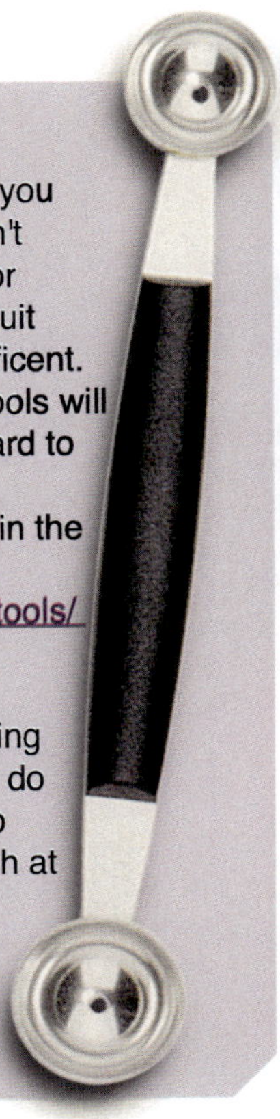

It might take you a little practice to perfect the art of scooping balls of fruit, but once you do you'll have what it takes to make the prettiest fruit dish at the party.

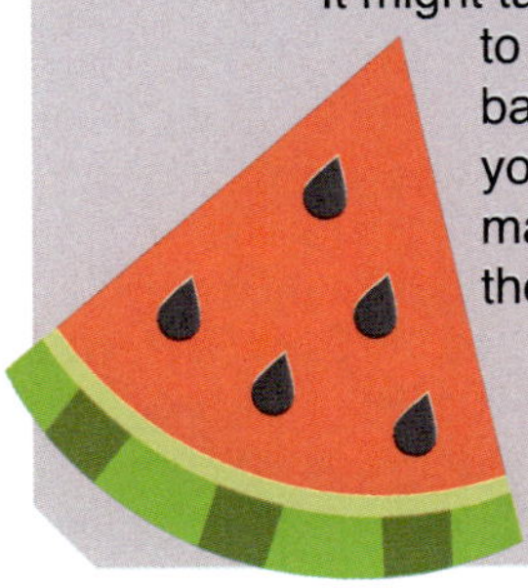

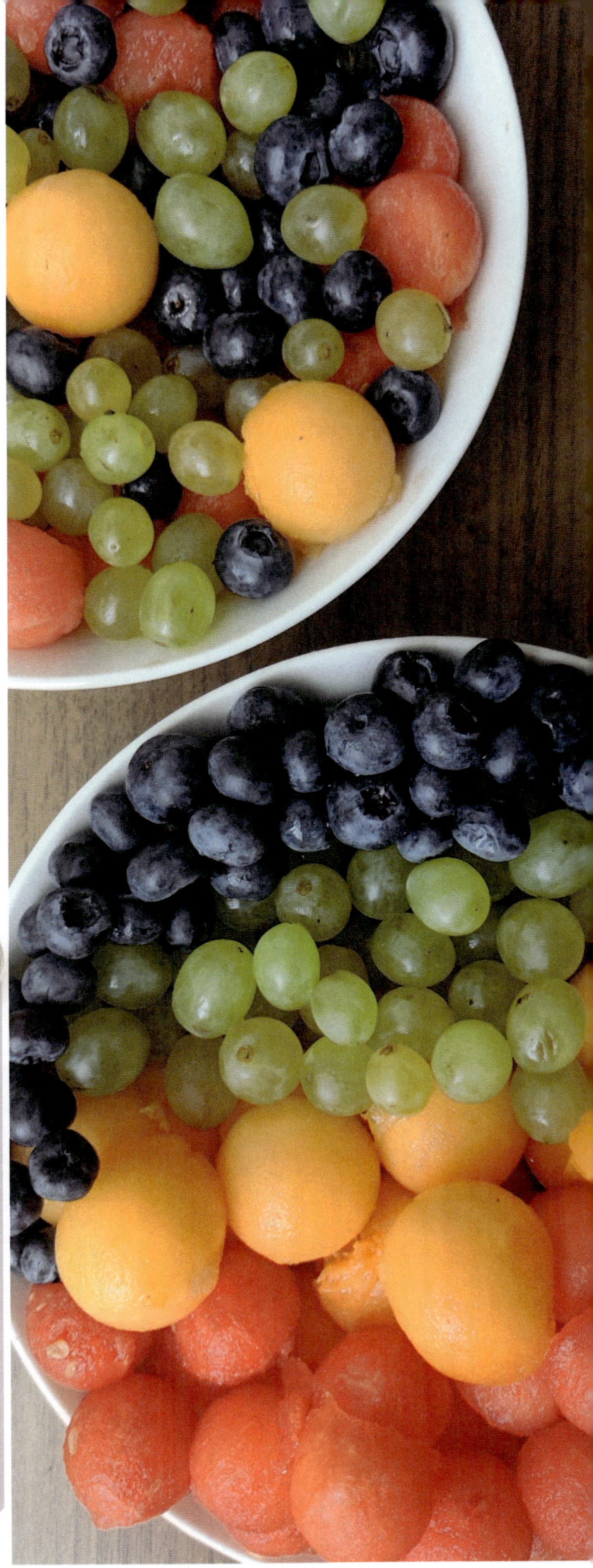

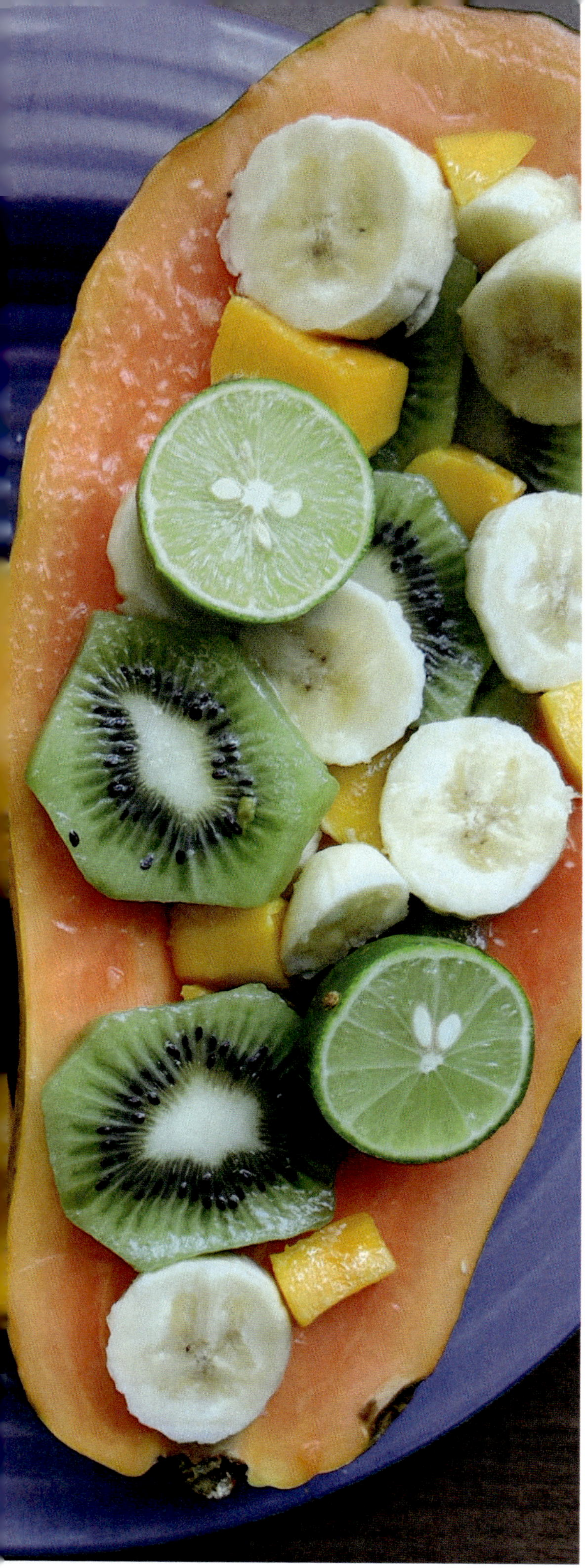

PAPAYA BOATS

These sweet, nutritious, fruit-filled boats will have you floating on the sea of wellness.

Serves: 2

INGREDIENTS:

- 1 papaya
- 3–4 kiwi
- 1–2 mangoes
- 2 lime
- 2 banana

STEPS:

1. Slice papaya in half lengthwise and scoop out seeds.
2. Remove skin from kiwis and slice flesh into rounds.
3. Peel bananas and slice into thin rounds.
4. Dice mangoes into bite-sized pieces.
5. Slice limes in half or into squeezable wedges.
6. Combine bananas, kiwi, and mangoes into the papaya boats.
7. Add lime as garnish to squeeze on top. Enjoy!

DELICIOUS WITH:

- Substitute any of the fruits in the papaya boat with your favorite seasonal fruit varieties.
- Pineapple, blueberries, and strawberries are a nice compliment to papaya.
- Serve these sweet, fruit-filled boats at any family feast.

Papaya Packs The Nutrients

These are the nutrients in just one cup of papaya:

- Water, 128 g
- Energy, 62.4 calories
- Protein, 0.681 g
- Fat, 0.377 g
- Carbohydrate, 15.7 g
- Fiber, 2.46 g
- Glucose, 5.93 g
- Fructose, 5.41 g
- Calcium, Ca, 29 mg
- Iron, Fe, 0.362 mg
- Magnesium, Mg, 30.4 mg
- Phosphorus, P, 14.5 mg
- Potassium, K, 264 mg
- Sodium, Na,11.6 mg
- Zinc, Zn, 0.116 mg
- Copper, Cu, 0.065 mg
- Manganese, Mn, 0.058 mg
- Selenium, Se, 0.87 μg
- Vitamin C, 88.3 mg
- Thiamin, 0.033 mg
- Riboflavin, 0.039 mg
- Niacin, 0.518 mg
- Pantothenic acid, 0.277 mg
- Vitamin B-6, 0.055 mg
- Folate, 53.6 μg
- Choline, 8.84 mg
- Carotene, beta, 397 μg
- Carotene, alpha, 2.9 μg
- Cryptoxanthin, beta, 854 μg
- Vitamin A, IU, 1380 IU
- Lycopene, 2650 μg
- Lutein + zeaxanthin, 129 μg
- Vitamin E, 0.435 mg
- Vitamin K, 3.77 μg

+More!!! Yes, that's not all folks. I couldn't list all the phytonutrients found in papaya. Soooo much goodness in whole foods!

PERSIMMON SMOOTHIE BOWL

Persimmon nice-cream is a truly special treat reserved for that special time of year when the sweet orange tree fruits come in season.

Serves: 1

INGREDIENTS:

- 1 Hachiya persimmon, frozen, or 2–3 Fuyu persimmons
- 1 banana, frozen
- 1 cup of coconut milk (almond milk works great,too)

STEPS:

1. Peel and freeze banana ahead of time. Prepare and freeze persimmon ahead of time also.
2. Put ingredients into blender and blend until well combined.
3. Serve in a bowl, or a large cup if you prefer.
4. Enjoy!

DELICIOUS WITH:

- Garnish with a round slice of a crisp persimmon.
- Add some fresh, sliced fruit, or a handful of shredded coconut, or nuts on top.
- Add some more plant milk to make it thinner for a smoothie and fill up a glass.

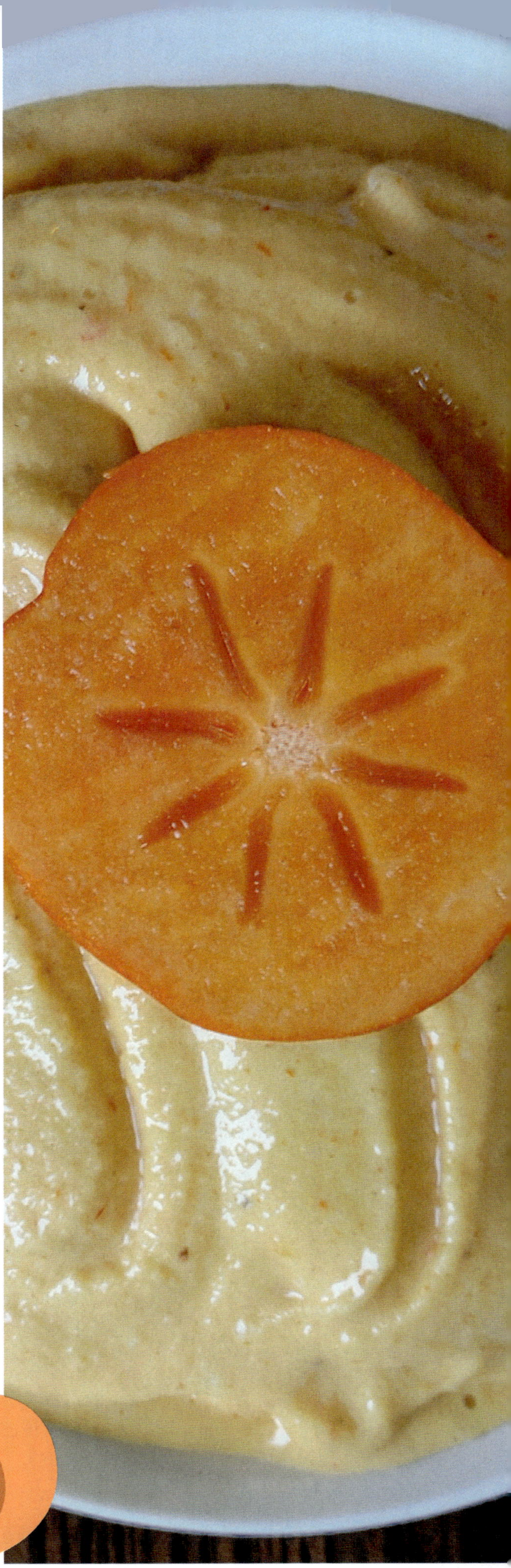

How to Pick a Persimmon

There are two main types of persimmons often referred to as Japanese and American. The American persimmons, also known as Fuyus, are referred to as non-astringent and can be eaten while crisp like apples. The Japanese persimmons, also known as Hachiyas, are referred to as astringent because their unripened flesh contains high levels of tannins which cause a very unpleasant sensation in the mouth if you bite into one before its time is right. Once they are ripe, the taste is all sweet-fruity-goodness. While Fuyu persimmons could be called a "dry fruit" and can be eaten much like an apple or crisp pear, the Hachiya variety is super juicy when it's ripe, to the point of being pudding-like. Because of this sloppy consistency when ripe, I prefer using Hachiyas for smoothies or to make preserves. They could also be used in baking or to make a persimmon pudding. If you are persimmon shopping at the store, you will spot a Hachiya for its acorn-like shape. Fuyus, the American variety, are more squat and could be mistaken for the cousin of a tomato.

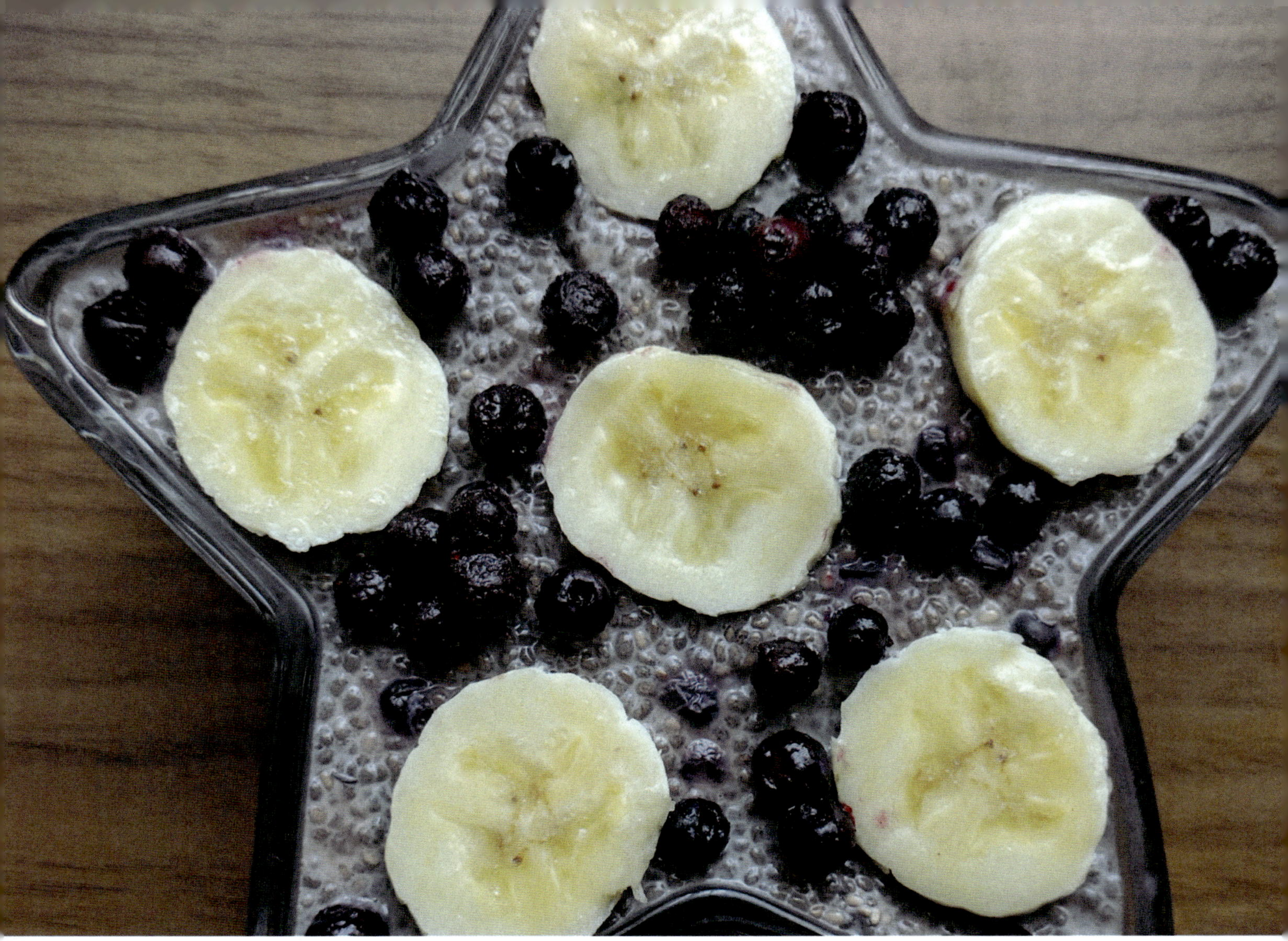

☀BLUEBERRY BANANA CHIA PUDDING☀

A cool, sweet, and creamy pudding that's purely plants and pleasantly pleasing to the palate.

Serves: 4

INGREDIENTS:

- 4 cups vanilla almond milk
- 1 cup chia seeds
- 12 oz. blueberries, fresh or frozen
- 3–4 bananas, large
  or 10–12 baby bananas sliced
- 3 tbsp. agave syrup

STEPS:

1. Mix all the ingredients together in a large bowl.
2. Pull out your favorite glasses and bowls to pour individual pudding servings into.
3. Make sure to stir out any clumps of chia seeds so that you have an evenly mixed pudding. (Your pudding should be a brilliant purple color at this point.)
4. Spoon pudding into serving dishes and set in fridge overnight.
5. Wake up the next morning, pull out your pudding, and top with more fresh banana slices and frozen blueberries, or whatever toppings you desire.
6. Share with the ones you love and enjoy!

✅ DELICIOUS WITH:

Add some fresh, sliced fruit, a handful of shredded coconut or nuts on top, or add some more plant milk to make it thinner for a smoothie and fill up a glass.

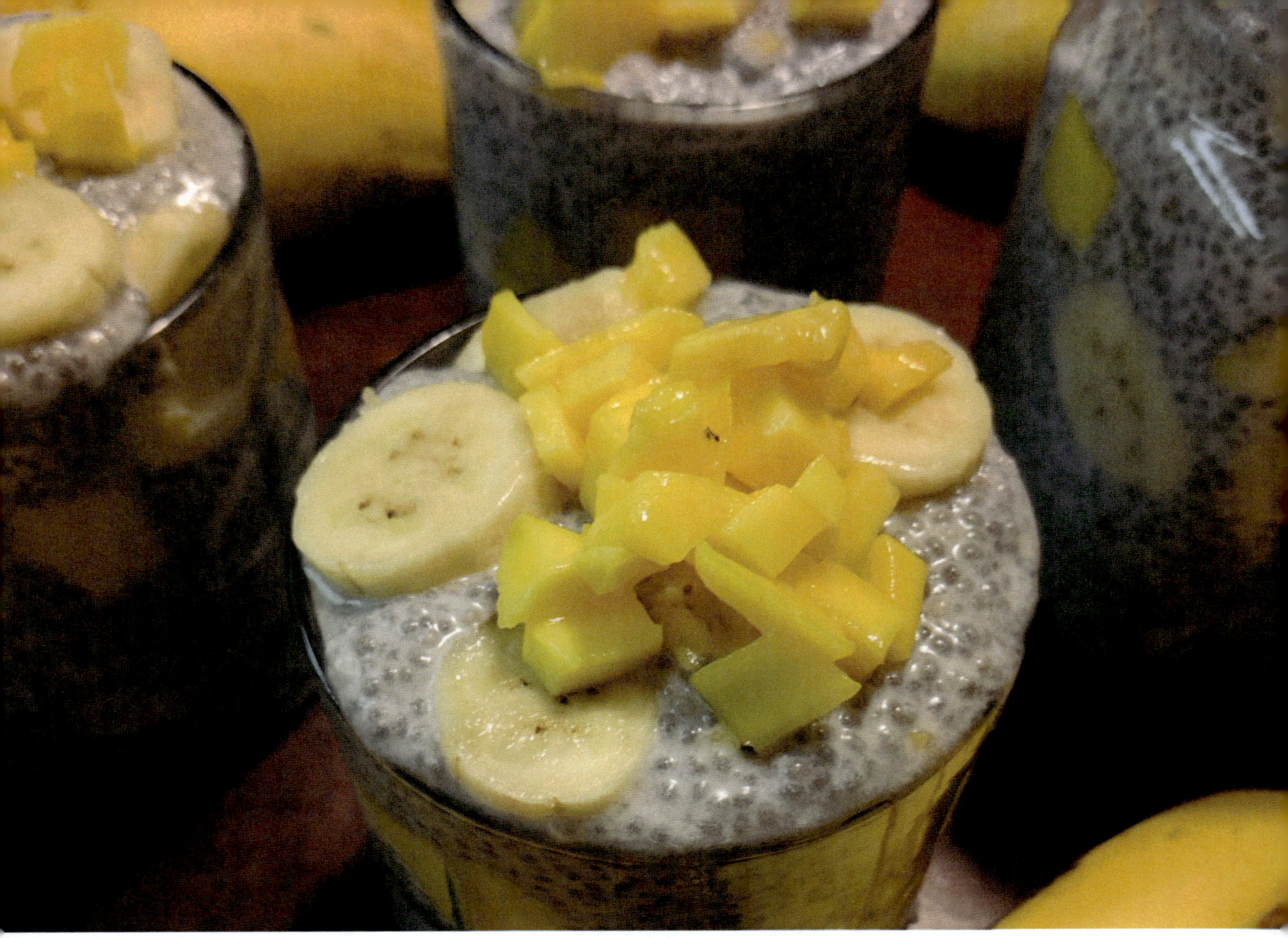

☀OVERNIGHT MANGO CHIA PUDDING☀

An easy, creamy, and sweet breakfast of purely seeds, fruits, and plant nectar.

Serves: 4

INGREDIENTS:

- 1 cup chia seeds
- 4 cups almond milk
- 4 bananas, medium or 12 baby bananas
- 2 mangoes, diced
- 3 tbsp. agave nectar

✅ **DELICIOUS WITH:** Add some fresh sliced fruit, a handful of shredded coconut, or nuts on top.

STEPS:

1. Combine first three ingredients in large bowl and stir out any clumps so mixture is even and all seeds are evenly coated in the seed milk.
2. Chop fruit and get four serving glasses, jars, or bowls.
3. Stir half of mango into pudding mix.
4. Put some bananas at bottom of serving cups.
5. Pour pudding on top of the bananas and add more bananas. Continue layering until full.
6. Top with fresh, sliced bananas and the other half of the diced mangoes.
7. Put pudding cups in fridge overnight.
8. Remove from fridge the next morning and enjoy!

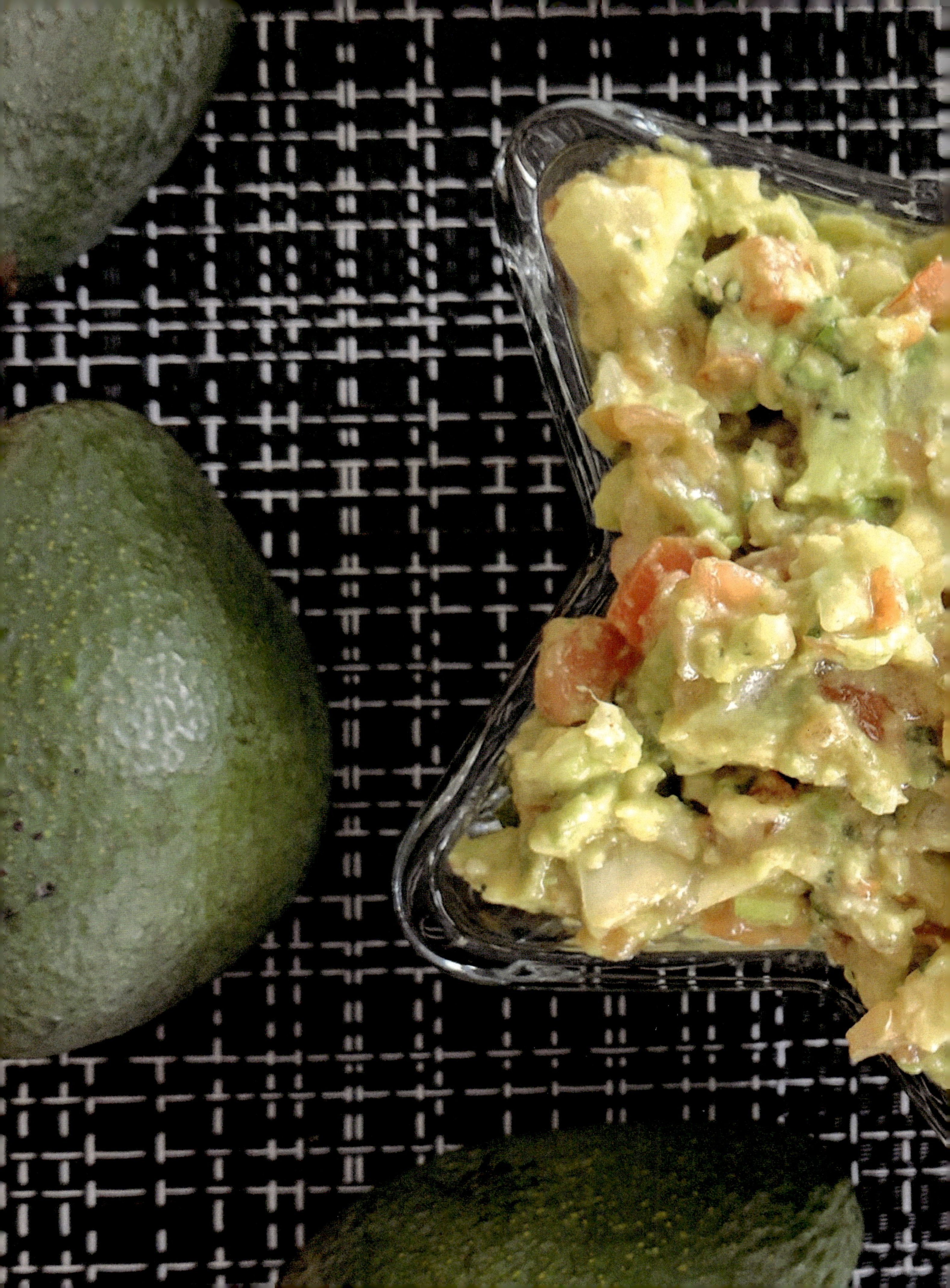

Dips, Dressings, and Sauces

BLEND, STIR, SHAKE

These dips, dressings, sauces, and sandwich spreads are made purely of whole plants ingredients. Simply seeds, shoots, fruits, and roots blend together in these recipes that make sandwiches, salads, pastas, and other plantiful plates more scrumptious.

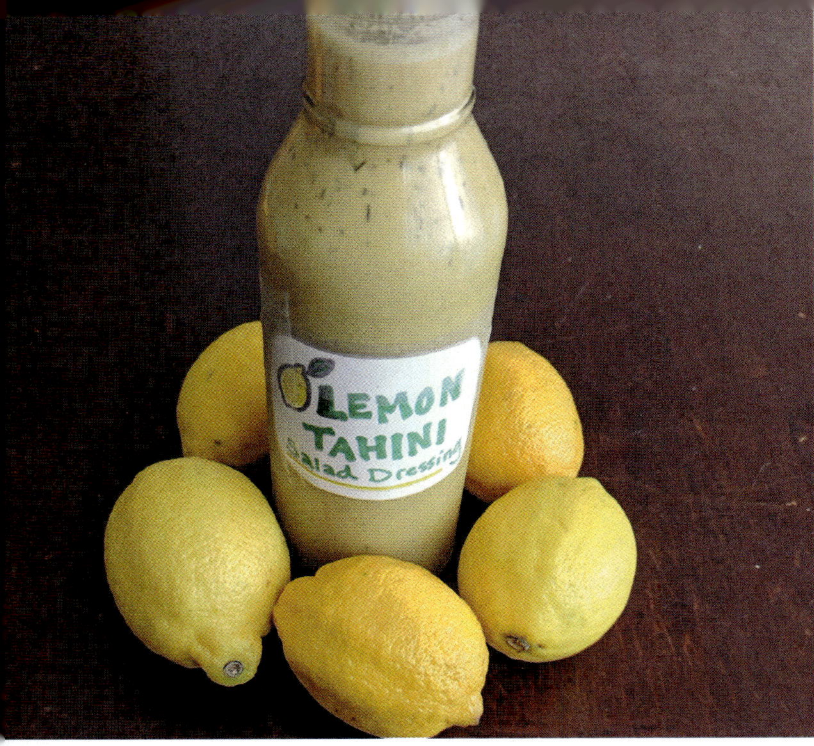

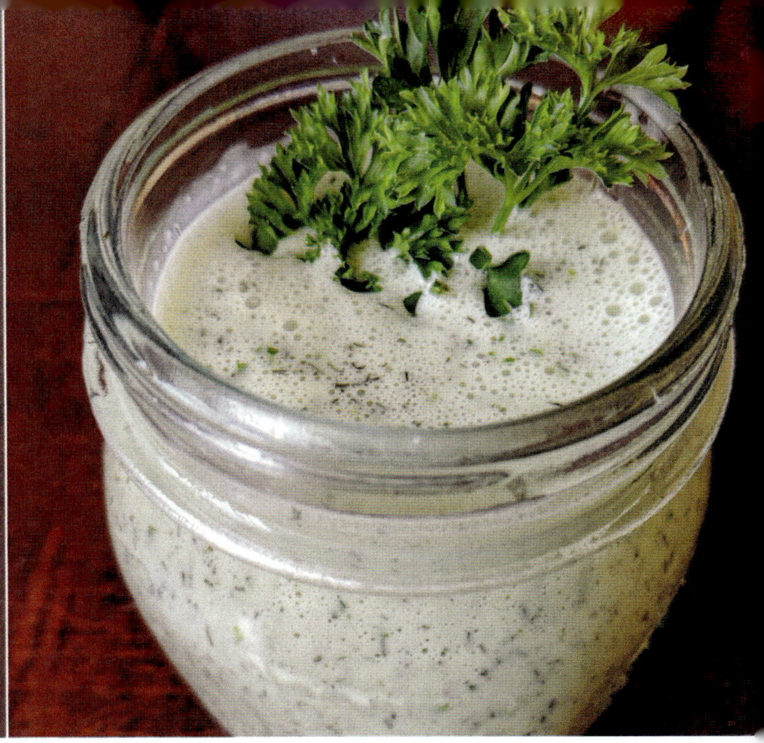

LEMON TAHINI

A savory blend of crushed sesame seeds, fresh citrus juice, and herbs that makes any salad more spectacular.

INGREDIENTS:

- 1/4 cup tahini
- 3 lemons, juiced
- 2 tbsp. apple cider vinegar
- 1 tbsp. liquid aminos (soy sauce)
- 1/2 tsp. dill
- 1/2 tbsp. garlic
- 1/2 cup nutritional yeast
- few twists of black pepper
- 1/2 cup water

STEPS:

1. Combine ingredients in mixing bowl or in a jar with a lid.
2. Whisk ingredients together or shake in jar with the lid on tight.
3. Enjoy on top of any salad or as a dip for fresh veggies.

DELICIOUS WITH:

- Dress any salad.
- Dip fresh veggies into this sauce.

COCONUT RANCH

A creamy herb-flavored dressing.

INGREDIENTS:

- 1 cup full-fat coconut milk/cream
- 1 garlic clove
- 2 green onions
- 1 tbsp. dill
- 2 tbsp. fresh parsley
- 3 tbsp. fresh herbs: basil, dill, or chives.
- 2 tbsp. apple cider vinegar
- 1 tsp. salt

STEPS:

1. Scoop the firm white coconut cream off the top of the can. Measure 1 cup. Use less of liquid coconut water to achieve thick creamy dressing consistency.
2. Rinse fresh herbs.
3. Add coconut milk, herbs, and vinegar to blender.
4. Blend until well combined.
5. Store leftovers in the refrigerator.

DELICIOUS WITH:

- Serve on top of salad or baked potato.
- Use as a dip for Perfect Potato Wedges.

The Preserving Power of Lemons

Lemon's are known for their high vitamin C content. Vitamin C is also known as ascorbic acid and is a powerful antioxidant that prevents rotting and spoilage. Lemon juice can be squeezed on fresh cut fruits and veggies to keep them looking fresh longer and will reduce any appearance of brown spots caused by exposure to the air. When you include lemon in your salad dressing it will also extend its refrigerator shelf life.

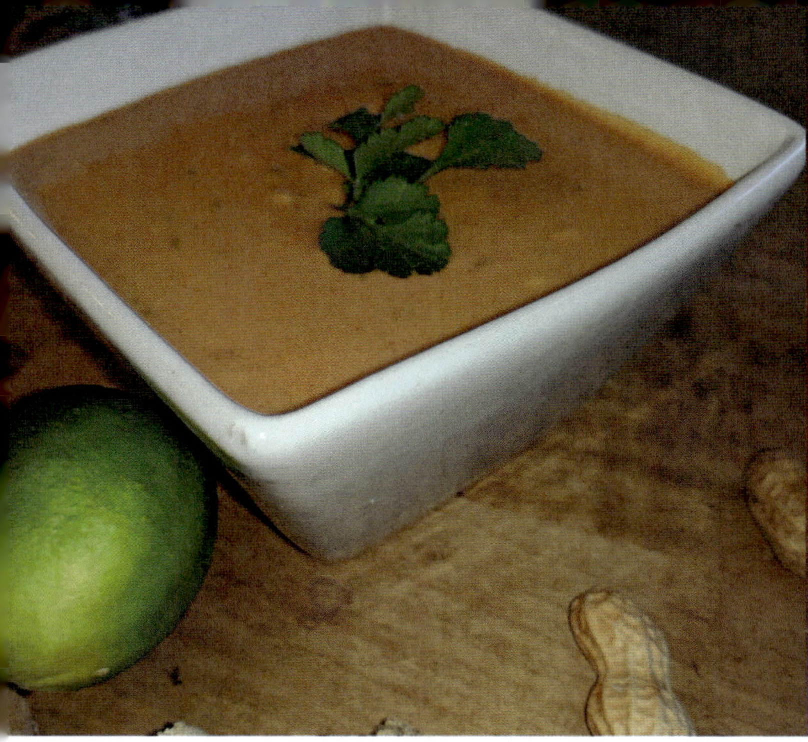

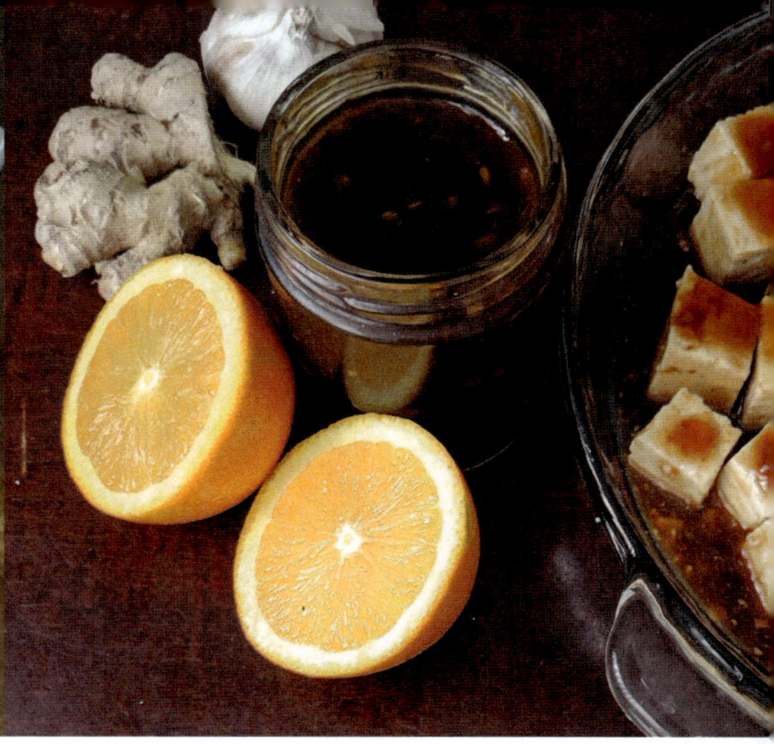

SPICY PEANUT SAUCE

A spicy goober sauce that goes perfect with spring rolls, tofu, kabobs, or salad.

INGREDIENTS:

- 1 cup peanut butter
- 2 limes, small
- 1/4 cup soy sauce
- 2 tbsp. vinegar
- 2 tbsp. ketchup
- 2 tbsp. sriracha
- 3 garlic cloves, diced small
- 5 green onions, diced small
- 1 tbsp. garlic powder
- 1.5 tsp. ginger powder
- 1 cup water

STEPS:

1. Combine ingredients in a large bowl or jar with lid.
2. Shake jar or whisk ingredients in a bowl until well combined.
3. Store leftovers in sealed jar in the refrigerator.

DELICIOUS WITH:

- Serve on top of salad.
- Use as a marinade for tofu.
- Use as a dip for spring rolls or fresh veggies.

TERIYAKI SAUCE

A sweet and savory sauce for marinating tofu and vegetables.

INGREDIENTS:

- 1/2 cup soy sauce
- 1 orange
- 1 cup water
- 3 garlic cloves
- 2 tbsp. corn starch
- 1 tbsp. ginger, fresh*
- 1 tbsp. agave

STEPS:

1. In a small pot combine soy sauce, water, agave, and cornstarch.
2. Juice orange into pot using a citrus juicer or strain seeds.
3. Chop garlic cloves and ginger into small pieces and add to pot.
4. Warm on medium heat stirring constantly until sauce thickens.
5. Remove from heat. Enjoy!

DELICIOUS WITH:

- Serve on top of salad.
- Use as a marinade for tofu.
- Dip spring rolls or fresh veggies into this flavorful sauce.

Peanut Power!

This beloved seed that grows underground and makes kids' bellies happy at lunchtime across America goes by many names including goober, groundnut, or monkey nut. Like other dried seeds—such as almonds, sunflower seeds, and cashews—ground peanuts make a thick paste that can be an excellent base for oil-free salad dressings and sauces. The natural oil in peanuts make sauces and sandwiches more satisfying. Try sprinkling a few on top of your next rice and veggie dish—so much crunchy yum!

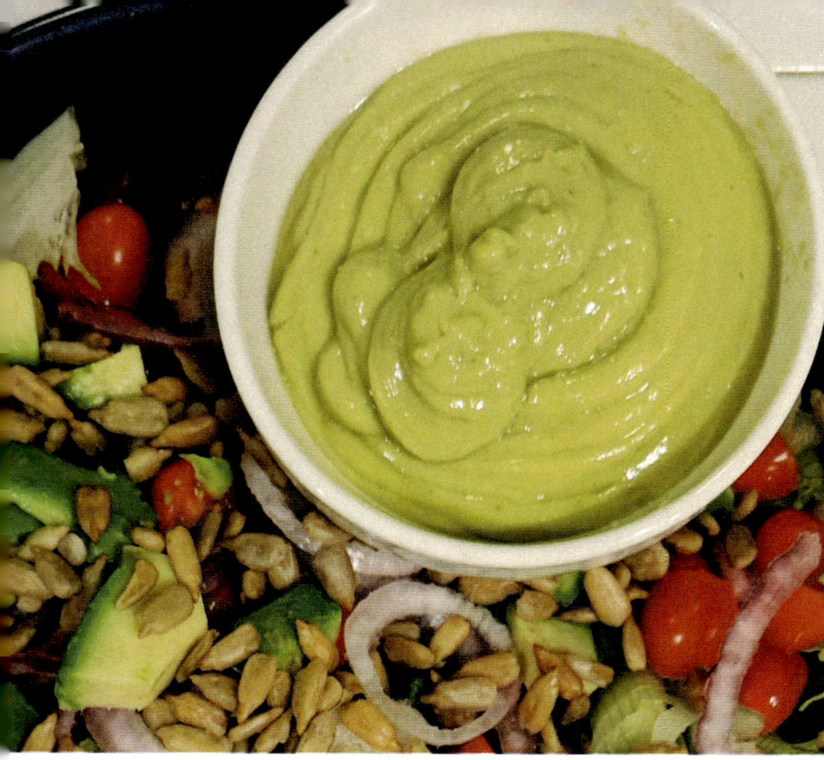

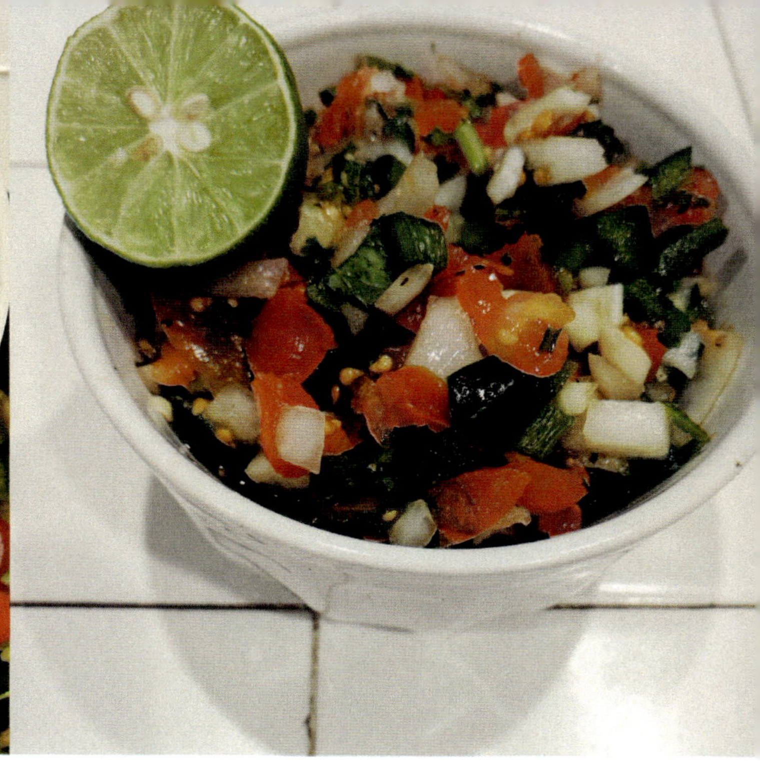

AVOCADO LIME SAUCE

A creamy dressing or dip with a cayenne pepper kick.

INGREDIENTS:

- 2 avocados
- 1 lime
- 1 garlic clove
- 1/2 tsp. salt
- 1/4 tsp. cayenne pepper
- 1/2 cup water
- optional: cilantro, small sprig

STEPS:

1. Wash avocado, lime, and cilantro.
2. Remove avocado pulp from skin and pit and place into blender.
3. Put all ingredients into blender and blend until smooth.
4. Blend until well combined.
5. Pour into serving vessel or store in jar with tight lid in the fridge. Best served immediately, or leftovers are good for 3–4 days.

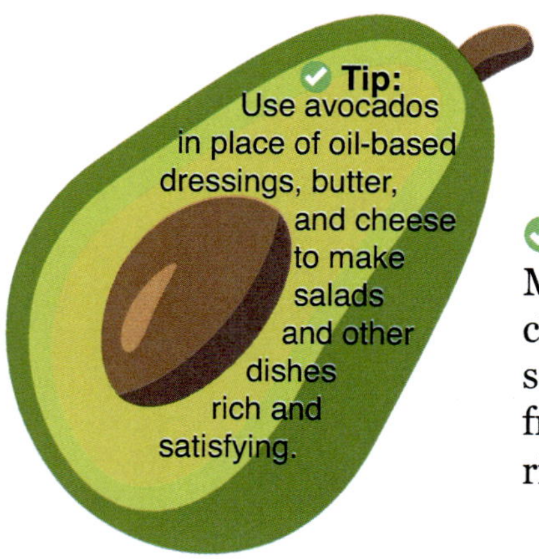
Tip:
Use avocados in place of oil-based dressings, butter, and cheese to make salads and other dishes rich and satisfying.

DELICIOUS WITH:

Make this sauce your tortilla chip dip, taco topper, burrito sauce, salad dressing, dip for fresh veggies, or sauce for rice.

PICO DE GALLO

A fresh yummy topping for tacos, potatoes, and more!

INGREDIENTS:

- 1 cup cherry tomatoes or 2 medium tomatoes
- 1/2 yellow onion, medium
- 3 garlic cloves
- 1 lime
- 1/2 poblano chili pepper (sub: 1 green pepper)
- 2 tbsp. cilantro
- 1 tsp. salt
- generous twists of black pepper

STEPS:

1. Wash fresh veggies.
2. Chop onions, garlic, pepper, tomatoes, and cilantro into small pieces and add to small mixing bowl.
3. Squeeze juice of one lime into bowl and add salt.
4. Stir until well combined.
5. Store leftovers in sealed jar in the refrigerator.

DELICIOUS WITH:

- Serve on top of tacos, Baked Potato (pg. 89), or salad.
- Use as a dip for tortilla chips.

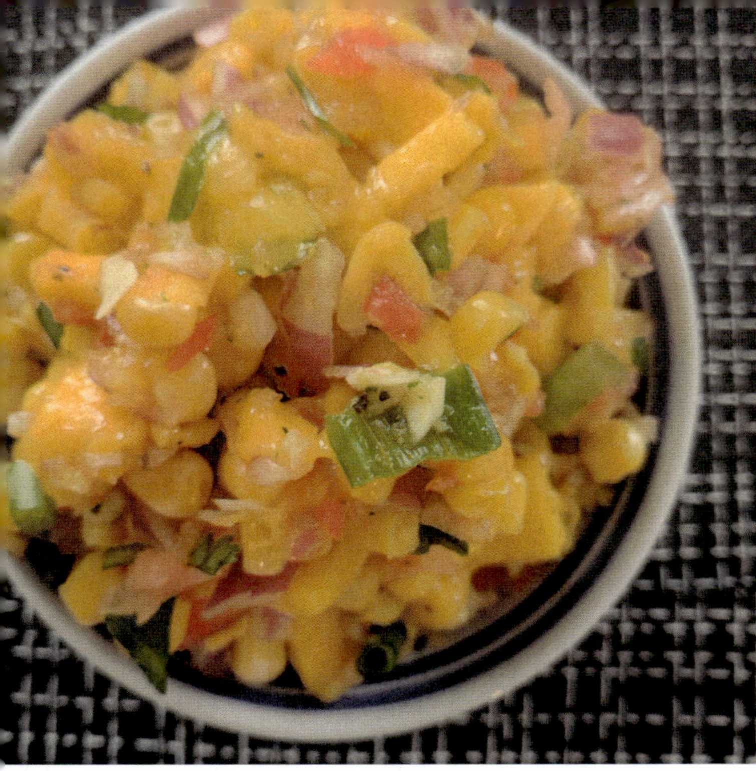

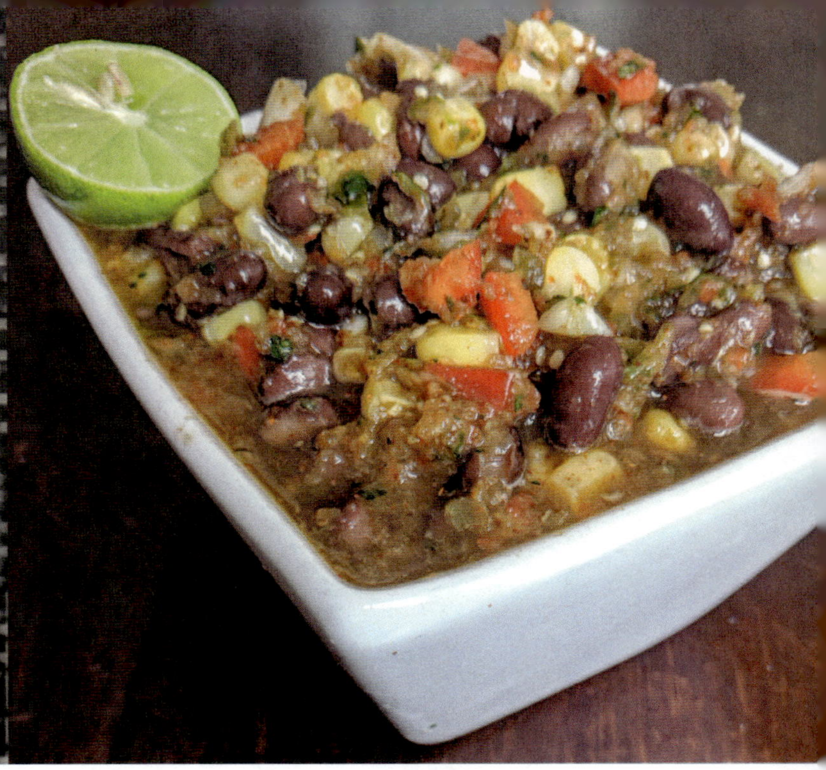

MANGO CORN SALSA

A crunchy and sweet, sun-colored salsa.

INGREDIENTS:

- 2 mangoes
- 1 Roma tomato
- 1 cup corn
- 2 green onions
- 2 tbsp. red onion, chopped
- 1 garlic clove
- 1 cilantro sprig
- 1 tsp. onion salt

STEPS:

1. Wash fresh fruits and veggies.
2. Place tomato, red onion, garlic, and cilantro into food processor of high speed blender for 15–30 seconds until mostly chopped into small pieces.
3. Dice mango into small chunks.
4. Chop green onions into small thin rounds.
5. Combine mango, corn, green onion, and remaining chopped ingredients.
6. Stir well. Enjoy!

DELICIOUS WITH: Tortilla chips, salad, Red Rice (pg.83), burrito, Chickpea Tacos (pg.111), or Taquitos (pg.110).

CHUNKY BLACK BEAN & CORN SALSA

A chunky chip dip or taco-topper with a nice spice.

INGREDIENTS:

- 1 cup corn
- 1 15 oz. can black beans, liquid drained
- 4 large tomatillos
- 4 garlic cloves
- 2 large green onions
- 1 large red or yellow bell pepper
- 1/2 medium yellow onion
- 2 tbsp. fresh cilantro, chopped
- 1 lime, juice
- 1 tbsp. chipotle powder seasoning

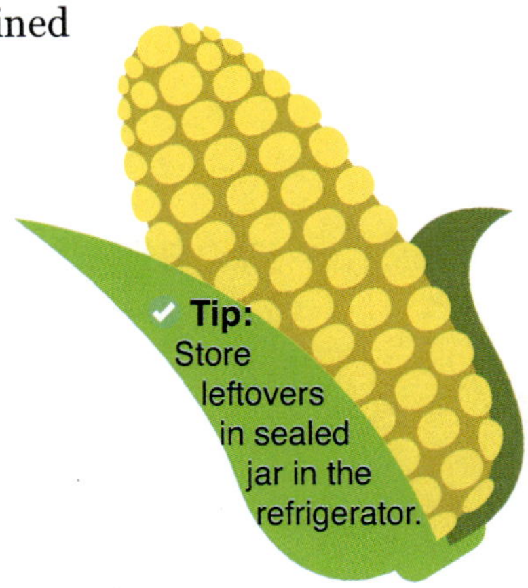

STEPS:

1. Wash fresh veggies.
2. Chop onions, garlic, bell peppers, and cilantro into small pieces.
3. Remove tomatillo skin and tough top, dice into quarters, and place into high speed blender.
4. Add half of chopped onions, bell pepper, garlic, and cilantro to blender with juice of lime.
5. Blend for 5–10 seconds or just until tomatillos have been reduced.
6. In a medium bowl, mix blender contents with remaining chopped veggies, corn, black beans, and spice. Enjoy!

DELICIOUS WITH: Serve on top of salad or Baked Potato (pg.89). Use as a dip for Perfect Potato Wedges (pg.93).

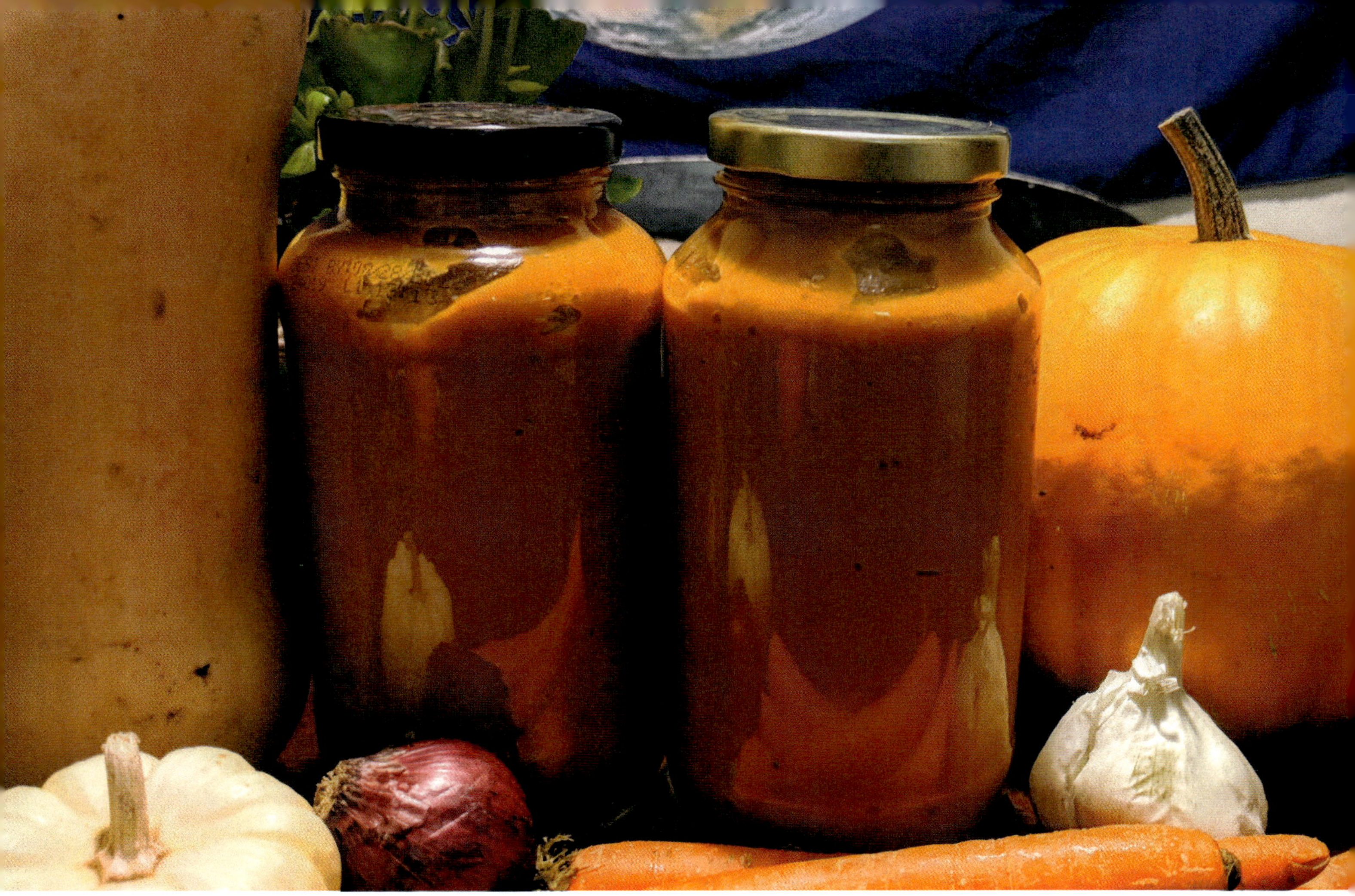

HARVEST PASTA SAUCE

Harvest Pasta Sauce is a 100% whole-plant food sauce that's vegan, oil-free, dairy-free, nutrient-rich, and so flavorful it will have you falling in love with fall over and over again.

INGREDIENTS:

- 1 whole pumpkin, baked
- 1 whole butternut squash flesh, baked
- 4 carrots
- 6 oz. tomato paste
- 1 can coconut milk (full-fat or coconut cream)
- 1 onion (red, yellow, or white)
- 8 garlic cloves, peeled
- 1 twig rosemary (or 1 tsp. dried)
- 2 sage leaves, fresh (or 1 tsp. dried)
- 2 tsp. salt
- 1/4 tsp. cayenne
- sprinkle black pepper
- 1 cup water

STEPS:

1. Place whole pumpkin and butternut squash on oven rack and bake at 375°F for about 40 minutes, or until soft enough to cut through easily with a knife.
2. Remove pumpkin and squash from oven. Cut in half and scoop out seeds with a large spoon. Scoop flesh of squashes into crockpot or into large pot on stovetop.
3. Dice carrots into large chunks and add to crockpot or large pot.
4. Peel onion and garlic cloves, chop into large chunks, and add to pot.
5. Add tomato paste, salt, pepper, cayenne, and water to the pot. Set crockpot to medium and allow to cook for 3–4 hours or until carrots, onion, and garlic are soft.
6. When contents of pot are all soft, add fresh herbs and coconut milk, stir contents, and turn off heat. Cover pot and allow to sit for 30–60 minutes for flavors to absorb and for contents to cool.
7. Add the contents of the pot to the blender and puree until smooth and well combined.
8. Enjoy on top pasta, pizza, or as a soup base.
9. Scoop any remaining sauce into clean empty jars and refrigerate for later use. Alternatively, freeze leftovers in tupperware.

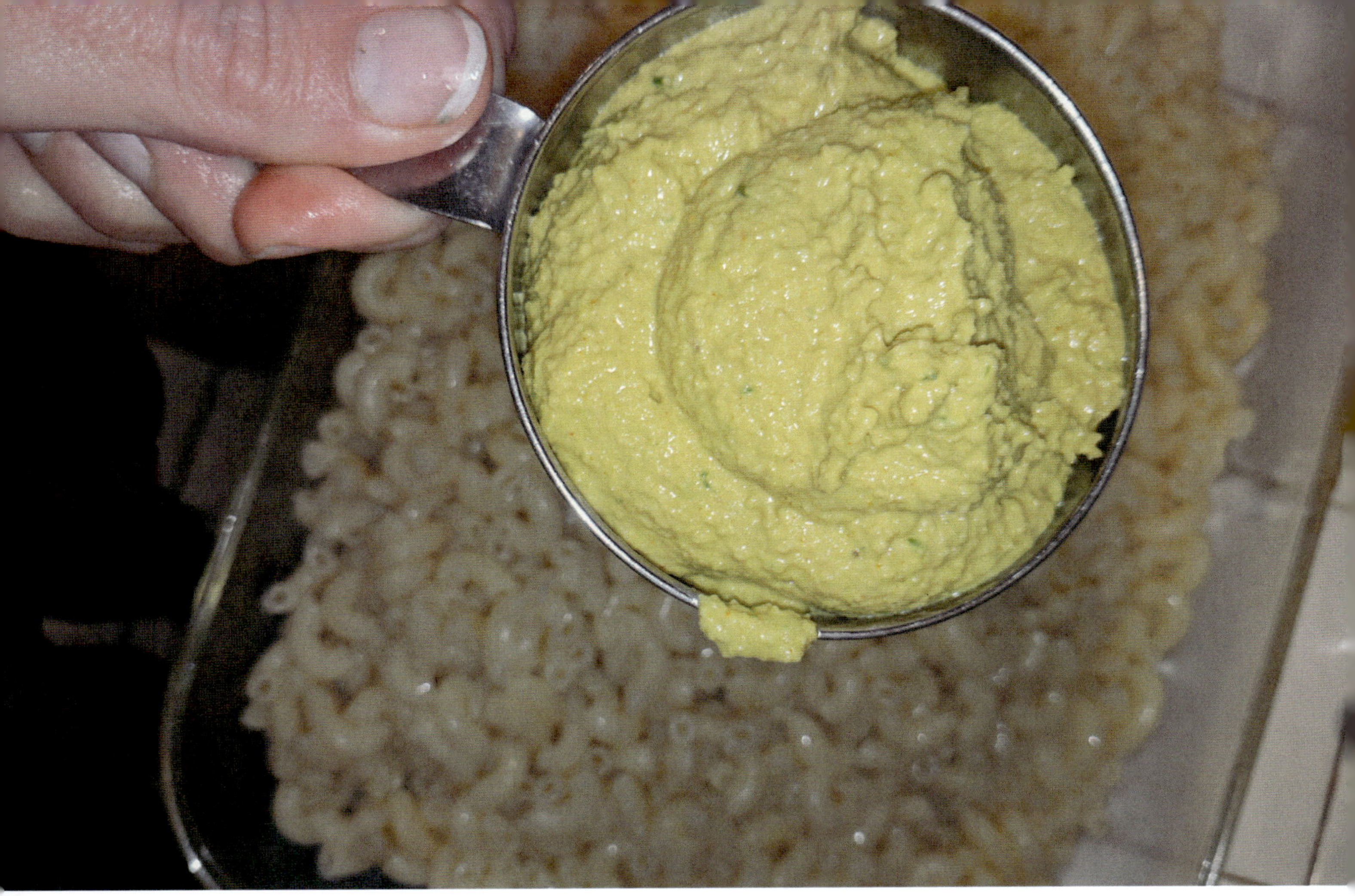

CH-EASY CASHEW SAUCE

An addictively creamy and easy-to-make sauce that makes tacos terrific and mac and ch-ease magnificent!

INGREDIENTS:

- 2 cups cashews, raw, soaked
- 10 garlic cloves, small/medium
- 1 cup nutritional yeast
- 2 tsp. salt
- 3 green onions
- 1 lemon or lime
- 1 tsp. ground mustard
- 1/2 tsp. cayenne pepper
- 1 cup water

STEPS:

1. Soak cashews for at least 1 hour and up to 24 hours.
2. Drain liquid from cashews and add to food processor.
3. Add other ingredients and spices and blend on high until smooth and well combined.

DELICIOUS WITH:

- Use to make a creamy, rich Ch-Easy Mac (pg.102).
- Top your tortilla chips and Chickpea Tacos (pg. 111) with this awesome sauce.
- Dip into with fresh veggies.
- Make it a sandwich spread.
- Top a Baked Potato (pg.89).

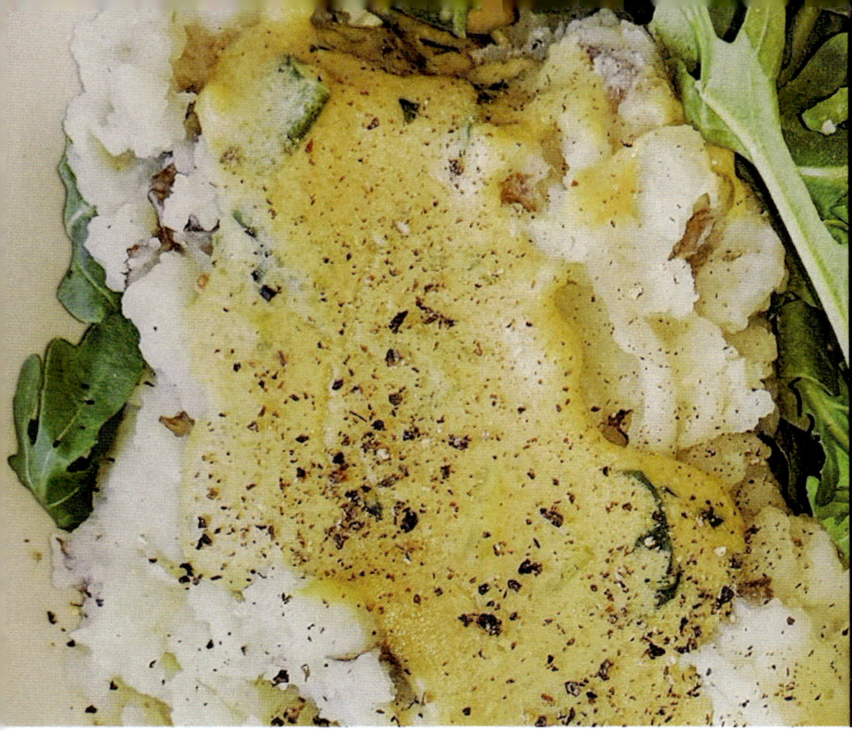

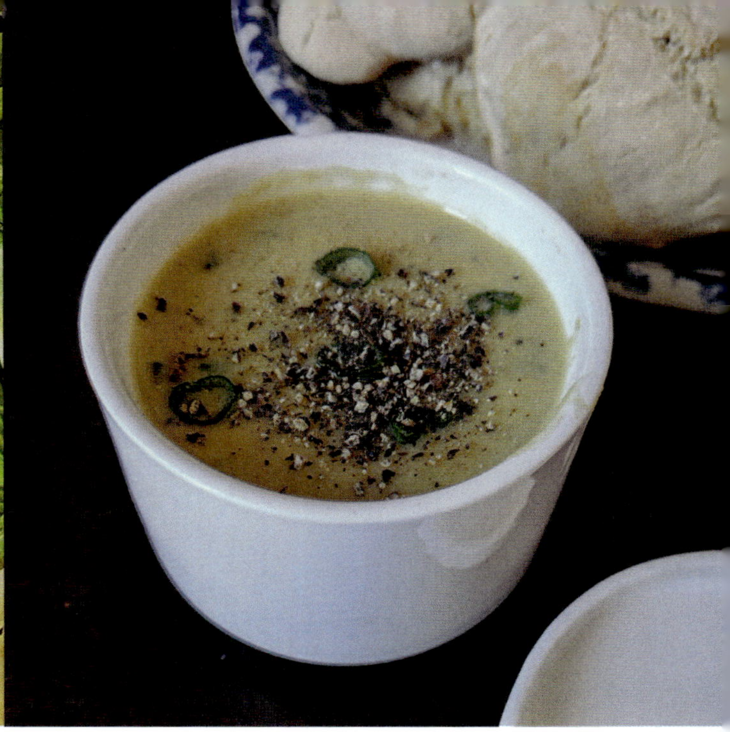

GARDEN GRAVY

A gravy so good it goes with almost anything.

INGREDIENTS:

- 1 cup nutritional yeast
- 1–2 green onions, chopped
- 1/4 cup cornmeal or 2 tbsp. corn starch
- 2.5 cup unsweetened almond milk
- 1/2 cup water
- 1 tbsp. liquid aminos/soy sauce
- 1 tsp. thyme, fresh is best
- 1 tsp. garlic, fresh minced is best
- 4 basil leaves, or 1 tsp. dried basil
- 1 tsp. rosemary, fresh chopped
- generous twists of black pepper

STEPS:

1. Combine ingredients in a saucepan.
2. Warm on low heat on the stovetop stirring frequently with a wire whisk.
3. Continue to heat and whisk gravy until desired thickness is achieved.
4. Enjoy!

BREAKFAST GRAVY

Green onion and pepper gravy that goes perfect with breakfast.

INGREDIENTS:

- 2.5 cup unsweetened almond milk
- 6 green onions, chopped small
- 1/2 cup nutritional yeast
- 1/2 cup water
- 1/4 cup flour or 2 tbsp. corn starch
- 1 tbsp. liquid aminos/soy sauce
- 1 tsp. sage (fresh is best)
- 1 tsp. garlic powder
- 1 tsp. onion powder
- 1 tsp. salt
- 1 tsp. black pepper

STEPS:

1. Combine ingredients in a saucepan.
2. Warm on low heat on the stovetop stirring frequently with a wire whisk.
3. Continue to heat and whisk gravy until desired thickness is achieved.
4. Enjoy!

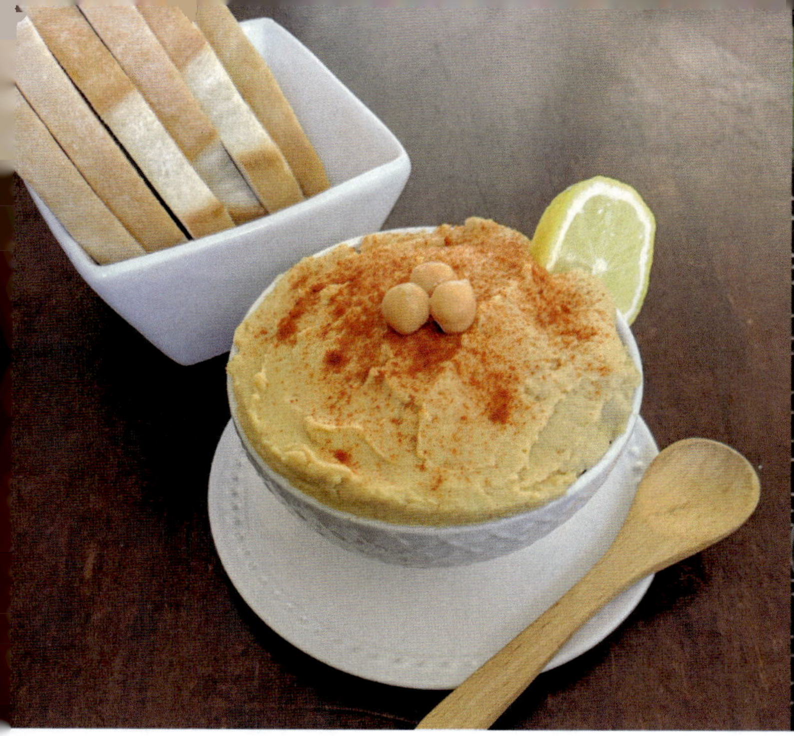

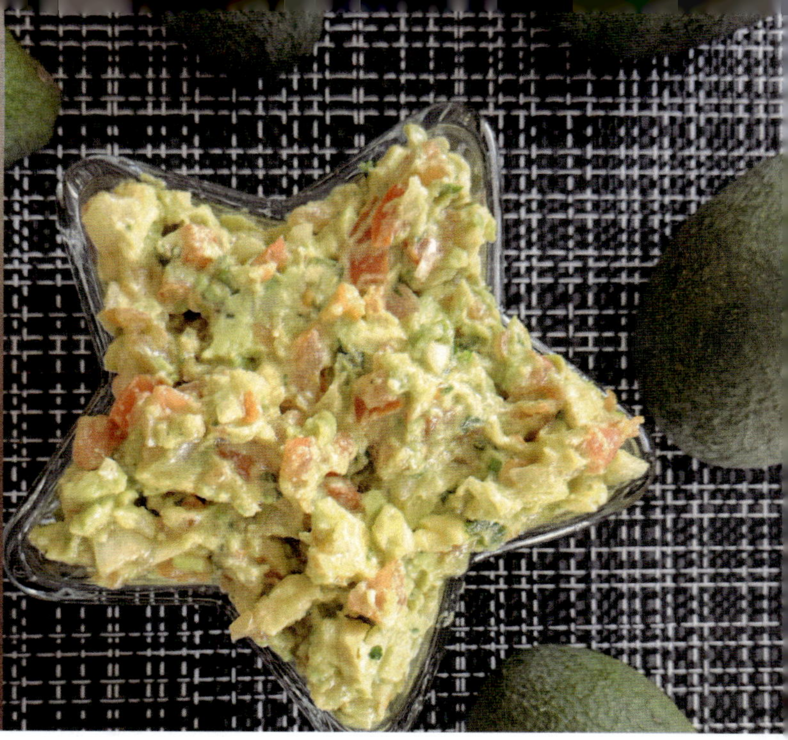

HEAVENLY GARLIC HUMMUS

Chickpeas and garlic pair up to please the palate in this satisfying sandwich spread.

INGREDIENTS:

- 5 cups garbanzo beans, rinsed, drained
- 3 garlic cloves
- 2 lemons
- 2 tbsp. tahini
- 1 tbsp. onion salt
- 1 tsp. cayenne pepper
- 1/2 cup water
- optional: paprika sprinkle

STEPS:

1. Place all ingredients into high-powered food processor and blend.
2. Add a tad more water to thin to desired consistency for dipping or spreading.
3. Enjoy!

DELICIOUS WITH:

- Spread on your sandwiches.
- Dip into with fresh carrot and celery sticks.
- Spread on thick cucumber slices or warmed pita bread.
- Dip into with tortilla chips.
- Enjoy on top of salad.

GARDEN GUACAMOLE

Avocados star in this creamy fresh dip.

INGREDIENTS:

- 4 ripe avocados
- 3 garlic cloves
- 1 large lime or 3–4 small key limes
- 1/2 small onion, diced
- 4 green onions
- 2 tomatoes
- 1 tsp. onion salt
- 1/4 tsp. cayenne pepper
- 1 tbsp. cilantro, chopped
- 1 tbsp. apple cider vinegar

STEPS:

1. Slice avocados in half, remove pits, and slice the flesh of fruit into chunks.
2. Scoop out avocado flesh into large mixing bowl.
3. Chop onions, garlic, cilantro, and tomatoes into small pieces and combine with avocado in bowl.
4. Add apple cider vinegar and spices.
5. Stir guacamole ingredients together aiming to slightly mash the avocados and leave some chunks remaining.
6. Enjoy!

DELICIOUS WITH:

- Top your tacos, burritos, and spicy soups.
- Dip into with tortilla chips.
- Enjoy on top of salad.

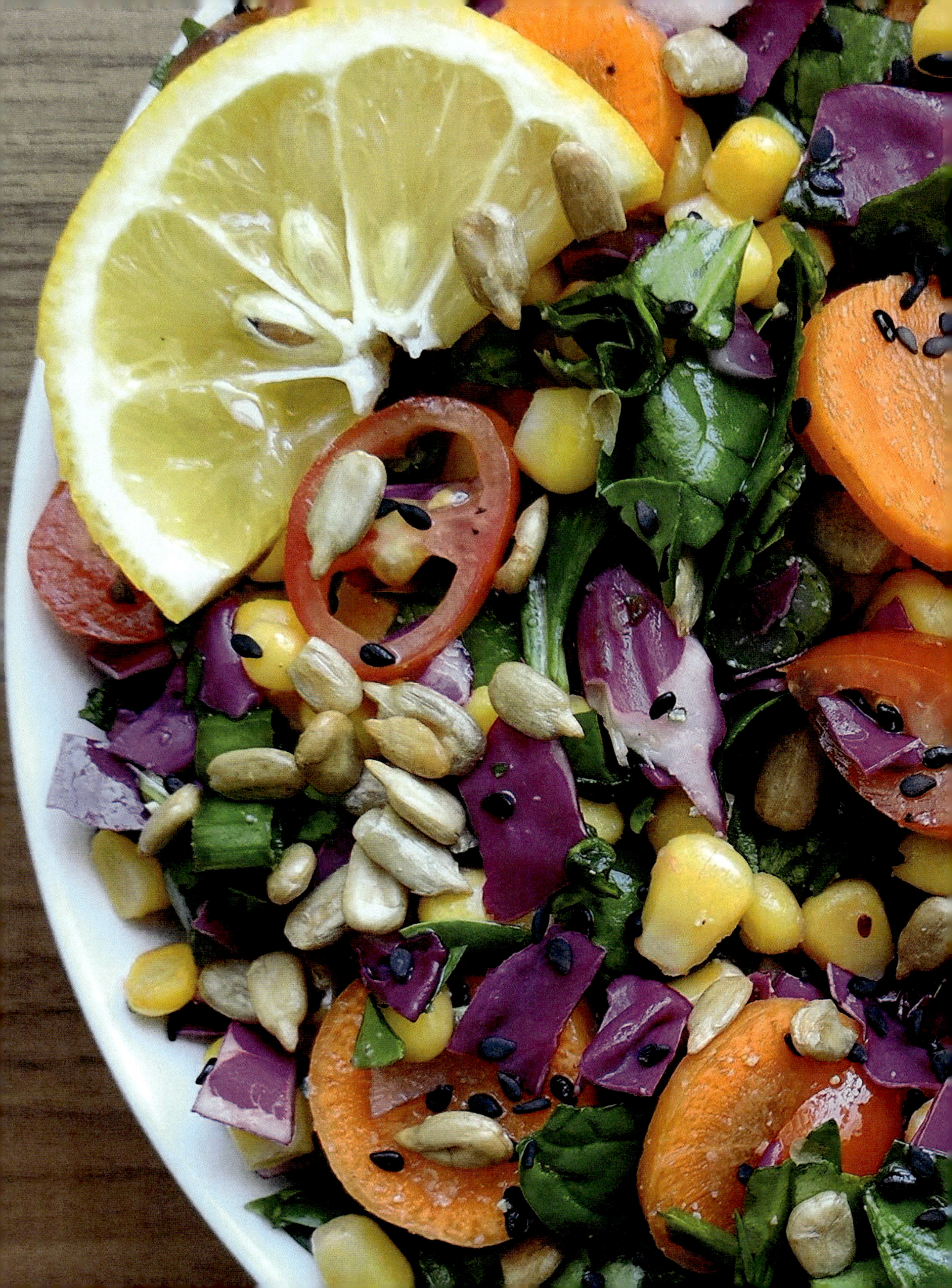

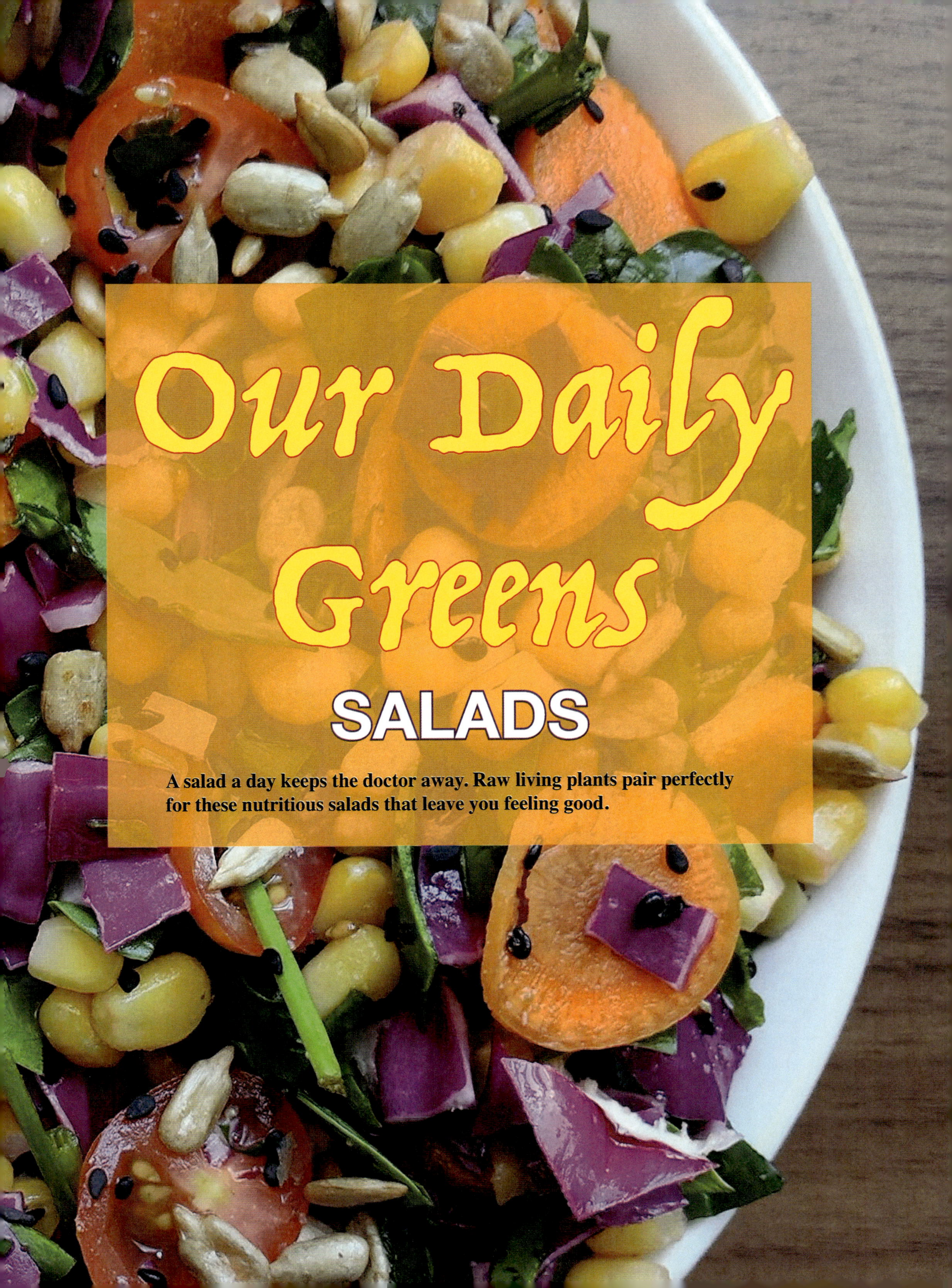

Our Daily Greens

SALADS

A salad a day keeps the doctor away. Raw living plants pair perfectly for these nutritious salads that leave you feeling good.

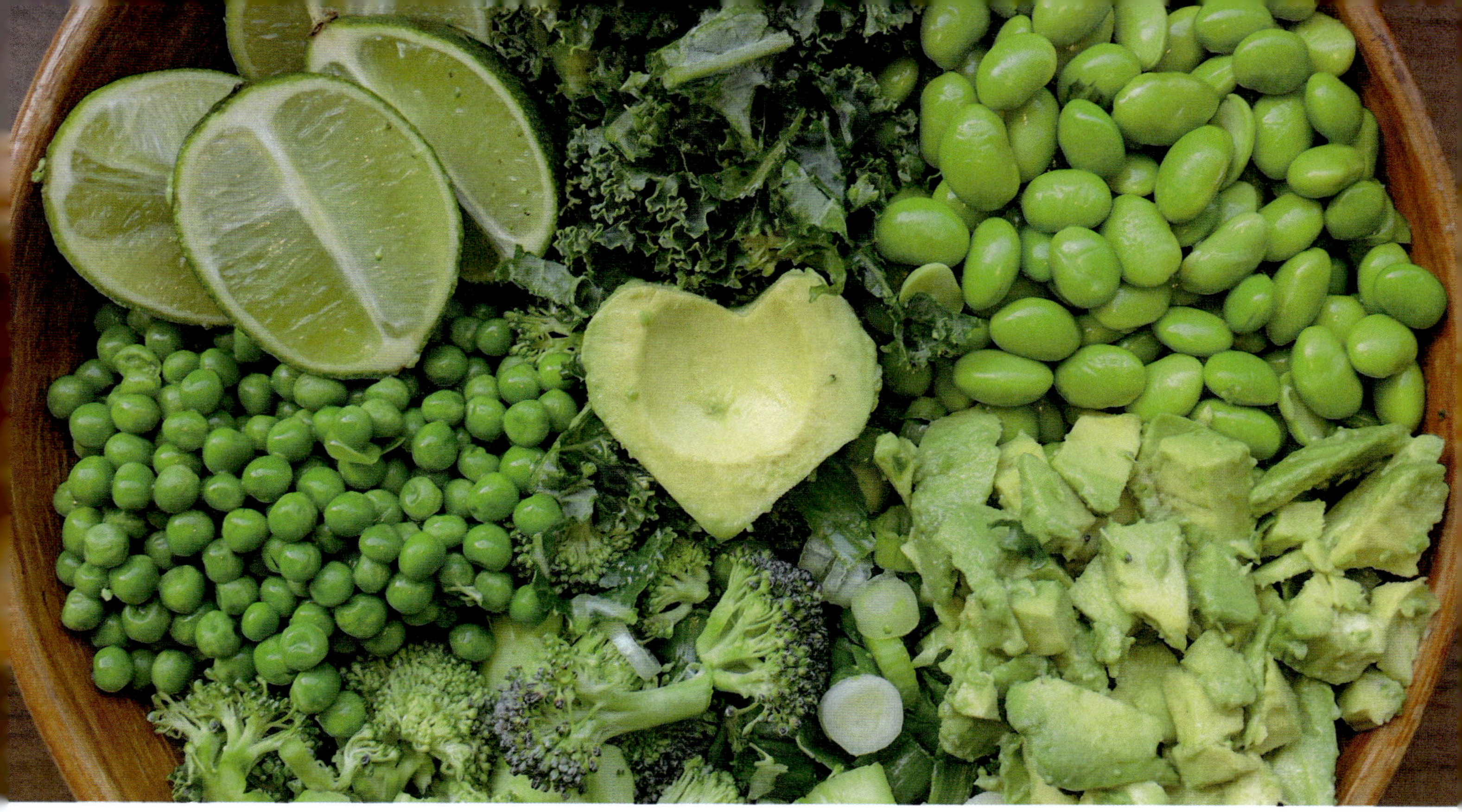

SEVEN GREENS SALAD

A tasty combination of flavors and textures that deliver all the nutritional goodness of greens.

INGREDIENTS:

- 2 cups kale, chopped
- 1 cup green peas, fresh or frozen and warmed
- 1 cup edamame beans, fresh or frozen and warmed
- 1 cup broccoli, chopped
- 5–7 green onions, diced
- 1–2 avocados, diced
- 1–2 limes, cut into wedges

DELICIOUS WITH: Lemon Tahini (pg. 56), Spicy Peanut Sauce (pg. 57), Baked Potato (pg.89), Steamed Quinoa (pg.84).

STEPS:

1. Chop up your fruits and shoots.
2. Combine green plants into a serving bowl.
3. Enjoy!

TIP: GET YOUR GREENS! Feel free to substitute any ingredient above with another green plant food. Arugula, celery, spinach, green lettuce, green apples, green grapes, green pear, micro-greens, sprouts, and snap peas are great options to try.

Why Greens Are Truly Great

Green foods are notorious for their antioxidant, anti-cancer, and other health-promoting benefits. The sharp color and odor of cruciferous vegetables—such as broccoli, kale, cabbage, and brussels sprouts—are thanks to the glucosinolates. The glucosinolates found abundantly in these crunchy plant foods are likely responsible for many of the health benefits they are known for. For starters, these phytonutrients help prevent the development and growth of cancer. According to Oregon State University,

> *"High intakes of cruciferous vegetables have been associated with lower risk of bladder, breast, colorectal, endometrial, gastric, lung, ovarian, pancreatic, prostate, and renal cancer."*

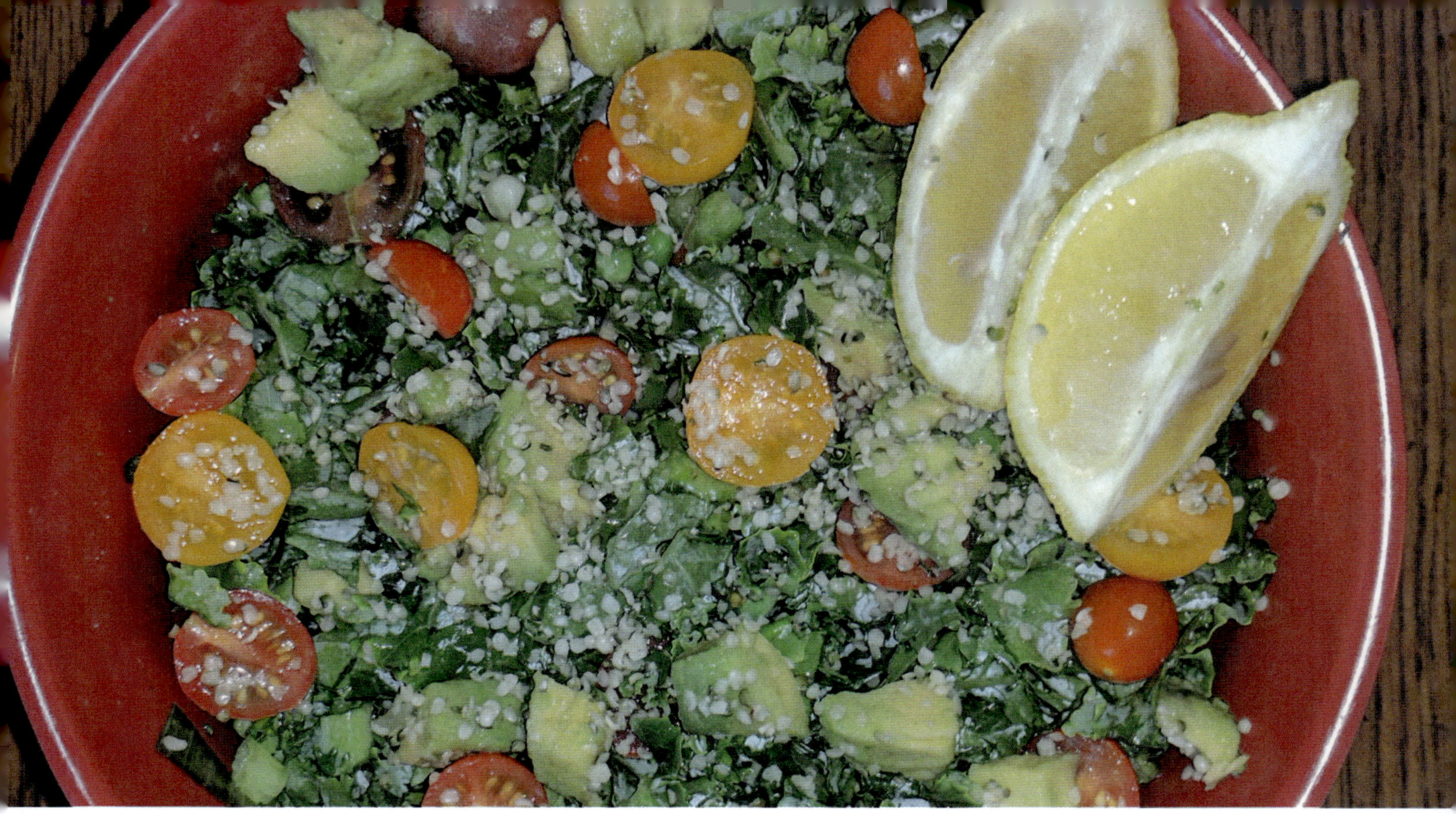

KING KALE SALAD

Kale reigns supreme for all the nutrients it delivers in this flavorful salad that pairs perfectly with soup, potatoes, or fresh baked bread.

INGREDIENTS:

- 4 cups kale, chopped small (about one bunch from market)
- 1 cup of cherry tomatoes
- 3–4 green onions, chopped small
- 1 avocado, diced
- 1/2 cup green peas
- 1/2 cup corn
- 1/4 cup hemp seeds
- 1 lemon

Kale is King

Kale has been hailed as one of the most nutrient dense foods known to Man, dubbed a "super food" for the extra large dose of protective phytonutrients, vitamins, and minerals it provides and the fact that it is super hardy and easy to grow. Any gardener will tell you that kale is a willing volunteer returning year after year without requiring reseeding. To receive all the health blessings King Kale has for you, chop it up small in salads like this one and add it to soups, stews, and casseroles.

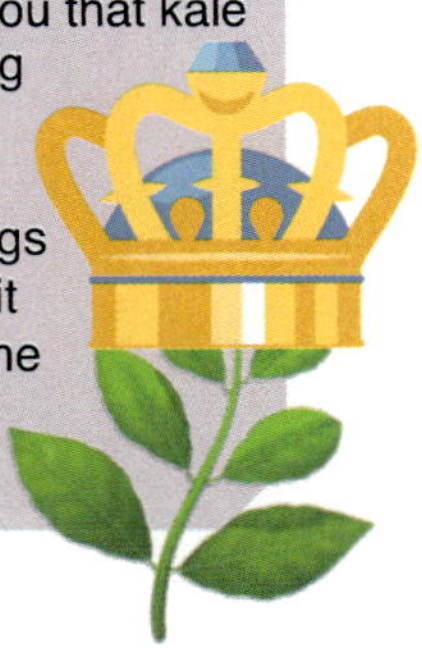

STEPS:

1. Rinse kale, tomatoes, onion, avocado, and lemon.
2. Remove kale leaves from tough stems. Discard stems.
3. Use a sharp knife to chop kale into small pieces.
4. Slice cherry tomatoes in half.
5. Dice avocado into small chunks. Chop green onions into small pieces.
6. Combine ingredients into large salad bowl.
7. Garnish with hemp seeds and lemon wedges.
8. Squeeze remaining lemon wedges over salad.
9. Share with your loved ones. Enjoy!

DELICIOUS WITH: Lemon Tahini Dressing (pg. 56), Spicy Peanut Sauce (pg. 57), Mashed Potatoes & Gravy (pg. 109), Steamed Quinoa (pg. 84), or a simple Baked Potato (pg. 89).

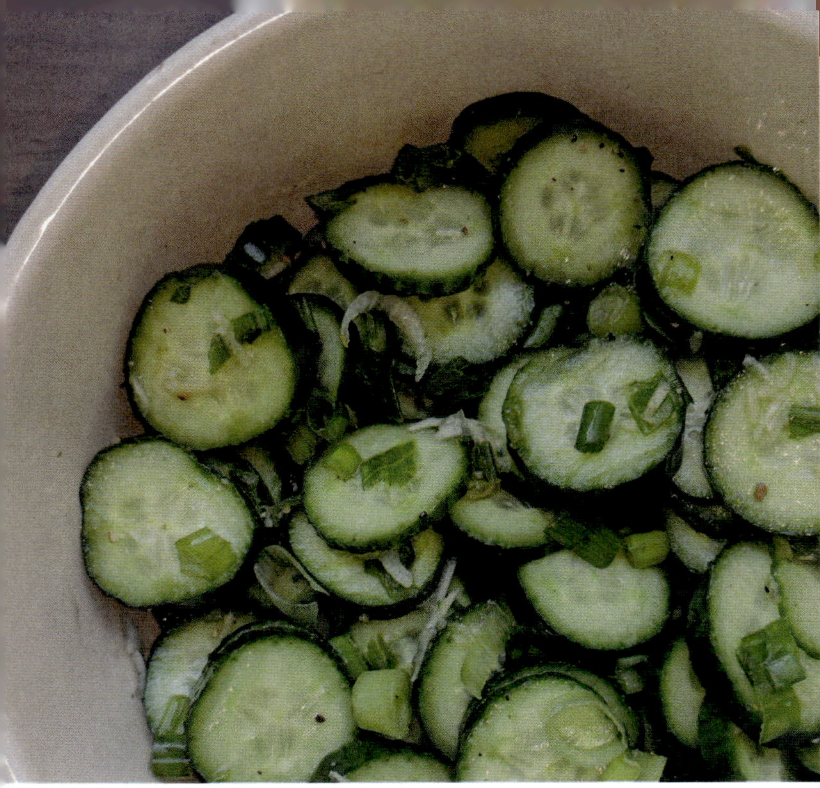

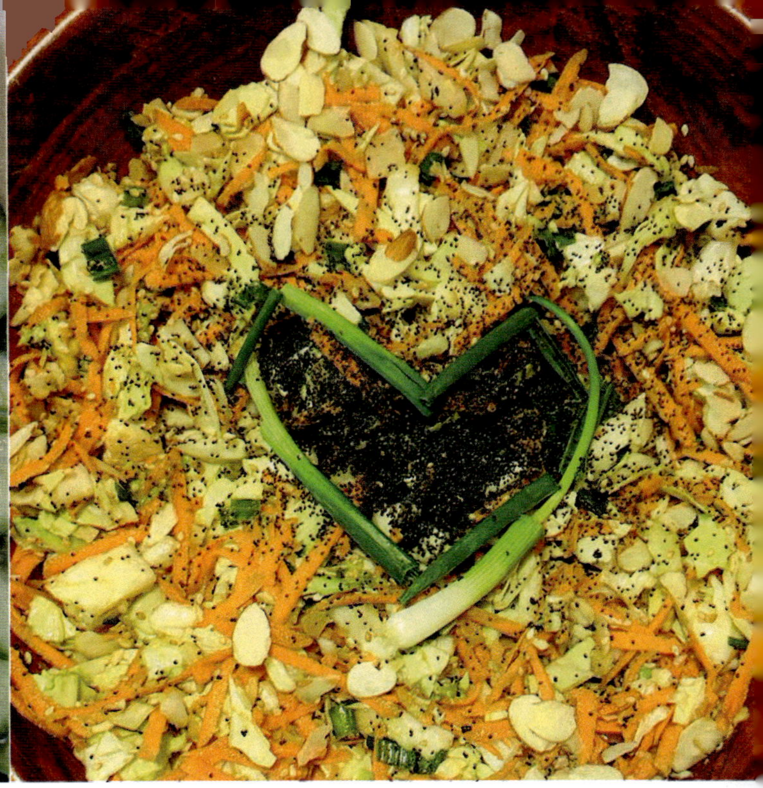

MARINATED CUCUMBERS

Marinated cucumbers are so simple and delicious on their own or as a side salad.

INGREDIENTS:

- 5 cucumbers, sliced
- 3 green onions, diced
- 2 large garlic cloves, minced
- big splash of apple cider vinegar
- little splash of Bragg Liquid Aminos or soy sauce
- dash of sea salt
- generous twists of ground black pepper

STEPS:

1. Slice cucumbers, dice green onions, mince garlic.
2. Mix and refrigerate before serving to allow flavors to further combine or serve immediately as we did this evening.
3. Enjoy!

DELICIOUS WITH: Red Rice N' Beans Bowl (pg. 98), Chickpeas N' Rice Bowl (pg.99), Go Garbanzos Bowl (pg. 101).

SERVING SUGGESTIONS:

- Serve on top of a garden salad.
- Make it a side dish for a veggie-packed meal.
- An excellent addition to a potluck or summer picnic.

SEEDY SLAW

A crisp and crunchy salad of cabbage and seeds.

INGREDIENTS:

- 5 cups green cabbage, shredded
- 3 carrots
- 5 green onion
- 1/4 cup almonds, sliced
- 1/8 cup poppy seeds
- 1/8 cup sesame seeds
- 1 tbsp. apple cider vinegar
- 1 tsp. garlic powder
- 1 tbsp. onion salt

STEPS:

1. Wash all fresh vegetables.
2. Shred cabbage or cut into small pieces.
3. Shred carrots.
4. Combine all ingredients into large salad bowl.
5. Top with poppy seeds, sesame seeds, and sliced almonds.
6. Enjoy!

DELICIOUS WITH: Diced avocado or a wedge of lime. Add dried cranberries, raisins, or a handful of chopped walnuts or pecans. Enjoy Seedy Slaw with Red Rice N' Beans Bowl (pg. 98), Ch-Easy Mac (pg. 102), Baked Potato (pg.89), Potato Wedges (pg. 93).

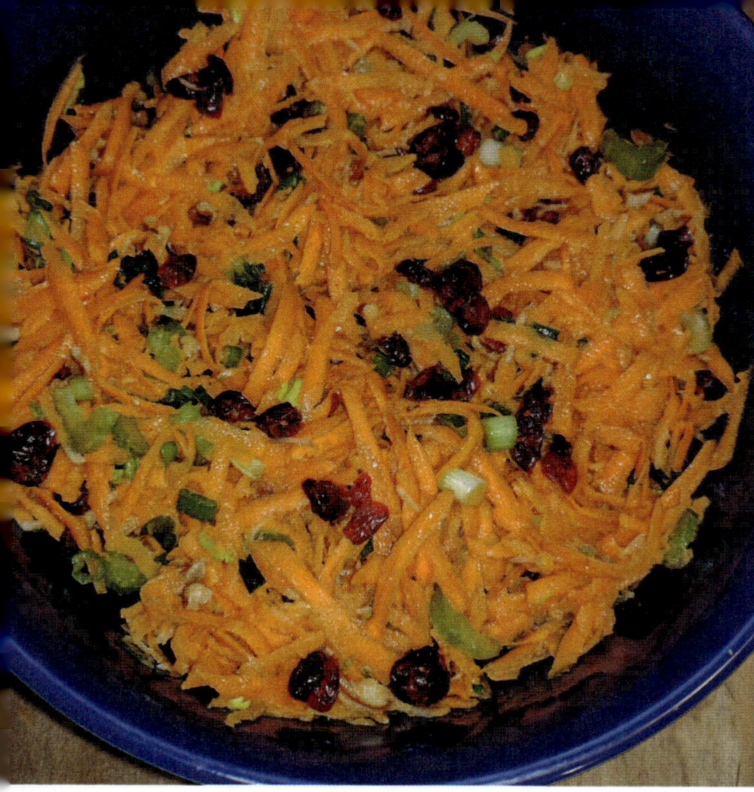

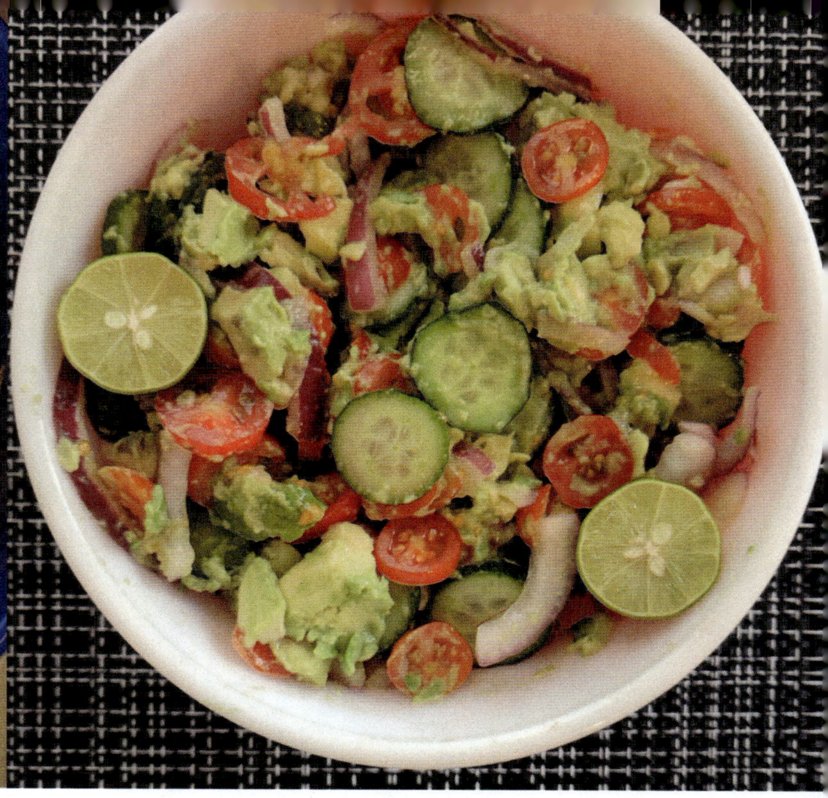

CARROT SALAD

Orange roots star in this sweet and spicy salad.

INGREDIENTS:

- 4–6 carrots (~4 cups shredded)
- 3 green onions
- 1/2 cup walnuts, chopped
- 1/4 cup dried cranberries
- 4 garlic cloves, small/medium
- 1 tbsp. agave syrup
- 1 tbsp. apple cider vinegar
- 1 tsp. mustard
- 1/4 tsp. ginger powder (or 1 tbsp. fresh)
- 1 tsp. salt

STEPS:

1. Wash carrots and green onions.
2. Shred carrots. Dice green onions. Chop walnuts into small pieces.
3. If you have a garlic press, press garlic into a large salad bowl. If not, shred garlic on fine shred setting. Or, chop as finely as possible.
4. Combine all ingredients into large salad bowl and stir well. Enjoy!

DELICIOUS WITH: Avocado or a wedge of lime.

- Substitute raisins for dried cranberries or chopped almonds or pecans for walnuts.
- Add a chopped apple for extra sweet crunch.
- Enjoy with Red Rice N' Beans Bowl (pg. 98), Baked Potato (pg.89), or as a side for soup.

CUCUMBER SALAD

A super refreshing and tasty salad that's perfect to enjoy all summer long.

INGREDIENTS:

- 3 fresh cucumbers, diced small
- large handful(s) of cherry tomatoes, chopped (I like them quartered)
- 1/4 red onion, chopped small
- 2–3 green onions, chopped small
- generous twists of ground black pepper
- spoonful of garlic, minced
- cayenne pepper to your taste (I include a teaspoonful for a nice kick)
- small dash of sea salt

STEPS:

1. Chop up your fruits and shoots.
2. Combine all ingredients and mix with a spoon.
3. Enjoy by itself straight from the bowl, use the cucumber salad to dress a bed of leafy greens, or use as a healthy topping for baked potatoes or rice.

DELICIOUS WITH: Avocado slices, tomato slices, red onion slices, leafy greens, Red Rice N' Beans Bowl (pg. 98).

SERVING SUGGESTIONS:

- Enjoy by itself as a refreshing summertime meal. Makes an easy to-go meal or main course for school lunch.
- Add on top of a simple garden salad.

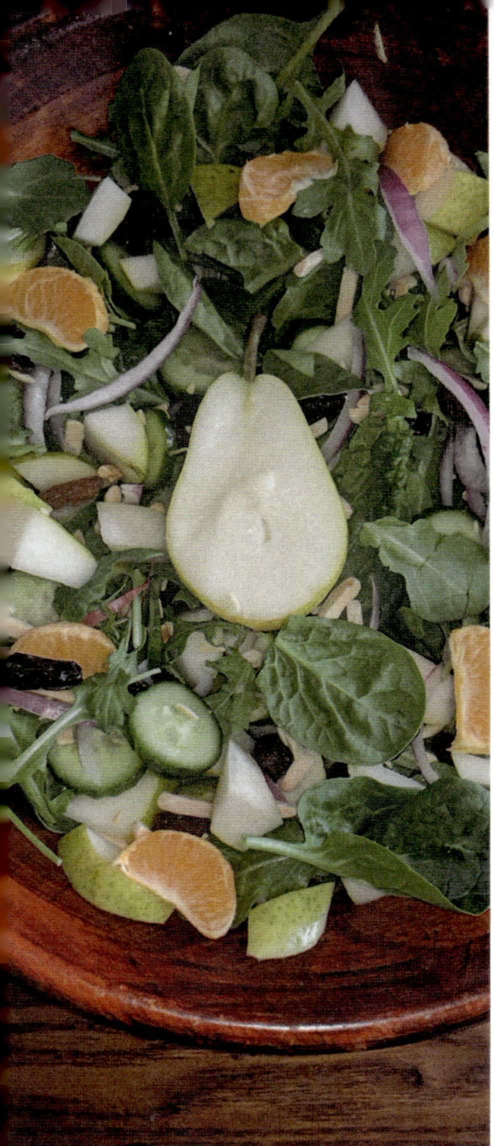

PEAR MANDARIN GREEN SALAD

A pear-fect combination of sweet fruits and tender and spicy greens to tantalize the taste buds and nourish the body.

INGREDIENTS:

- 2 cups baby spinach or large spinach leaves, torn
- 1 cup arugula
- 2 pears
- 3 mandarins
- 1/2 cup raisins
- 1/2 cup almonds, slivered
- 1/4 red onion, sliced thinly
- 1 Persian cucumber[1], sliced into thin rounds
- 1 lime

STEPS:

1. Wash, chop, and prepare veggies for salad.
2. Combine veggies in large salad bowl.
3. Garnish with
4. Enjoy!

DELICIOUS WITH: Lemon Tahini Dressing (pg. 56), Basic Bread (pg. 86)

1—Persian cucumbers are my favorite but any cucumber works fine!

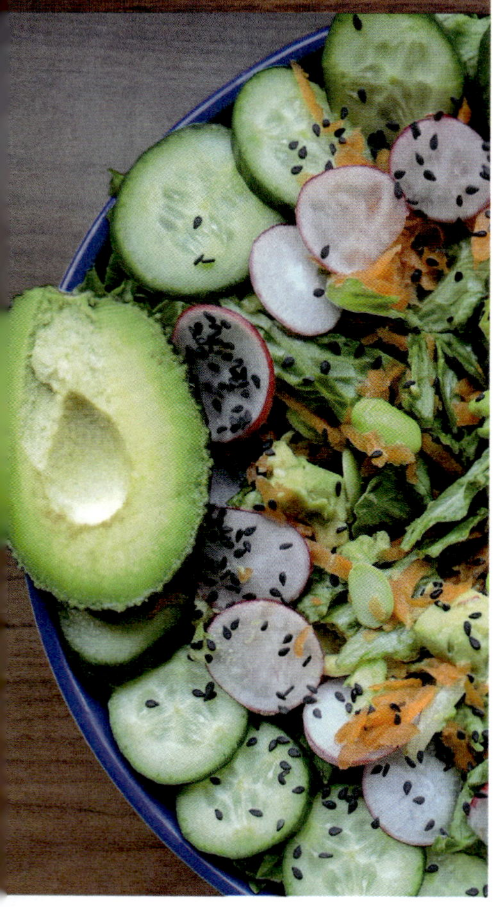

GARDEN SUSHI SALAD

A sushi-inspired salad that's 100% fresh delicious plants.

INGREDIENTS:

- head of green lettuce leaves, torn
- 1 avocado, diced
- 1 cucumber, sliced
- handful of radishes, sliced
- 1 carrot, shredded
- 1 cup of edamame (fresh soy beans)
- 1 tsp. apple cider vinegar
- 1 tbsp. Bragg Liquid Aminos/soy sauce
- sprinkle of black sesame seeds

STEPS:

1. Wash, chop, and prepare veggies for salad.
2. Combine veggies in large salad bowl and add apple cider vinegar, soy sauce, and sesame seeds.
3. Garnish with cucumber and radish slices.
4. Enjoy!

DELICIOUS WITH: Fresh mango diced, bits of dried seaweed, whole Basic Brown Rice (pg. 82).

PEANUT BUTTER TOFU SALAD

This simple salad made a delicious and nutritious lunch when topped with homemade peanut butter tofu.

INGREDIENTS:

SALAD:

- 1 head of romaine lettuce
- 2 carrots, small, shredded
- large handful of arugula, chopped
- 2 green onions
- handful of cherry tomatoes
- handful of chopped cilantro
- 1 lime quartered, with the juice squeezed on top

PEANUT DRESSING:

- heaping spoonful of peanut butter
- drizzle of Bragg Liquid Aminos or soy sauce
- 1/2 teaspoon of minced garlic
- dash of apple cider vinegar
- dash of nutritional yeast
- dash of sriracha hot sauce, and
- generous twists of fresh ground black pepper

Top this salad with baked peanut butter tofu. To make the peanut butter tofu I combine:

- 20 oz. extra firm tofu
- a few spoonfuls of peanut butter
- a swirl of Sriracha hot sauce
- a few swirls of Bragg Liquid Aminos or soy sauce, and 1 tsp. minced garlic

STEPS:

1. Stir these ingredients till they make a thickish paste.
2. Cut extra firm tofu into bite-sized cubes.
3. Pour tofu into bowl with peanut paste and stir until tofu is evenly coated with paste.
4. Pour into glass bake dish and bake at 350°F for 15–20 minutes.
5. Top salad with baked tofu and enjoy.

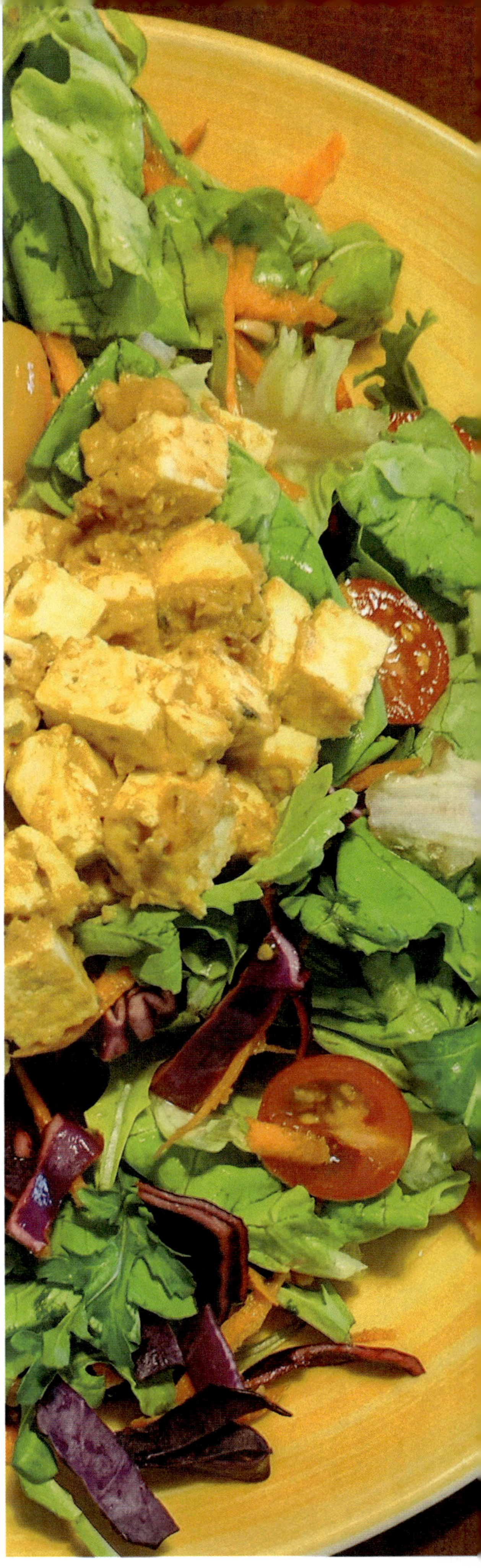

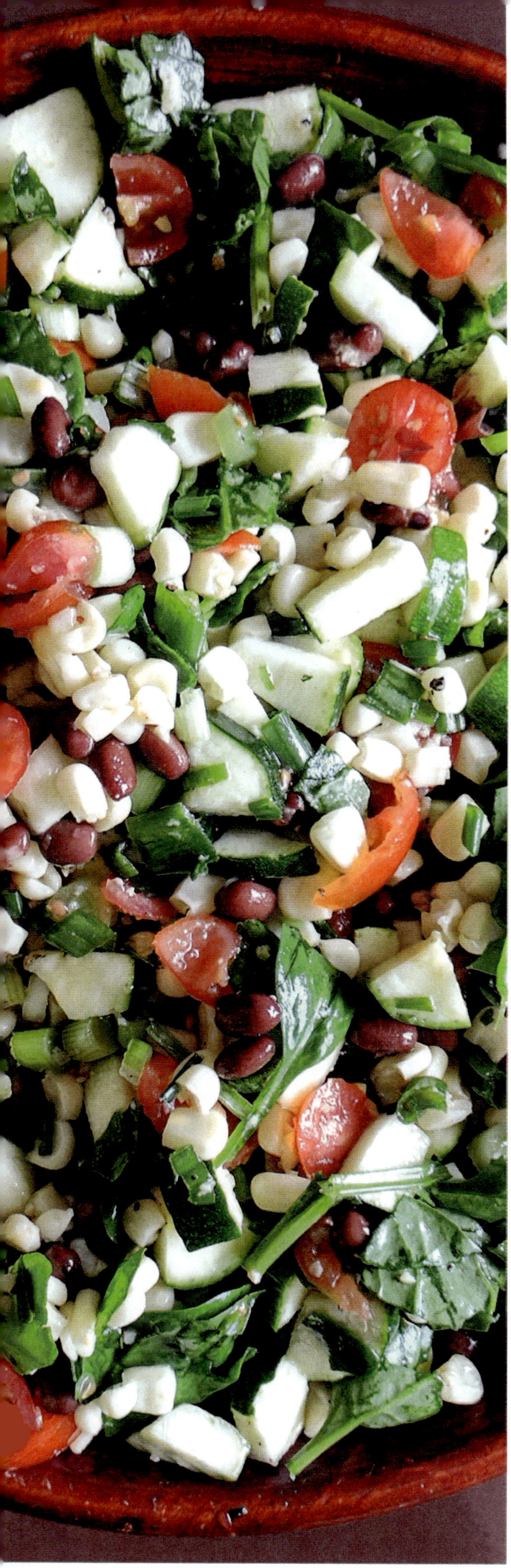

3 SISTERS SALAD

This recipe features the three sisters of Native American agriculture: corn, beans, and squash.

INGREDIENTS:

- 1 cup black beans with liquid drained
- 1 cup corn, fresh, frozen, or canned
- 1/2 zucchini, medium
- 2 green onions
- large tomato or handful of cherry tomatoes
- 1 cup greens—arugula, kale, spinach, or lettuce, chopped
- 1 lime
- 1/2 tbsp. garlic, minced
- 1/4 tsp. sea salt
- 1/4 tsp. black pepper
- optional: sprinkle of cayenne pepper

STEPS:

1. Wash fresh veggies.
2. Chop zucchini, tomato, onions, and greens into small pieces.
3. Combine beans, corn, and chopped veggies into bowl.
4. Cut lime in half and squeeze juice on top.
5. Add garlic, sea salt, black pepper, and cayenne pepper.
6. Stir until well combined.
7. Share with friends or family. Enjoy!

TIPS:

- Use any type of beans. Pinto, white, garbanzo, kidney, navy, lima, or edamame soy beans would all work nice with this recipe.
- Use fresh corn off the cob. Peel the corn, remove the silky threads, and use a sharp knife to carefully cut away the corn kernels from the cob.
- Try adding a jalapeno pepper with seeds removed and chopped into small pieces.
- Add 1/4 green, red, or yellow bell pepper chopped small.
- Try different types of greens. Besides the ones mentioned above mustard greens, dandelion greens, endive, and cabbage would all go well chopped into small pieces for this salad. Notice how different greens have distinct flavors that add a new flavor to your recipe.
- For a different flavor try cilantro chopped small instead of garlic.
- Red onion chopped small is a good substitute for green onion. Onion powder can also work to help season your salad.
- Try adding a splash of apple cider vinegar or hot sauce if you like extra spice.
- Add one chopped avocado—so delicious!

RAINBOW SALAD

A nutrient-packed flavorful salad featuring all the colors of the rainbow.

INGREDIENTS:

- Red—1–2 large tomato, diced or ~20–30 cherry tomatoes, halved or sliced
- Orange—2 carrots, diced into thin rounds
- Yellow—2 cups corn
- Yellow—1 lemon (juice of)
- Green—2 cups spinach or kale leaves, torn or cut into small pieces
- Green/White—2 green onions, diced small with white part too!
- Blue/Purple—~4 large purple cabbage leaves, chopped into small pieces
- Blue/Purple—1/4 cup red onion, chopped very small
- Brown—1/4 cup roasted sunflower seeds (kernels)
- Black—2 tsp. black sesame seeds

Spices

- 1/4 tsp. sea salt
- 1/4 tsp. black pepper
- 1/4 tsp. garlic powder

STEPS:

1. Chop all fresh plants and combine in bowl.
2. Add spices to bowl, squeeze lemon on top, and stir.
3. Serve Rainbow Salad next to or on top of steamed quinoa or rice or mix the grains together with your salad. Try it different ways.
4. Share with your loved ones, enjoy!

DELICIOUS WITH: Diced avocado, pickled beets, Lemon Tahini dressing (pg. 56), Spicy Peanut Sauce (pg. 57), Mashed Potatoes & Gravy (pg. 109), Steamed Quinoa (pg. 84), Mushroom Risotto (pg. 85).

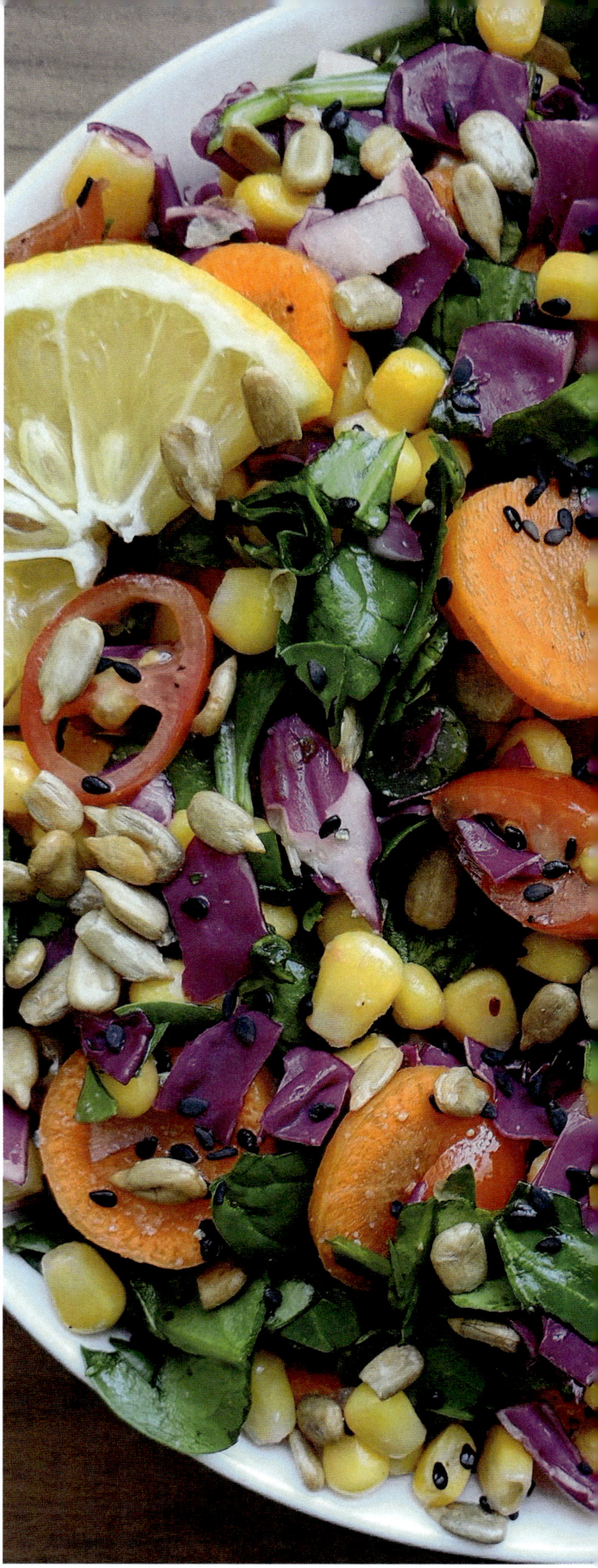

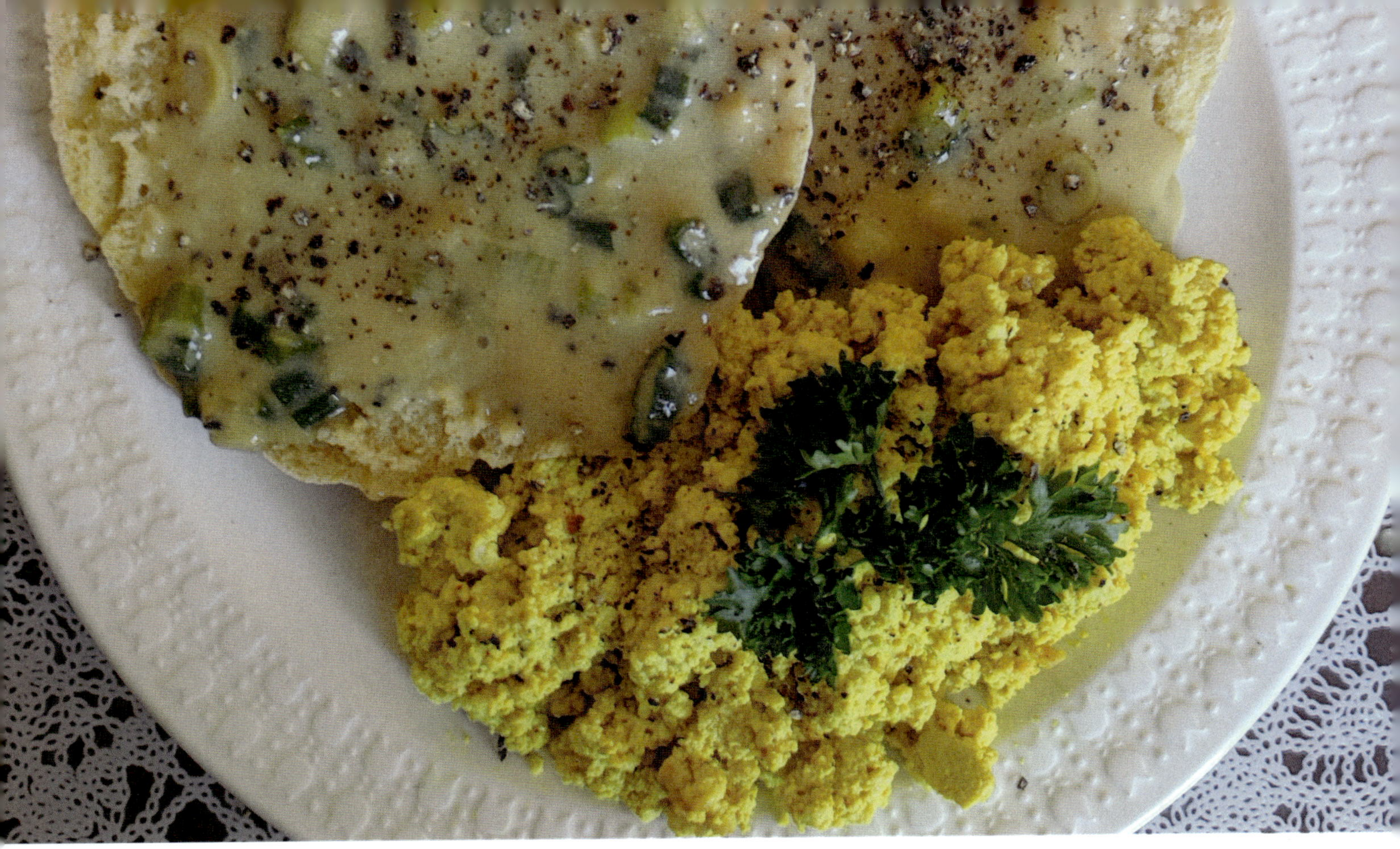

SCRAMBLED TOFU

A purely plants take on scrambled eggs that is a satisfying breakfast or sandwich topper.

SERVINGS: 4

INGREDIENTS:

- 16 oz. extra firm tofu
- 1 tsp. onion salt
- 1 tsp. mustard
- 1 tsp. turmeric
- 1 tsp. nutritional yeast
- 1 tsp. soy sauce
- 1/2 tsp. garlic powder
- 1/2 tsp. salt
- optional: 1/2 tsp. coconut oil (to grease pan only if needed)

STEPS:

1. Combine spices in a large bowl with tofu.
2. Use a large wooden spoon or a potato masher to mash tofu into a crumbly texture.
3. Continue to mash tofu until spices are well combined and the tofu has a uniform golden hue.
4. **Oil-Free Bake:** Bake at 425°F for 20 minutes in a glass baking dish. Stir and bake another 10 minutes until deep golden color is achieved. Or, spread out scrambled tofu in a layer ~1 inch thick onto parchment paper on a baking sheet and bake for 15 minutes, then stir/flip and bake for another 10 minutes until a golden color is achieved. **Stovetop:** Place cocount oil into a skillet and warm pan to medium heat. When oil is melted and coating the pan add tofu mix and allow to cook until color deepens, stirring occasionally.
5. Enjoy!

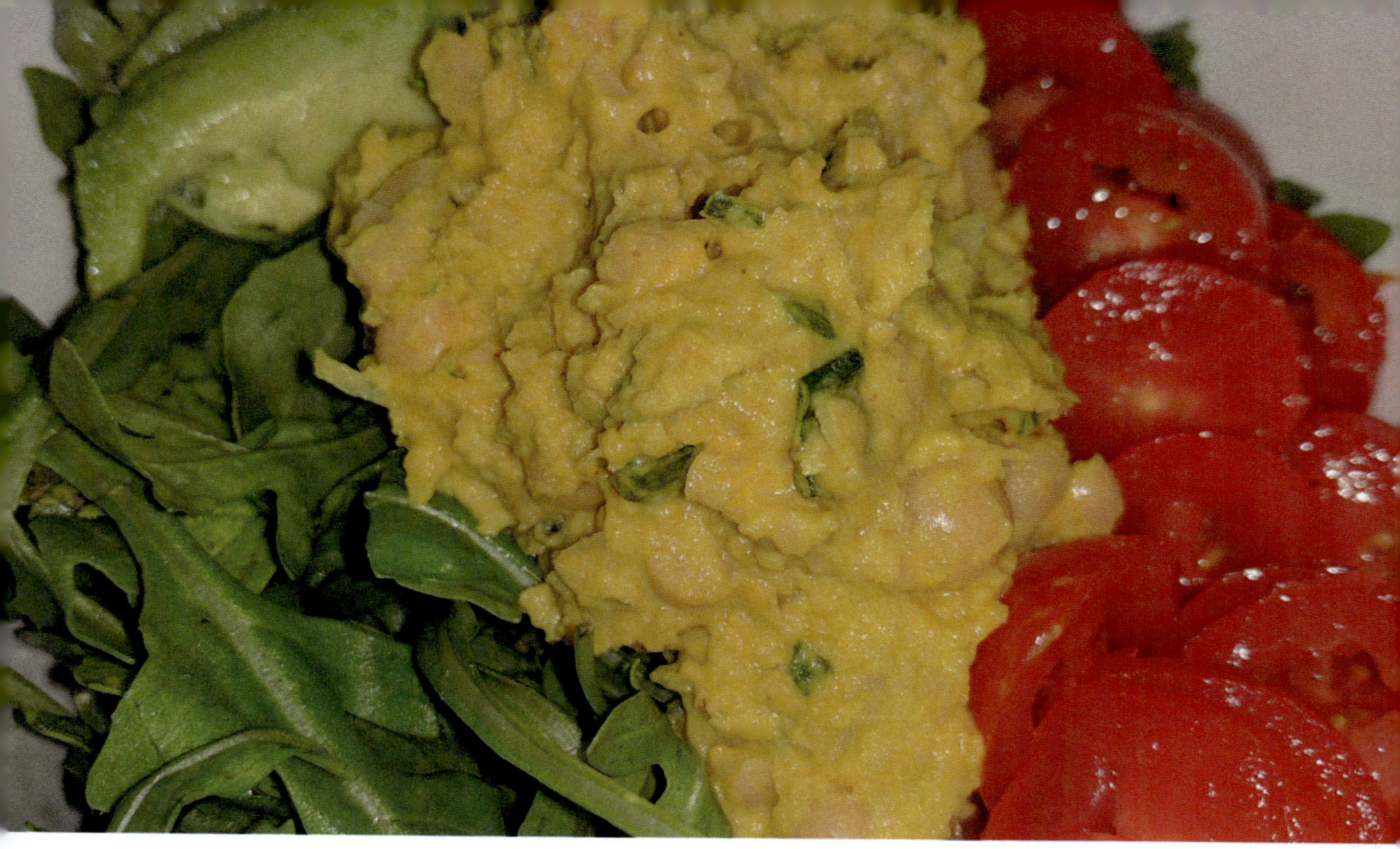

CHICKPEA OF THE SEA SALAD

Go garbanzos over this 100% whole plants version of classic Tuna Salad.

SERVINGS: 3

INGREDIENTS:

- 1 can of garbanzo beans
- 3 green onions
- 2 tbsp. red onion or shallots, minced
- 1 tbsp. apple cider vinegar
- 1 tbsp. whole grain mustard
- 1 tsp. turmeric
- 1 tsp. garlic powder
- 1 tsp. sea salt
- generous twists ground black pepper
- optional: 1 celery stalk

STEPS:

1. Drain can of garbanzo beans, rinse, and strain.
2. Put garbanzos into large mixing bowl and mash with a fork or potato masher, allowing some small chunks of beans to remain.
3. Dice onions and add to mix.
4. Dice celery into small pieces for extra crunch.
5. Add all spices and stir until well combined.
6. Enjoy!

DELICIOUS WITH: Sliced tomato, arugula, lettuce, thinly sliced red onion.

SERVING SUGGESTIONS:

- Spread it on bread for a tasty sandwich.
- Enjoy on top of a simple green salad.
- Dip into this creamy dip with celery or carrot sticks, baked tortilla chips, or fresh bread.

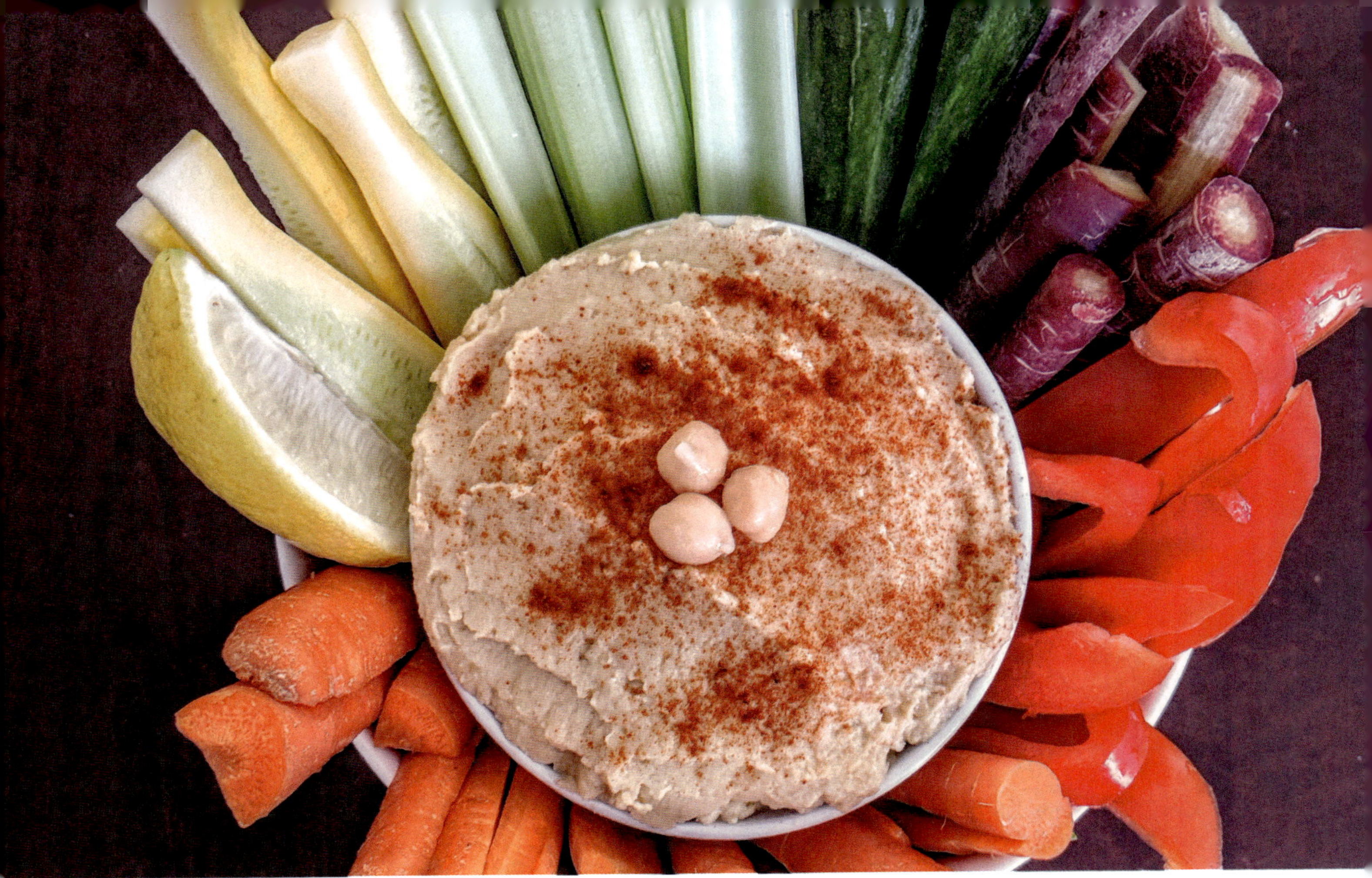

RAINBOW STICKS N' HUMMUS

A beautiful and healthy snack that features all the colors of the nutrition rainbow. Make it a platter for sharing at your next party or simply make it a nutrient-packed meal.

INGREDIENTS:

- Red **radishes** or **tomatoes**
- Red **bell peppers**, sliced lengthwise
- Orange **carrots**
- Yellow **summer squash**
- Green **cucumbers**, sliced into spears
- Green **celery**
- Purple **kale, carrots,** or **cauliflower**
- Heavenly Garlic Hummus (pg. 63)

STEPS:

1. Wash all fresh veggies.
2. Chop fresh veggies into dip-able sticks/pieces.
3. Arrange the rainbow of veggies into your serving bowls or on a platter.
4. Serve with Heavenly Garlic Hummus.

DELICIOUS WITH: Basic Bread (pg.86), crackers, or serve it on top of salad.

10 Good Reasons To Eat The Rainbow

1. **Beauty in the Bowl:** Who doesn't like their meal to be pleasing to the eyes as well as the taste buds? The eyes eat first, science says.
2. **Delightful aroma:** Breathe in deep and feel your senses react pleasantly to the smells of the food that humans evolved to thrive on.
3. **Tasty tasty:** So much flavor to please the palate! Humans naturally delight in fresh fruits and other plant foods in their natural state, no cooking, spicing, or masking identity with spices needed!
4. **Red food** nutrients protect against cancer and heart diseases.

5. **Satisfying:** Whole plants are full of fiber which leaves you feeling full and satisfied after your meal and promotes healthy digestion.
6. **Orange foods** protect healthy vision and support a healthy immune system.
7. **Hydrating:** Whole plant foods are an excellent source of pure water filtered through plants.
8. **Green foods** support healthy skin and hair and prevent damage to the body's cells.
9. **Blue and purple foods** are rich in antioxidants, good for the brain, and support healthy memory.
10. **Get ALL the nutrients!** Phytonutrients are found in the colorful parts of plants and so eating foods from all the color groups means that you get the whole rainbow of nutrients.

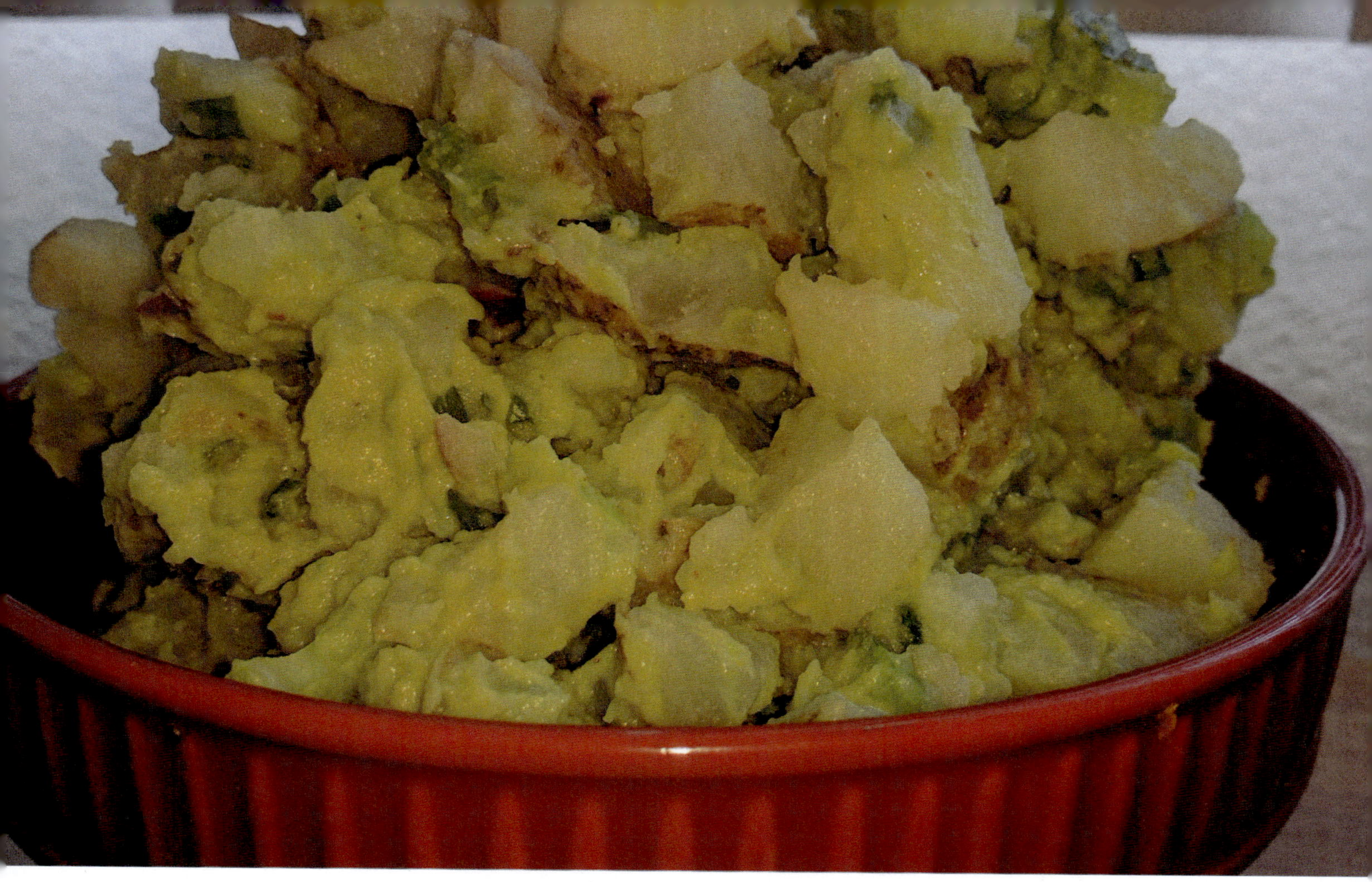

GREEN POTATO SALAD

Potato salad perfection without the mayo. Green Potato Salad is 100% oil-free and 100% whole plants—perfect for your summer picnic or potluck.

INGREDIENTS:

- 5–6 potatoes, large
- 5–6 green onions
- 2 avocados
- 1 tbsp. garlic powder
- 1 tbsp. onion salt
- 1 tbsp. dill, dried
- 1 tsp. salt
- 1 tsp. pepper

STEPS:

1. Wash potatoes, onion, and avocado.
2. Use a sharp knife to remove any bad spots on potatoes.
3. Chop potatoes into bite-sized chunks.
4. Put chopped potatoes into large pot and cover with water.
5. Bring potatoes to boil on stovetop on high, then reduce heat and leave pot covered.
6. Boil potatoes just long enough to where they get soft but are still firm and don't fall apart easily.
7. Strain potatoes in colander.
8. Cut avocados in half, remove pits, scoop the ripe green flesh into a large bowl, and mash with spices.
9. Dice green onions into small pieces (scissors work great).
10. Add potatoes and onions and mix together until potatoes are evenly coated with avocado and spice mash.
11. Enjoy!

SERVING SUGGESTIONS:

- Perfect for a summer picnic or potluck.
- Goes well with a fresh fruit salad.
- Make it a sidekick for your favorite plantiful sandwich.

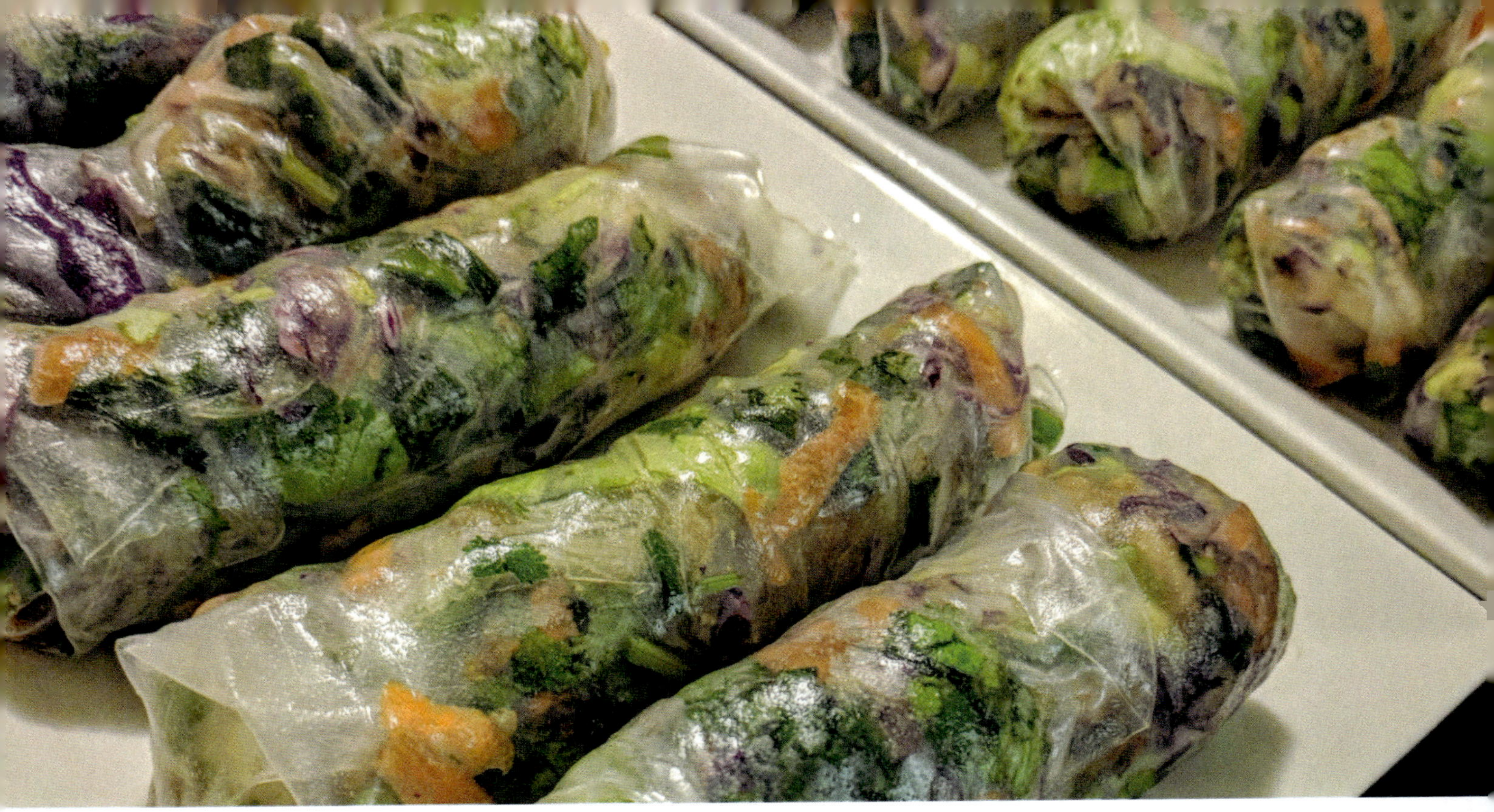

FRESH SPRING ROLLS

A tasty mix of raw plants rolled up to please your palate.

INGREDIENTS:

Use any assortment of fresh plants that you like. Here I used:

- red cabbage, shredded
- carrots, shredded
- arugula greens, chopped small
- green onions, diced
- radishes, sliced
- cilantro
- extra firm tofu
- Bragg Liquid Aminos or soy sauce
- rice paper rolls

STEPS:

1. Chop raw tofu[1] into squares and put in a shallow glass pan with a splash of soy sauce.
2. Slice, shred, and dice ingredients to fill your rolls.
3. In a large bowl, mix fresh veggies together with a splash of soy sauce and add tofu.
4. Add water to a shallow plate for dipping the rice papers.
5. Wet each rice paper roll completely, then put it onto a dry plate.
6. Allow rice paper wrap to sit for about 1 minute until no longer stiff, but before it becomes too gummy.
7. After 1 minute, put a large spoonful of filling into the middle and quickly roll up like a burrito tucking in the edges of the wrap.
8. After rolling, place wraps on a plate, not touching each other.
9. Enjoy them soon—these are best eaten fresh!

DELICIOUS WITH: Spicy Peanut Sauce (pg. 57), avocado slices, green cabbage or lettuce leaves as filling, Everything But the Bagel.

1—I use raw tofu for these but marinated or baked tofu would also work well.

Learning To Roll With Rice Paper

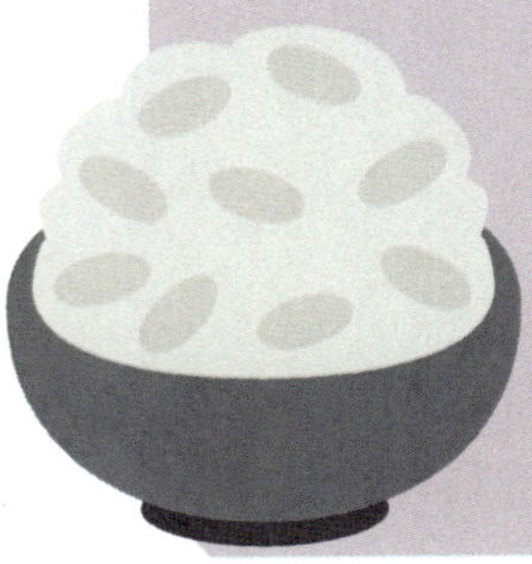

I once had the privilege of hosting a kind-hearted monk from Vietnam who taught me to roll with rice paper for the first time. The thin translucent sheets of rice paper had always intimidated me before, but he made it look so easy and once I started practicing I found I could create fresh veggie spring rolls too. Mine might not be as perfectly constructed as the ones you will find at a Thai restaurant, but I think I do OK and they are definitely a delightful meal. My kids and I enjoy fresh spring rolls dipped in Spicy Peanut Sauce (recipe on pg. 57). While a couple spring rolls can easily cost you $5 at a local market or restaurant, homemade spring rolls are super affordable. When I make these I generally make a big bowl of the filling and roll just the right amount we will enjoy immediately. Since spring rolls are definitely best eaten fresh right after preparing, I save any leftover filling and wrap more spring rolls later.

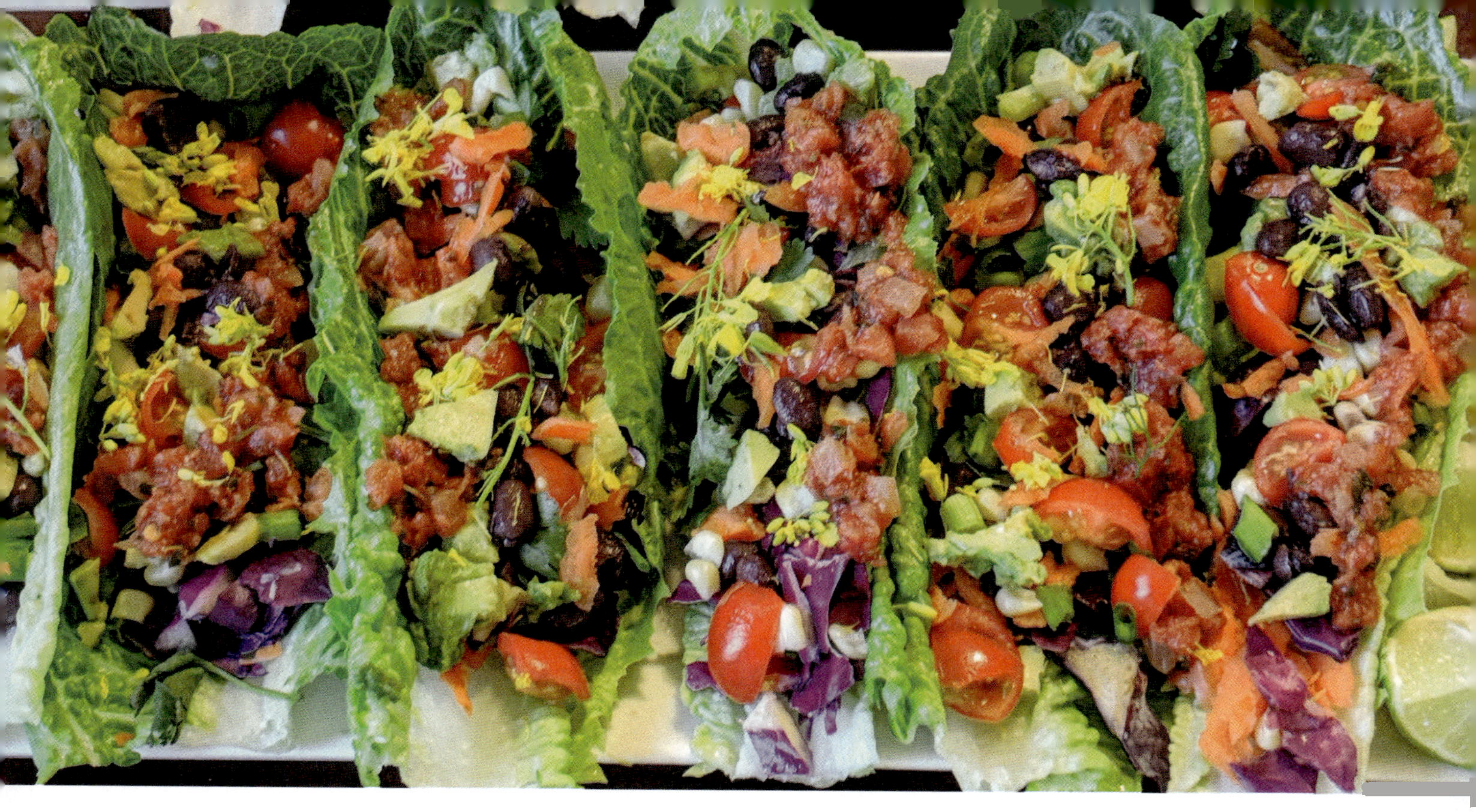

RAW RAINBOW TACOS

100% raw and ridiculously tasty tacos.

INGREDIENTS:

- romaine lettuce leaves, large unbroken (for taco shells)
- red cherry tomatoes
- red bell pepper
- carrots
- yellow corn
- avocado
- cilantro
- red cabbage
- purple kale
- salsa
- black beans

STEPS:

1. Wash all fresh fruits and veggies.
2. Break off large romaine lettuce leaves for taco shells and set aside.
3. Shred carrots and purple cabbage.
4. Cut purple kale, cilantro, and bell pepper into small pieces.
5. Slice cherry tomatoes into thin round slices.
6. Warm black beans.
7. Dice avocado.
8. Combine fresh taco ingredients onto center of romaine leaves.
9. Enjoy your Raw Rainbow Tacos!

DELICIOUS WITH: Garden Guacamole (pg. 63), beans.

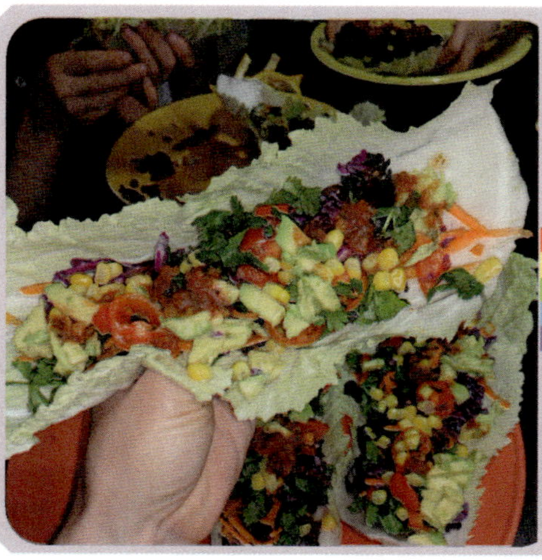

The Eat the Rainbow Every Day

Nutrition science is a fairly young field. We have only known what vitamins are for just over 100 years. In the last couple decades there have been thousands of new nutrients discovered and many experts believe there's thousands more undiscovered still. These newest nutrients on the block are the phytonutrients ("phyto"="plant") and are concentrated in the colorful parts of the plants. The newest, most up-to-date advice in the field of nutrition says to focus on eating a rainbow of whole foods every day, rather than on counting calories. If you make sure you get all the colors of the rainbow you are also getting all the nutrition found in the colors—all the protective health benefits nature has to offer you!

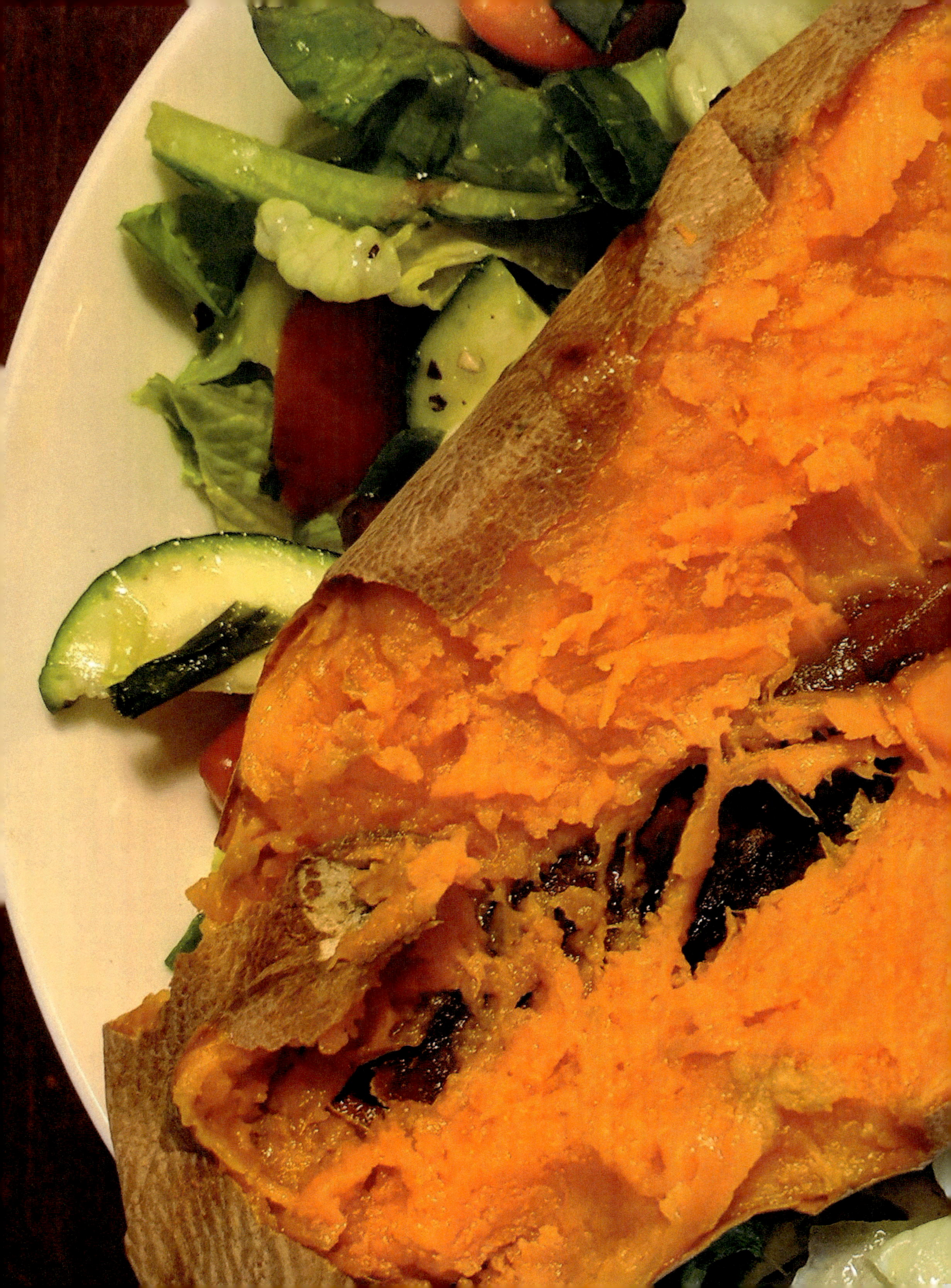

Savory Sidekicks

SIMPLE SIDE DISHES

Pair these simple side dishes with the soups, salads, and bountiful bowls in this recipe book to make a perfect meal. Or, make one of these sidekicks the star of supper—a flavorful rice or basic baked potato can be a tasty and nutritous centerpiece.

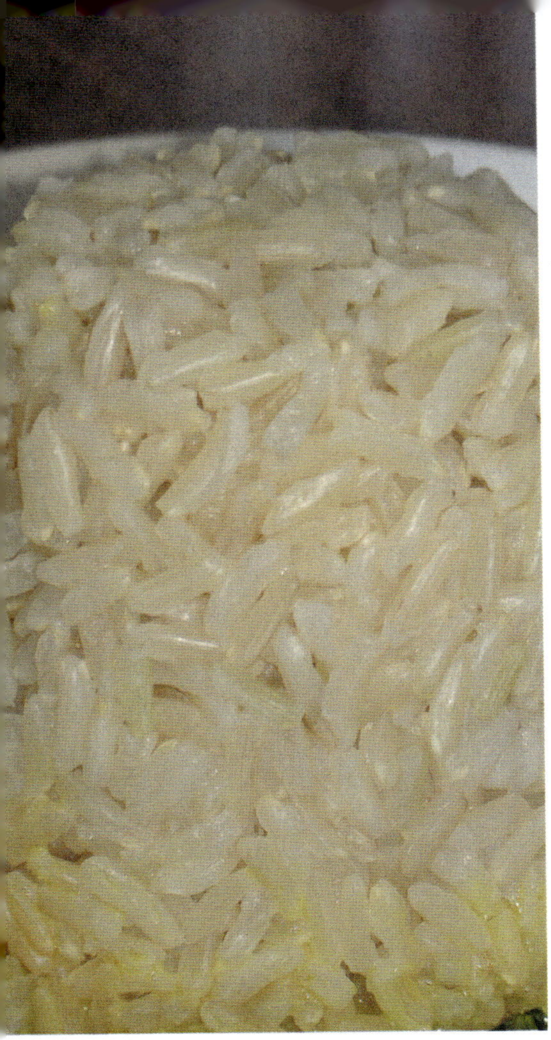

BASIC BROWN RICE

Try whole grain brown rice to get 100% of the nutrients this seed food has to offer!

Serves: 4

TIP!
Leftover rice stores well in the fridge for up to a week. Freeze leftover rice for up to a month!

INGREDIENTS:

- 2 cups brown rice
- 4 cups water
- pinch of sea salt

STEPS:

1. Rinse rice with cold water until water runs clear. Use a fine mesh strainer or you can do this in your cooking pot being careful not to pour out your rice.
2. Place rice into a pot with a tight-fitting lid and bring water to a boil over high heat.
3. As water begins to boil stir rice, cover, and reduce heat to low,
4. Allow rice to steam to perfection which usually takes about 45–50 minutes. Stir rice to check that it is almost completely soft before turning off heat.
5. Remove rice from heat and keep lid on for another 10 minutes to allow it to steam the rest of the way to perfection.
6. Remove lid, fluff rice with large spoon or fork, and serve.

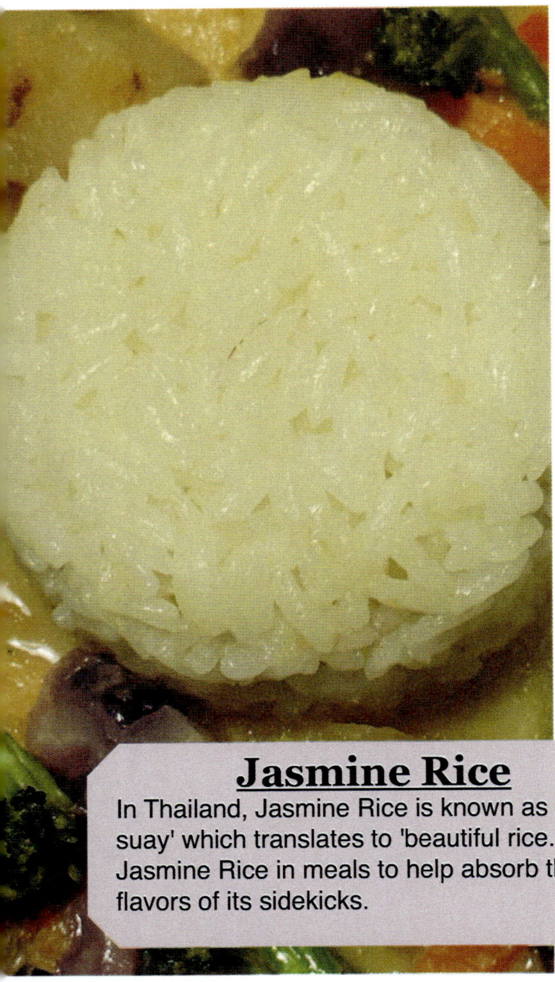

STEAMED JASMINE RICE

Fragrant and lovely steamed rice with a more delicate texture.

Serves: 2–3

INGREDIENTS:

- 2.5 cups Jasmine rice
- 3 cups water

STEPS:

1. Remove excess starch from rice by rinsing rice with cold water until water runs clear. Use a fine mesh strainer to catch rice or carefully strain in your cooking pot.
2. Place rice into a pot with a tight-fitting lid.
3. Add enough water to cover the rice with about 1/2 inch of water above level of rice. Use your finger to test. It should be approx 3 cups of water.
4. Bring water to a boil over medium/high heat.
5. As water begins to boil stir rice, cover, and reduce heat.
6. Allow rice to simmer until it has absorbed all the water, which usually takes about 10 minutes.
7. Stir rice to check that it is almost completely soft before turning off heat.
8. Remove rice from heat and keep lid on for another 10 minutes to allow it to steam the rest of the way to perfection.
9. Remove lid, fluff rice with large spoon or fork, and serve.

Jasmine Rice

In Thailand, Jasmine Rice is known as 'khao suay' which translates to 'beautiful rice." Use Jasmine Rice in meals to help absorb the flavors of its sidekicks.

RED RICE

Slightly sweet and spicy red rice goes great with beans.
Serves: 4

INGREDIENTS:

- 2 cups whole grain rice
- 5 cups water
- 4 garlic cloves
- 1 bell pepper
- 3 green onions
- 1 tbsp. onion salt
- 1 tbsp. garlic powder
- 1/2 cup corn
- 1/4 tsp. cayenne
- 4.6 oz. tomato paste

STEPS:

1. Wash veggies.
2. Chop bell pepper, green onions, and garlic into small pieces.
3. Sauté onions, garlic, and bell pepper with 1 tbsp. water on medium heat 5–10 minutes until peppers, onions, and garlic are tender and have released their sweet aroma.
4. Add rice and spices to pan with the onions, peppers, and garlic for a few minutes. Stir to mix and avoid sticking.
5. Add water, cover, and bring to a boil.
6. When water is boiling, reduce heat and leave covered stirring occasionally.
7. Turn heat off when rice is almost cooked and almost all the water is absorbed.
8. Leave rice covered for another 10–15 minutes to allow it to steam the rest of the way to perfection.
9. Fluff rice with a large fork before serving.

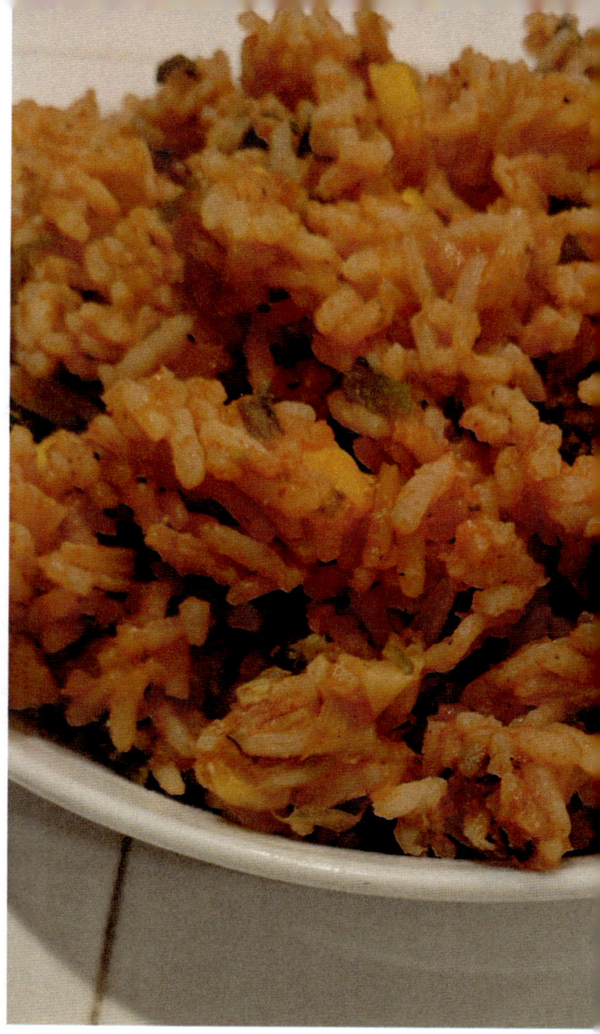

YELLOW RICE

Fragrant, herb-seasoned rice with a gorgeous golden hue.
Servings: 8

INGREDIENTS:

- 2 cup dry, white Jasmine rice
- 4 cups vegetable broth (I prefer low-sodium)
- 3 tbsp. nutritional yeast
- 1 tbsp. salt
- 2 tsp. garlic powder
- 1.5 tsp. turmeric
- 1 tsp. onion powder
- 1 tsp. ground sage
- 1 tsp. dried thyme
- sprig of fresh rosemary chopped small (or 1 tsp. dried rosemary)

STEPS:

1. Rinse rice until water comes out clear to remove excess starch.
2. Add rinsed rice to large pan with a tight fitting lid and add vegetable broth and spices.
3. Prepare rice in typical fashion (see Steamed Jasmine Rice pg.82).

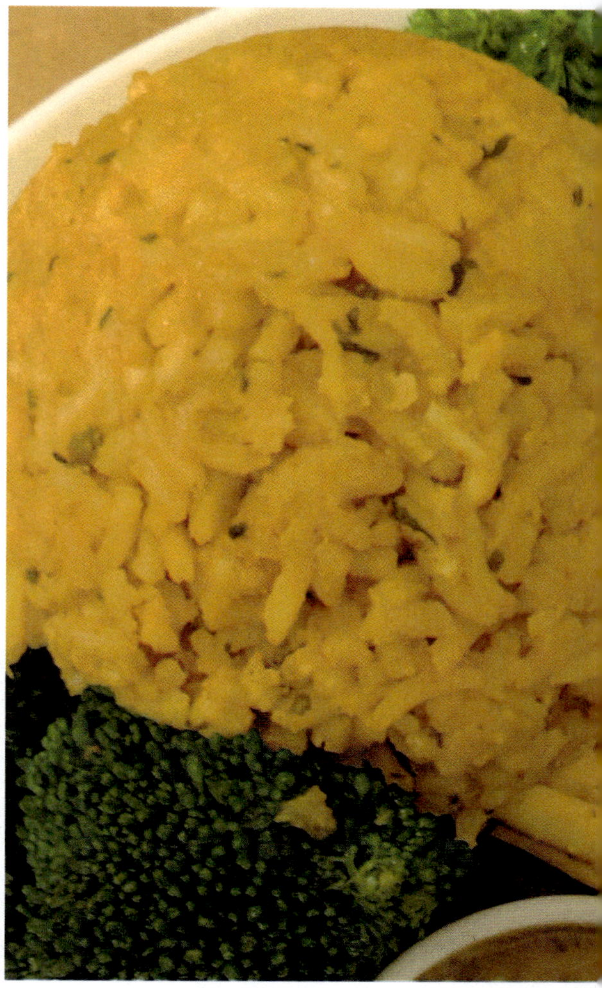

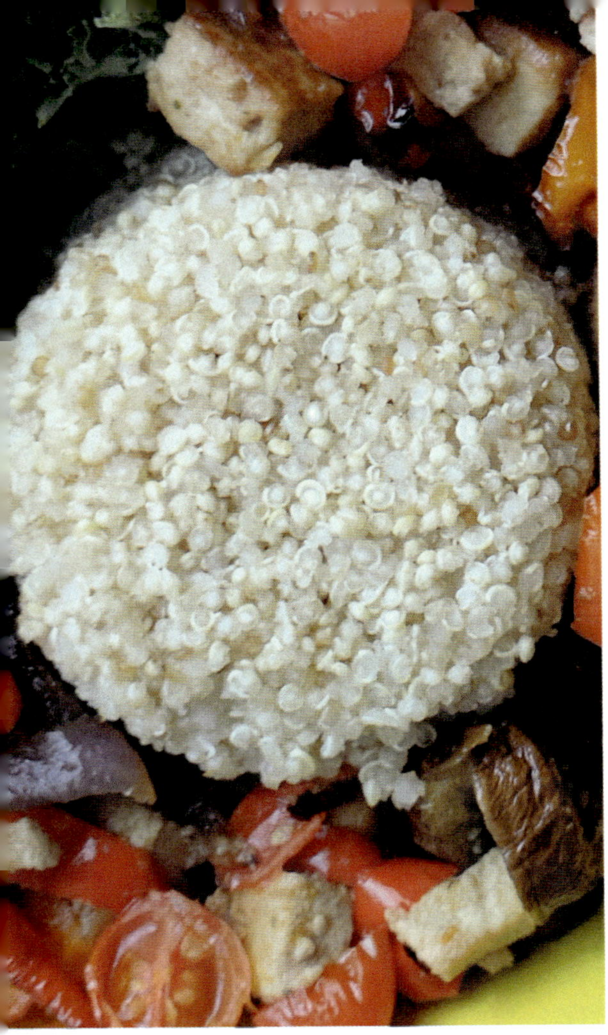

STEAMED QUINOA

Fluffy and nutty seeds steamed to delicious perfection.
Serves: 4

INGREDIENTS:

- 2 cups quinoa, dry
- 4 cups water
- 1/2 tsp. salt

STEPS:

1. Place quinoa into a bowl and cover with water. Allow to sit for 5–10 minutes before rinsing, or agitate grains with your hands and rinse immediately using a strainer to not lose the grains down the drain.
2. Add quinoa and water to large pot with a lid.
3. Bring water to a boil and add salt.
4. When water returns to a boil, reduce heat and allow to simmer on low, stirring occasionally until most of the liquid is absorbed and quinoa becomes a translucent color, about 15 minutes.
5. Remove pot from heat, cover, and allow to steam the rest of the way to perfection, about 10–15 minutes.

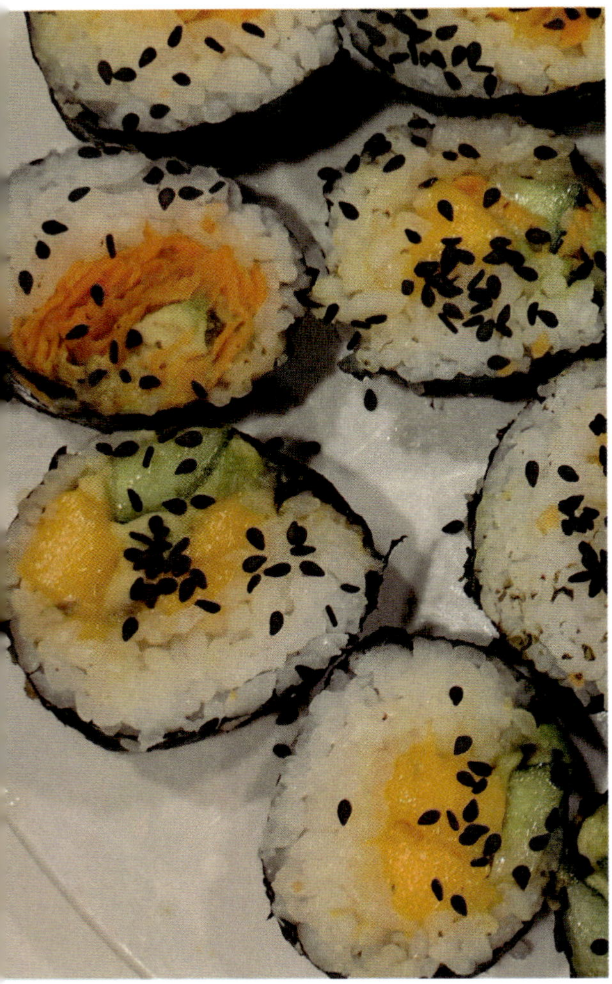

SUSHI RICE

The gooiest rice for stick-together sushi.
Serves: 4

INGREDIENTS:

- 2 cups sushi rice[1]
- 2.25 cups water
- 1 tsp. salt

DELICIOUS WITH:

Garden Sushi Cups (pg.106)

STEPS:

1. Rinse rice in large pot or bowl 2–3 times until water is mostly clear.
2. Bring rice to boil with water and salt on stovetop and reduce heat.
3. Allow rice to cook on a low boil for ten minutes. Turn off flame.
4. Allow rice to remain in pot for 1 hour with tight fitting lid. Enjoy!

1—While you can use regular white rice, sushi rice is preferrable because of its high stickiness factor. If using regular white rice, use more water than normal to make it more sticky.

Sticky Rice

Sushi rice is sometimes called "sticky rice" because of its high starch content which results in a more sticky-textured rice. This is the ideal rice for perfect slice-able sushi rolls.

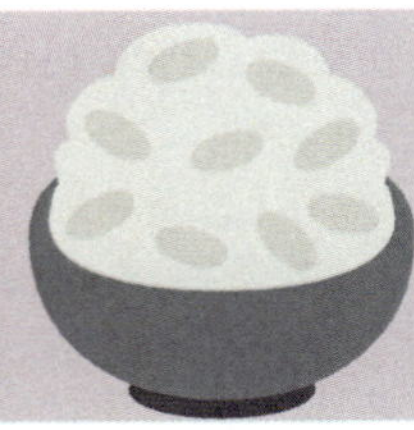

MUSHROOM RISOTTO

Mellow mushrooms make a sidekick of rice even more mouthwatering.

Serves: 4

INGREDIENTS:

- 2 cups whole grain rice
- 10 garlic cloves
- 1/2 yellow onion
- 1/2 cup nutritional yeast
- 1.5 cups almond milk
- 8 oz. white mushrooms
- optional: 1 tbsp. mushroom seasoning
- 1 tsp. salt

STEPS:

1. Rinse rice until water comes out clear to remove excess starch.
2. Dice fresh garlic cloves, yellow onion, and mushrooms into small pieces.
3. Warm pan on stovetop with 1 tbsp. of water and add garlic and onion.
4. Add rinsed rice and remaining spices to pan.
5. Prepare rice in typical fashion (see Steamed Jasmine Rice pg. 82).

DELICIOUS WITH: Fresh arugula, steamed mixed vegetables, Basic Baked Tofu (pg. 92), asparagus, fresh diced tomatoes.

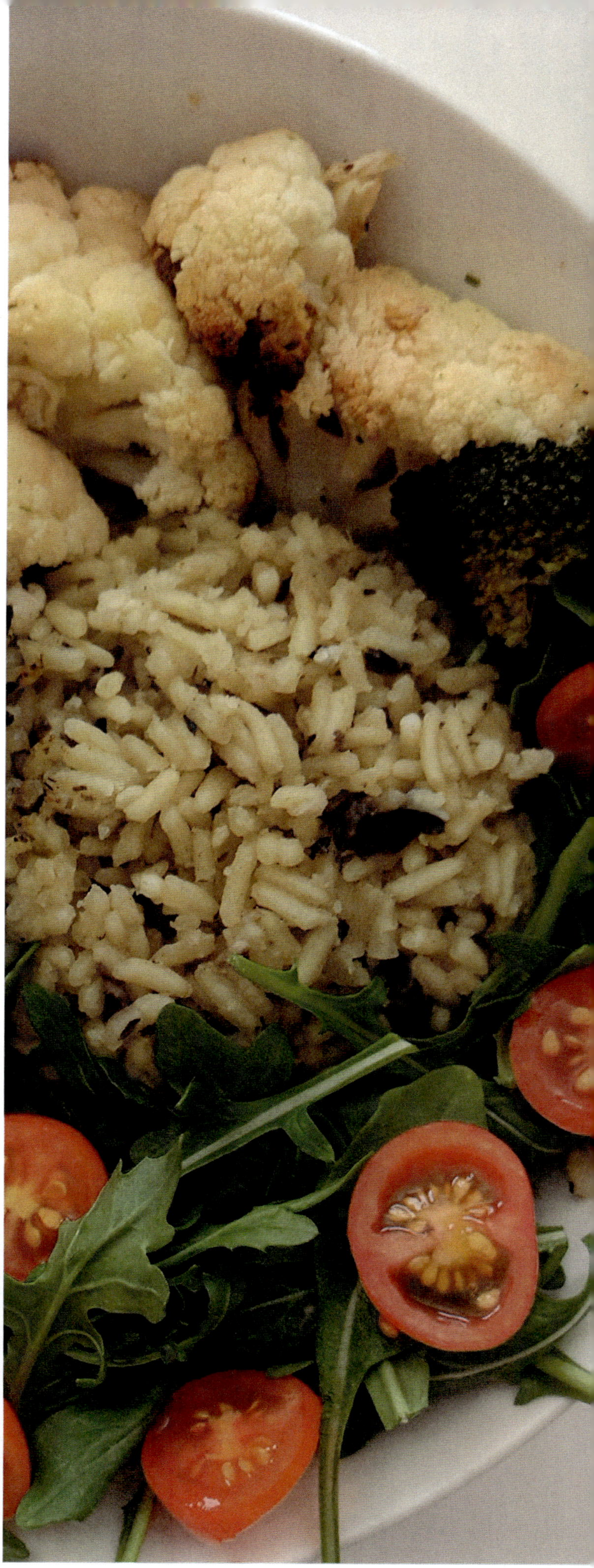

The Exception to the Rule

Mushrooms are an exception to the Golden Rule of the Frugivore Diet which says to simply eat whole plants. Mushrooms are not plants, they belong to the Fungi Kingdom of life. Mushrooms are actually more closely related to animals than to plants. Still, mushrooms are rich in nutrients such as B vitamins and make a delicious addition to an otherwise whole plant foods diet. Find another recipe featuring fungi—Mushroom Barley Soup—on page 119.

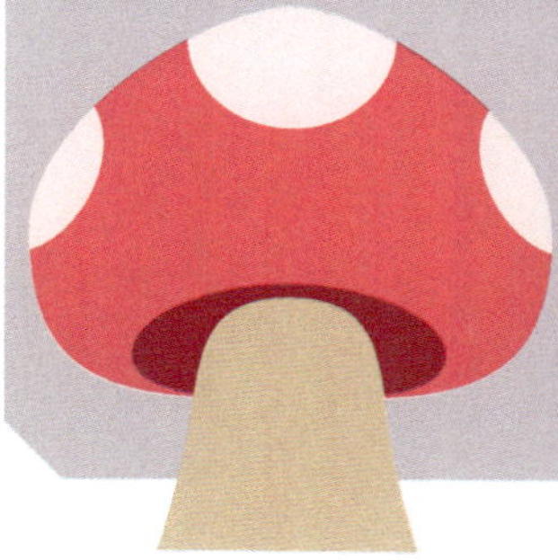

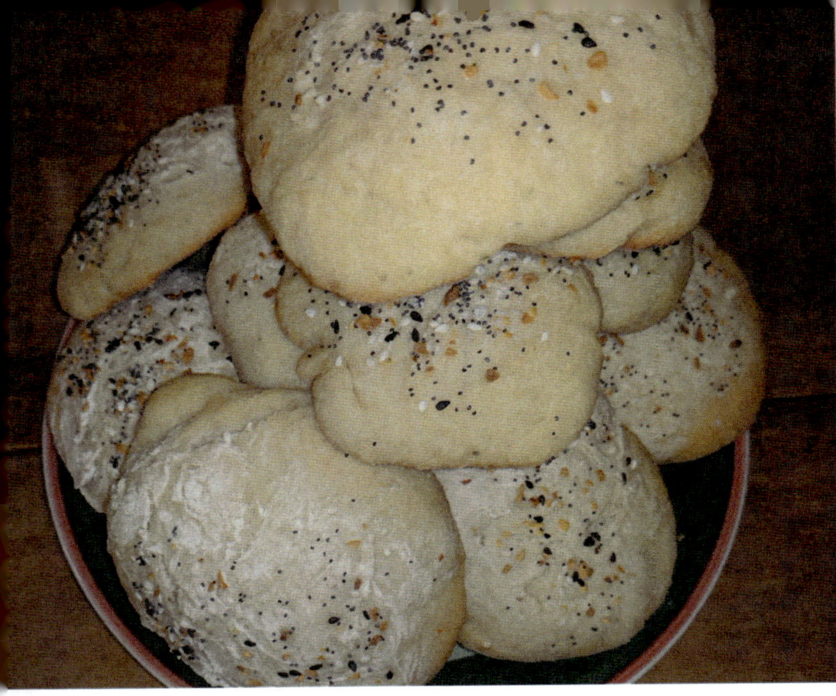

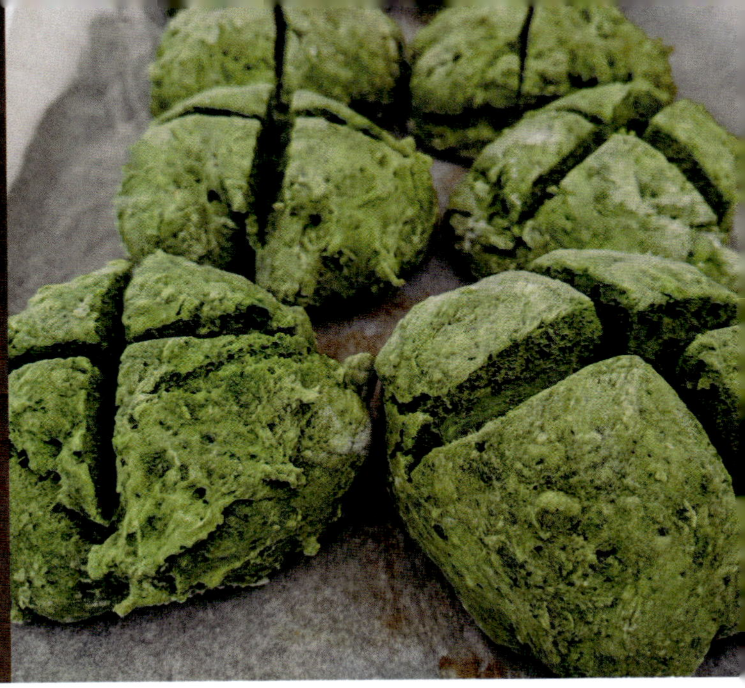

BASIC BREAD

A simple bread that can be formed into loaves, rolls, bread sticks, or any shape you desire.

Yields: 16 rolls or two loaves

INGREDIENTS:

- 6.5 cups flour (whole wheat or white)[1]
- 1 package active yeast
- 2.25 cups warm water
- 3 tbsp. sugar
- 1 tbsp. salt

STEPS:

1. In a large bowl, combine yeast and warm water. Stir until yeast dissolves.
2. Add sugar into warm water and yeast mix and stir until dissolved. Allow to sit for 5 minutes.
3. Add flour and salt. Stir until well mixed.
4. Sprinkle flour on your clean dry hands and use to knead dough into a large well combined ball.
5. Knead dough, cover, and allow to rise for 1–1.5 hrs or until it doubles in size.
6. Bake at 375°F for 30–35 minutes until the top and bottoms of the bread turn golden.
7. Remove bread from pan. Place on wire rack to cool.

1—I use white whole wheat flour from Trader Joe's. This flour is delicate like white flour and good for baking. While whole grains are preferred, you can substitute with white flour for a softer texture.

GREEN SODA BREAD

A gorgeously green no-yeast bread that packs a nutritious dose of fresh spinach.

Serves: 8 large dinner rolls or two small loaves

INGREDIENTS:

- 3 cups flour
- 2 cups spinach, packed
- 1 cup almond milk (or non-dairy milk)
- 1 tsp. baking powder
- 1 tsp. baking soda
- 1 tsp. salt
- 1.5 tbsp. apple cider vinegar

STEPS:

1. Preheat oven to 450°F.
2. Combine dry ingredients in large bowl.
3. Place spinach, vinegar, and almond milk into blender and blend until well combined.
4. Mix wet ingredients in bowl with dry ingredients until well combined.
5. Divide dough into eight pieces to make dinner rolls or into two to make two smaller loaves.
6. Shape loaves and place on baking sheet.
7. Bake for 30 minutes or until bottom of rolls are slightly golden and crisp.
8. Remove from oven and cover with towel before serving to keep rolls tender.

Good Luck With Irish Soda Bread

Soda bread is a traditional Irish food made with the most basic ingredients—flour and baking soda. Though the Irish didn't invent the idea of using soda to leaven bread, they have become most associated with this simple bread. Soda bread was the easiest and most affordable bread to put on the table for many Irish during times of poverty. I like making Green Soda Bread for St. Patrick's Day in March along with other traditional Irish foods including Irish Garden Stew, featured on page 115.

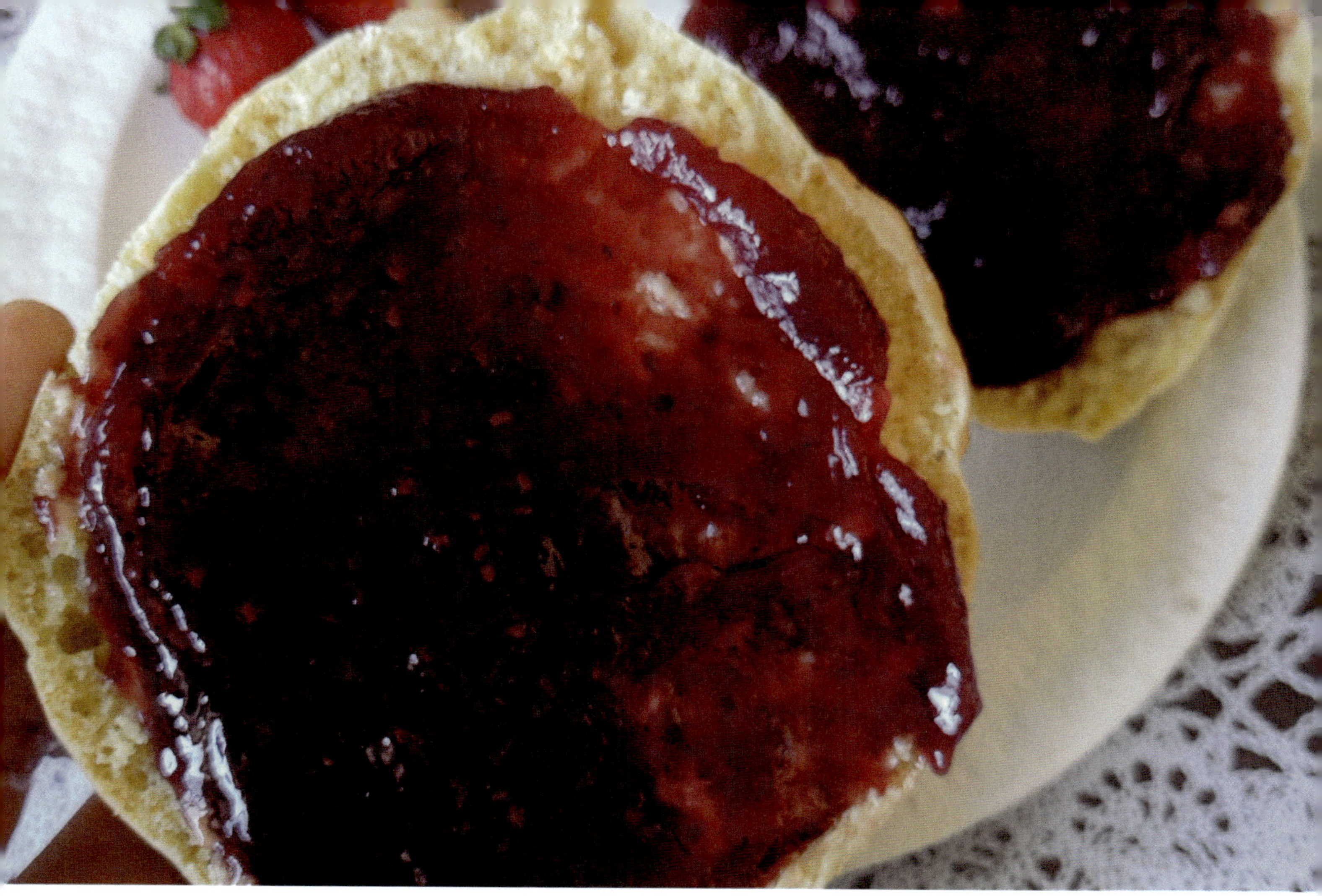

CORNMEAL ALMOND MILK BISCUITS

Make breakfast better with these fluffy, moist biscuits that are perfect with a fruit spread, doused in Breakfast Gravy, topped with Scrambled Tofu, or enjoyed straight from the oven.

Serves: 10 large biscuits, the perfect size for a breakfast sandwich

INGREDIENTS:

- 2.5 cups flour
- 1/2 cup cornmeal, finely ground
- 2 cups almond milk
- 1/4 cup corn starch
- 2 tbsp. baking powder
- 1 tbsp. apple cider vinegar
- 1 tsp. salt
- 1/2 tsp. baking soda
- optional: 2 tbsp. nutritional yeast

DELICIOUS WITH: Scrambled Tofu (pg.74), Breakfast Gravy (pg. 87), fruit preserves, avocado slices, arugula.

STEPS:

1. Combine dry ingredients in large mixing bowl.
2. Add almond milk and apple cider vinegar to the bowl.
3. Mix just until dough is well combined (don't overmix![1]) and place in the freezer for 20 minutes.
4. Preheat oven to 425°F.
5. Remove dough from freezer and scoop out large spoonfuls onto a stick-free, parchment-paper lined, or lightly-oiled baking sheet.
6. Bake for 20 minutes until biscuits have risen and their bottoms are lightly browned.

1—Overmixing quick breads can result in a more dense and chewy texture. Biscuits require more gentle kneading than yeast dough so that they do not turn out tough and so that you achieve a light airy texture when they are fresh out of the oven.

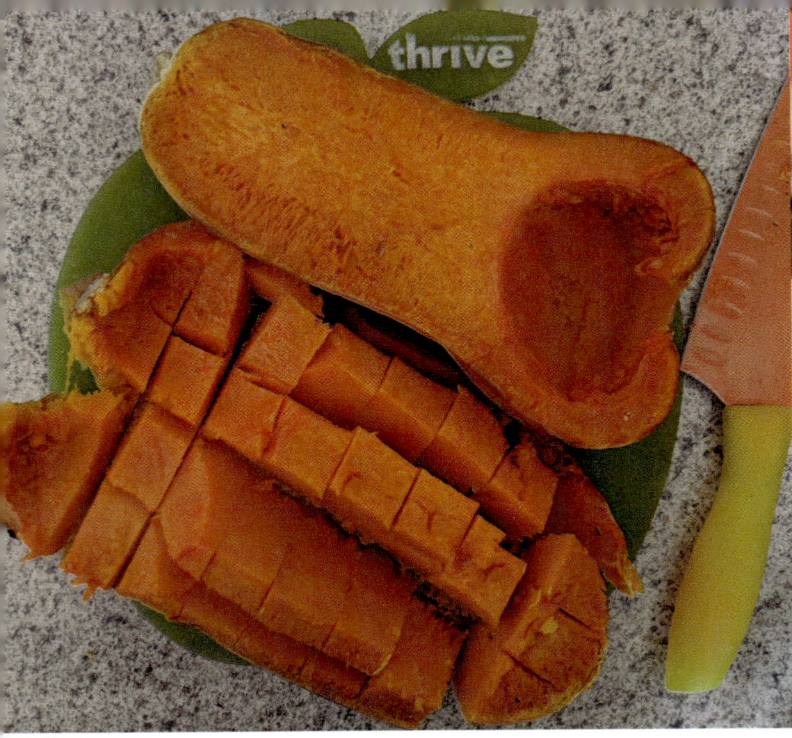

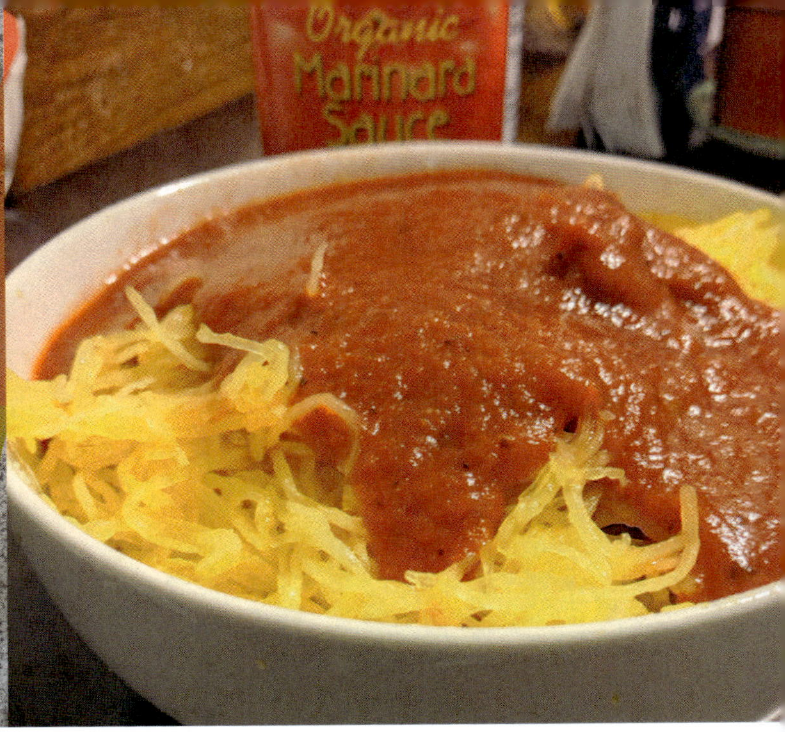

BAKED BUTTERNUT SQUASH

Savor this sweet and succulent winter squash as main course or side dish.[1]

Serves: 4

INGREDIENTS:

- 1 butternut squash, large

STEPS:

1. Preheat oven to 400°F.
2. Rinse squash to remove any debris.
3. Put the whole uncut squash on your oven's middle rack. (see caption below).
4. Bake for 40–60 minutes, more or less depending on size of your squash and how hot your oven runs. Check squash after 30 minutes and every 10 minutes after. You will know the squash is done when you can easily slice through it with a knife. The outer skin should begin to brown and some of the squash sugars may seep out while baking.

DELICIOUS WITH: Salad, marinara sauce, Harvest Pasta Sauce (pg.86).

1—Baked squash makes a great soup thickener or can be hidden in pasta sauce for extra flavor and nutrition.

BAKED SPAGHETTI SQUASH

When baked, this squash with noodle-like guts is a nutrient-rich, lighter alternative to spaghetti.

Serves: 4

INGREDIENTS:

- 1 spaghetti squash

STEPS:

1. Preheat oven to 400°F.
2. Put the whole, uncut squash on your oven's middle rack. (see tip box below)
3. Bake squash for 30–40 minutes, more or less depending on size of your squash and how hot your oven gets. Aim for al dente style squash strands so they will hold their spaghetti-shape and not turn into mush.
4. Cut squash in half, remove seeds with a spoon, carefully scoop out squash strands into a serving bowl or dish, and fluff with a fork to separate strands without breaking their shape.
5. Enjoy! Top with your favorite sauce.

DELICIOUS WITH: Squash on Squash (pg. 100).

Cutting Into Squash With Ease

Squash does not need to be cut before baking. If you prefer you can slice down the middle and remove the seeds before baking. If so, you can add spices such as salt, pepper, garlic powder, and dill to squash before baking. Because I have weak wrists due to carpal tunnel (the price of spending countless hours editing and formatting books on the computer!), I bake my squash whole and cut it in half after baking. I used to struggle to get a knife through an unbaked squash until I learned that pre-cutting squash was not a requirement. After your squash is properly baked you will be able to slice into it with ease and can easily remove the seeds at that stage.

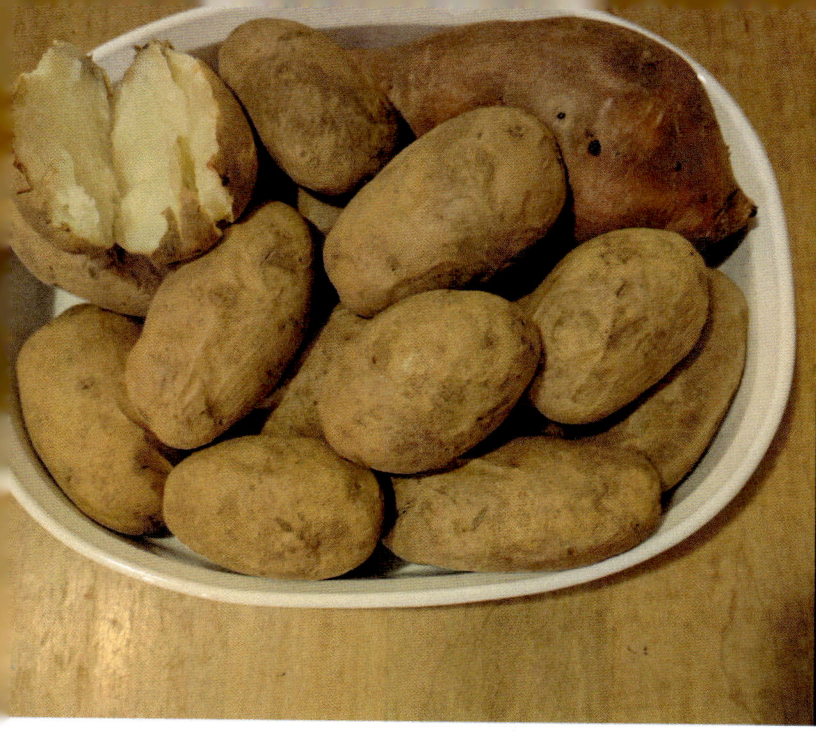

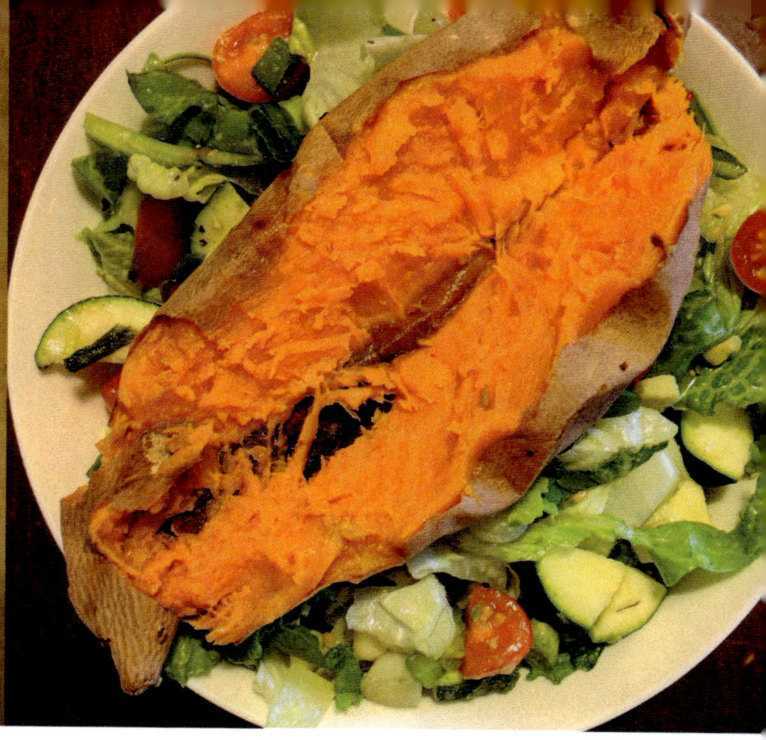

BAKED POTATO

It's hard to find an easier, more nutrient-rich, more-satisfying, and more affordable meal than the basic baked potato. This super spud makes a superb sidekick for numerous other salads, sauces, and sautéed vegetables.

Serves: 4

INGREDIENTS:

4 Russet potatoes, large

STEPS:

1. Preheat oven to 400°F.
2. Scrub any debris off of potatoes.
3. Use a fork to poke a few holes in the potatoes to prevent them from bursting.
4. Bake potatoes for 45–60 minutes. Baking time varies along with variation in potato size and oven. You may need to cook them a little more or less depending. Check your potatoes after 30 minutes. You will know they are done when you can easily stick a fork or knife into them. If you are baking other things in the oven, you can bake potatoes at the same time at a slightly lower or greater temperature. Adjust baking time accordingly.

BAKED SWEET POTATO

A sweet root baked to creamy deliciousness.

Serves: 4

INGREDIENTS:

4 sweet potatoes, medium/large

STEPS:

1. Preheat oven to 400°F.
2. Scrub sweet potatoes to remove debris.
3. Use a fork to poke a few holes in your potatoes to prevent them from bursting.
4. Bake sweet potatoes for 45–60 minutes.[1] Due to variation in potato size and ovens, you may need to cook them a little longer or a little less depending. You will know they are done when you can easily stick a fork or knife into them. It is normal for them to bleed a little sugar when they are thoroughly baked.

DELICIOUS WITH: Seven Greens Salad (pg. 66), King Kale Salad (pg. 67), Marinated Cucumbers (pg. 68), Seedy Slaw (pg. 68), 3 Sisters Salad (pg. 72), Rainbow Salad (pg. 73), Red Pepper Corn (pg. 91).

1—You can bake right on your oven's rack or on a pan to prevent juices dripping.

Potato vs. Sweet Potato: What's the Difference?

Although these two stars of the Frugivore Diet both share the "potato" name, they actually belong to two different families. Potatoes belong to the nightshade family of plants and are more closely related to tomatoes and peppers, while sweet potatoes belong to the morning glory family and have the beautiful star-shaped flowers to prove it. While both are packed with healthy carbohydrate energy and a full spectrum of nutrients, their nutrition profile does differ. Sweet potatoes contain more sugar and fiber per gram, while potatoes contain more starch. Both tubers are the underground storage organs of plants. These dense packages of nutrition will leave you feeling satisfied and energized throughout your day.

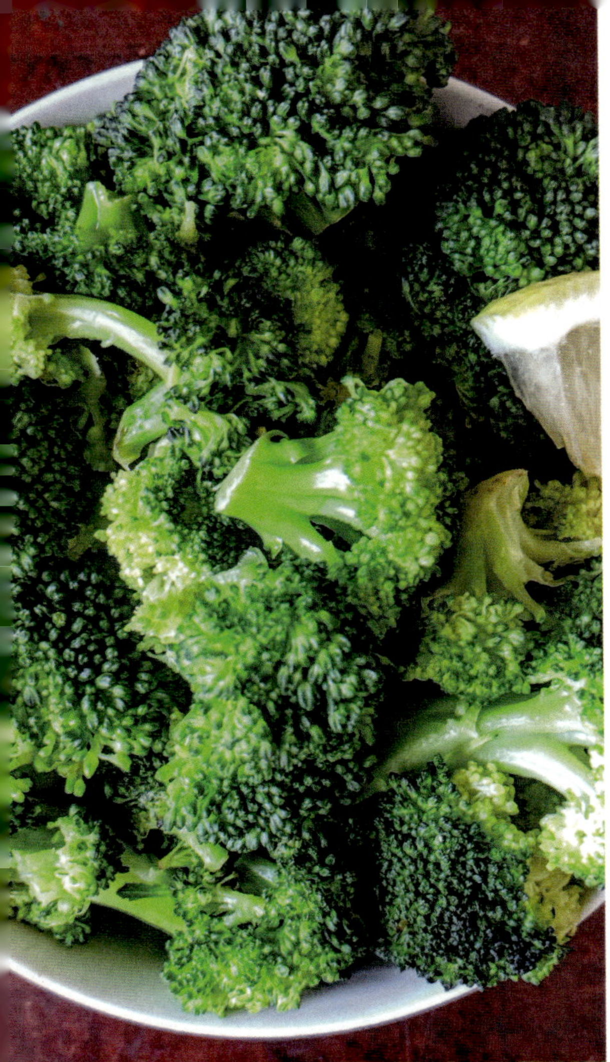

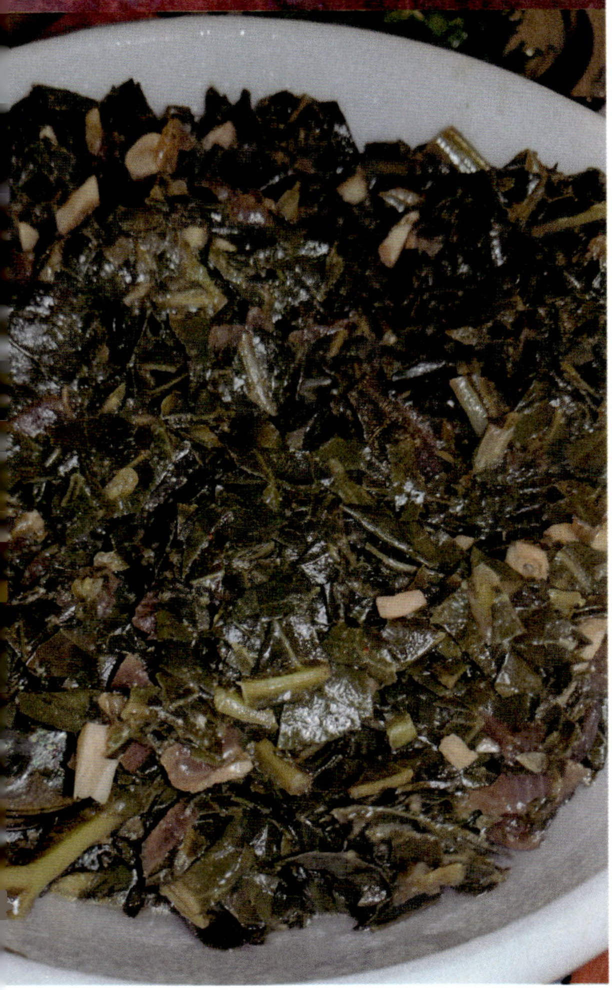

STEAMED BROCCOLI

Flavorful flowers steamed to a soft, yet still-crisp, superbness.

Serves: 4

INGREDIENTS:

- 4–6 cups broccoli, chopped
- 1 lemon (or 1/3 cup water)
- sea salt to taste
- fresh ground black pepper to taste

STEPS:

1. Wash broccoli and chop into bite-sized pieces.
2. Add water or squeeze juice of lemon into your pot, pan, or steamer, and bring to a low boil.
3. Add broccoli, reduce heat, and cover.
4. Steam broccoli for 5–7 minutes to retain vibrant green color, crunch, and nutrition. Keep a close eye to not overcook as mushy brocolli has lost the goodness of taste and nutrition.
5. Serve immediately. Sprinkle on salt and pepper. Enjoy!

DELICIOUS WITH: Yellow Rice (pg. 83), Mushroom Risotto (pg. 85), Broccoli Bowl (pg. 100), Basic Baked Tofu (pg.92).

SOUTHERN STYLE COLLARD GREENS

South Carolina-style seasoned and boiled greens.

Serves: 6

INGREDIENTS:

- 32 oz. collard greens
- 5 garlic cloves
- 1 onion, small
- 3 tbsp. apple cider vinegar
- 2 tbsp. soy sauce, low sodium
- 1 tbsp. agave nectar (or another sweetener)
- 1/4 tsp. cayenne pepper
- 1 cup water
- generous twists of fresh ground black pepper

STEPS:

1. Wash collard greens and remove soft leaves from tough stems.
2. Chop collard green leaves into small, thin ribbons.
3. Dice onion and garlic into small pieces. Sauté in large pot on medium heat with soy sauce until tender. Add collard greens and other ingredients, and boil on low for about 15 minutes until collards have reduced and are tender.

DELICIOUS WITH: A squeeze of lemon juice, Steamed Quinoa (pg. 84), Mushroom Risotto (pg. 85), Basic Baked Tofu (pg. 92), Mashed Potatoes & Gravy (pg. 109).

PEAS AND CARROTS

Classic peas and carrots make the perfect pair.

Serves: 4

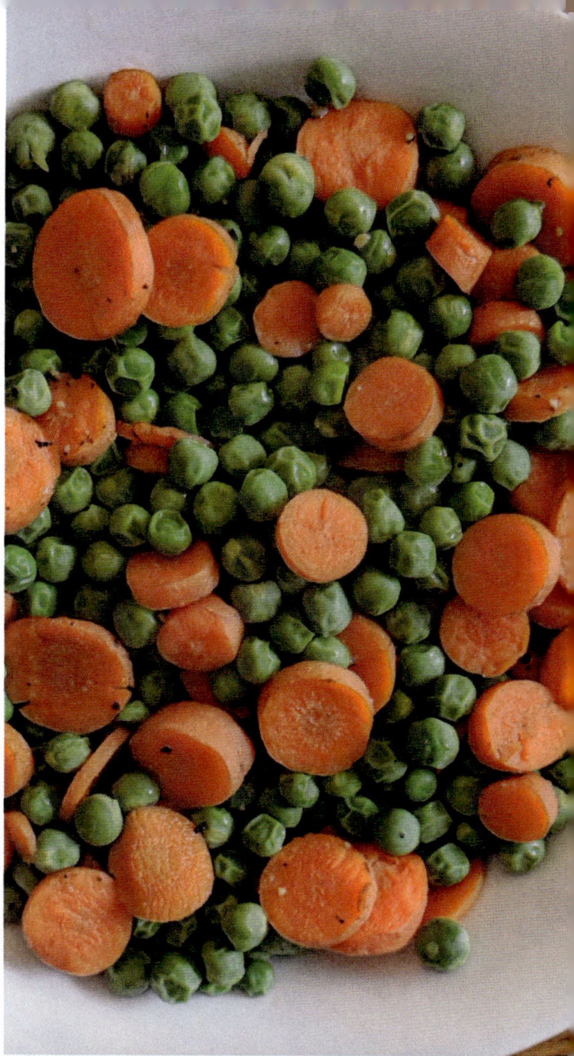

INGREDIENTS:

- 2 cups green peas, fresh or frozen
- 4 medium carrots[1]
- 1 tbsp. nutritional yeast
- 1 tsp. salt
- 1/2 tsp. black pepper
- 1/4 cup water

STEPS:

1. Wash carrots and slice into thin rounds.
2. Add carrots, water, and spices to small saucepan with a lid.
3. Bring water to boil and allow to boil for 2 minutes.
4. Reduce heat to low simmer and add green peas.
5. Simmer on low-medium heat for about 10 minutes or until carrots and peas are tender but not mushy. Remove from heat while orange and green colors are still vibrant. Enjoy!

DELICIOUS WITH: Yellow Rice (pg. 83), Broccoli Bowl (pg. 100).

1—I generally buy bags of whole carrots, but baby carrots are an easy-to-chop option.

RED PEPPER CORN

Sweet corn, red peppers, and edamame satisfy your savory side.

Serves: 4

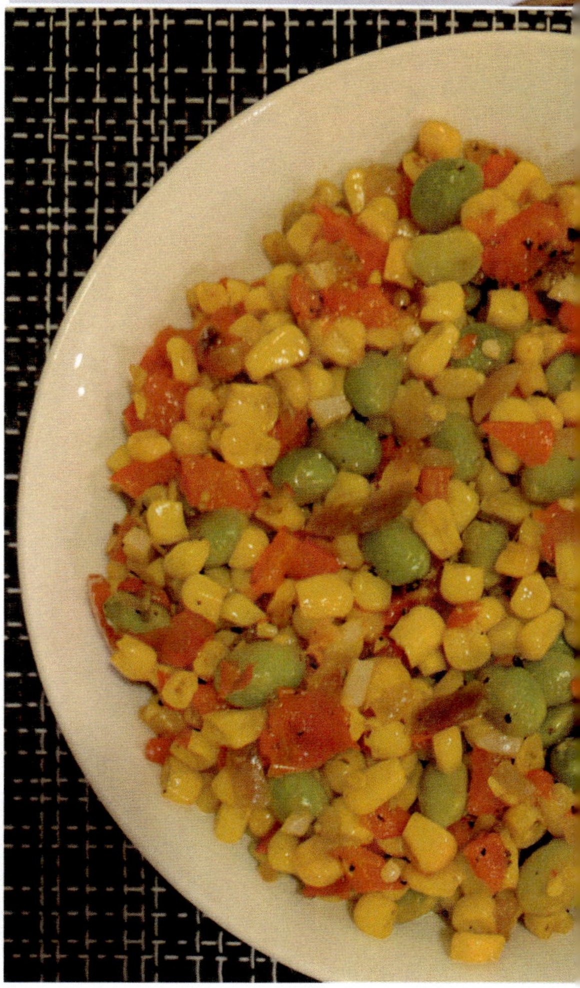

INGREDIENTS:

- 3 cups corn
- 1 cup edamame beans, shelled
- 1 red bell pepper
- 2 garlic cloves
- 2 tbsp. red onion, chopped small
- 1 tsp. salt
- 1/4 tsp. cayenne pepper
- generous twists of ground black pepper
- 1 tbsp. water

STEPS:

1. Chop red onion, garlic, and red bell pepper into small pieces.
2. Sauté onion, garlic, and bell pepper in 1 tbsp. water on medium heat until they begin to turn soft.
3. Add corn, edamame beans, and spices and continue to cook on medium heat for about 10 minutes.

DELICIOUS WITH: Baked Potato (pg. 89), Baked Butternut Squash (pg. 88), Basic Brown Rice (pg.82), Steamed Quinoa (pg. 84).

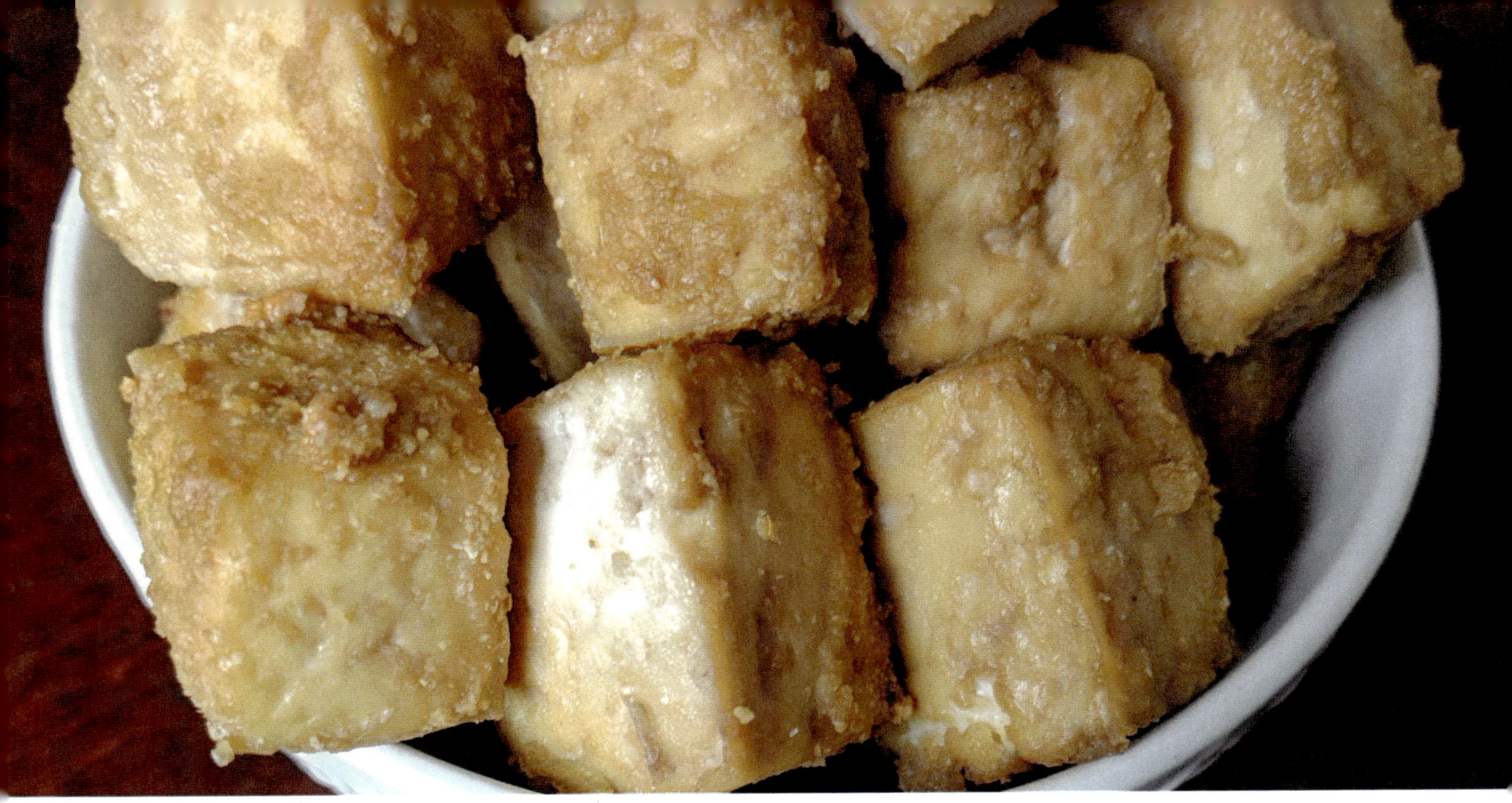

BASIC BAKED TOFU

An easy and pleasing baked tofu recipe.

Serves: 4

INGREDIENTS:

- 16 oz. extra firm tofu (1 standard-sized tofu block)
- 2 tbsp. soy sauce
- 1 tbsp. corn starch
- 1 tbsp. garlic powder
- 1 tbsp. nutritional yeast
- 1 tsp. salt

DELICIOUS WITH: Steamed Yellow Rice (pg. 83), Steamed Quinoa (pg. 84), roasted potatoes, Steamed Broccoli (pg. 90), Rainbow Salad (pg. 73).

1—Another method I use to help tofu absorb flavors and not crumble is to simply slice into cubes and place cubes, not touching each other, in a glass baking dish. Bake for 10–15 minutes to start to steam off some of the moisture. This will help tofu keep its shape.

STEPS:

1. Remove tofu from package and drain water.
2. Slice tofu into 1/2 inch slices with a sharp knife and place on a clean absorbent towel.
3. Cover tofu, place a heavy object on top, and apply slight pressure to help tofu drain extra water.[1]
4. Remove tofu from towel and cut into square cubes.
5. Place tofu in bowl, add spices, and stir carefully to coat the tofu evenly paying attention to maintain its cube shape.
6. Place tofu in ziploc bag or container and allow to marinate in the freezer for a couple hours, or in the fridge overnight.
7. Spread tofu out on a baking sheet. Use parchment paper to avoid tofu sticking to the pan.
8. Bake at 400°F for 30 minutes, turning occasionally so all sides brown evenly. Turn on your oven's broiler for an additional 5 minutes for extra crispy tofu squares.

Should You Be Scared of Soy?

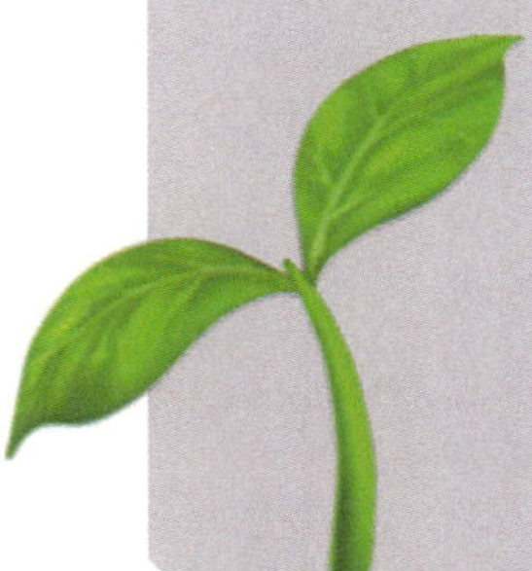

Many people are confused about whether or not to eat soy. On the one hand we hear about how diets high in soy can protect against cancer and other diseases. On the other hand we hear that soy can cause hormone imbalances putting your health at risk. The truth about soy is simple, thankfully. According to Dr. Neal Barnard, MD, president of the Physicians Committee for Responsible Medicine, there's "No Debate: Soy is Beneficial to Health." Yet there is a small but important caveat here—like most all plant foods today, to determine if soy foods are healthy for you follow this rule: Whole Plant Foods = GOOD FOR YOUR HEALTH. Processed Foods and animal foods = HAZARDOUS TO YOUR HEALTH. When it comes to soy, whole soybeans are a great food. Tofu, miso, tempeh, and soy milk are minimally processed foods which still maintain most of the nutrients in whole soy, so enjoy these foods in moderation to enrich your meals. For more on the science of soy visit: https://healingwithplants.us/topic/nutrition/.

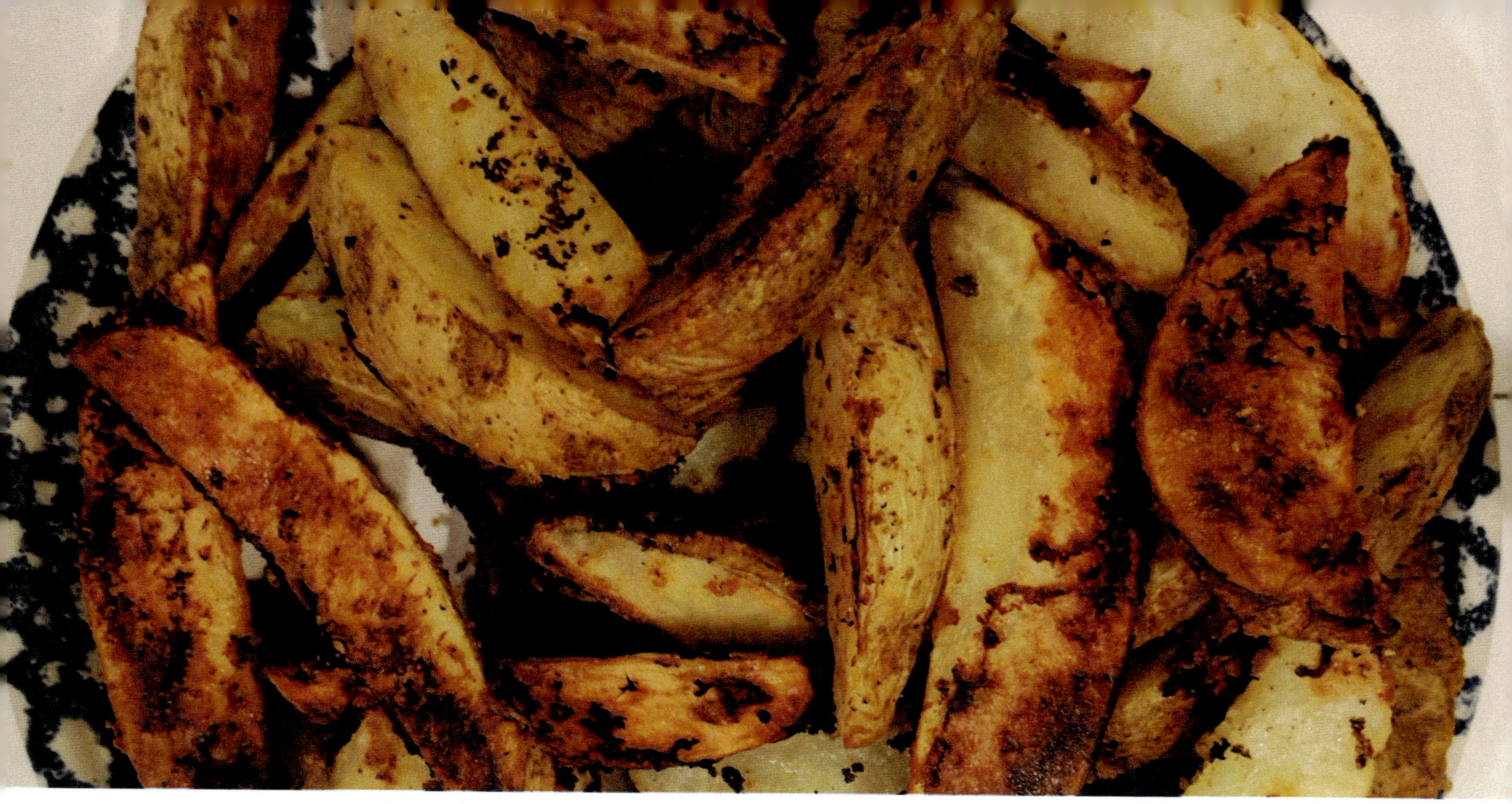

PERFECT POTATO WEDGES

Crispy baked spuds comfort the soul and nourish the body.

Serves: 4

INGREDIENTS:

- 6 baking potatoes, medium
- 1/4 cup nutritional yeast
- 2 tsp. corn starch
- 1 tsp. garlic powder
- 1 tsp. salt

Optional for more spice:

- 1 tbsp. garlic, minced
- 1–2 tbsp. fresh herbs (cilantro, basil, parsley, rosemary, dill, thyme)
- 1 tsp. chili powder (adds heat)
- generous twists of black pepper

DELICIOUS WITH: Salad, Coconut Ranch (pg. 56), Avocado Lime Dressing (pg. 58), King Kale Salad (pg. 67), Seedy Slaw (pg.68), Rainbow Salad (pg. 73).

STEPS:

1. Preheat oven to 450°F.
2. Slice potatoes into halves and then each half into quarters. Slice to achieve your desired thickness.
3. Place sliced potatoes into a metal colander and rinse well under cold water.
4. Place metal colander on top of pot with boiling water and cover with a lid. Allow the wedges to steam for 5 minutes until just slightly tender but not so long that they begin to break. (This could also be done in the pot.)
5. Place potato wedges into a large bowl, add spices, and stir to coat evenly.
6. Place potato wedges onto baking pan, ideally not touching each other to achieve maximum crispiness. Use parchment paper to avoid wedges sticking to pan.
7. Cook potatoes at 450°F for 20 minutes, then remove from oven and flip wedges.
8. Bake for another 10–15 minutes until edges are golden brown and slightly crispy.

Making a Perfect Potato Wedge

Potato wedges have always been one of my favorite foods. These will always remind me of Fridays during Lent when my family would go to the local fish and chips restaurant and I would order simply potato wedges. Creating the perfect potato wedge is possible, even without oil, because potatoes themselves are a rich and satisfying food. The secret is in the spice and what you coat your potatoes with. I use a little corn starch which makes the wedges crispier as it absorbs moisture and has a high percentage of amylose. Spreading your potatoes on a baking sheet so that they don't touch each other also helps maximize the crisp factor. How you spice your potato wedges is up to how fancy you want to get, and what ingredients you have to work with.

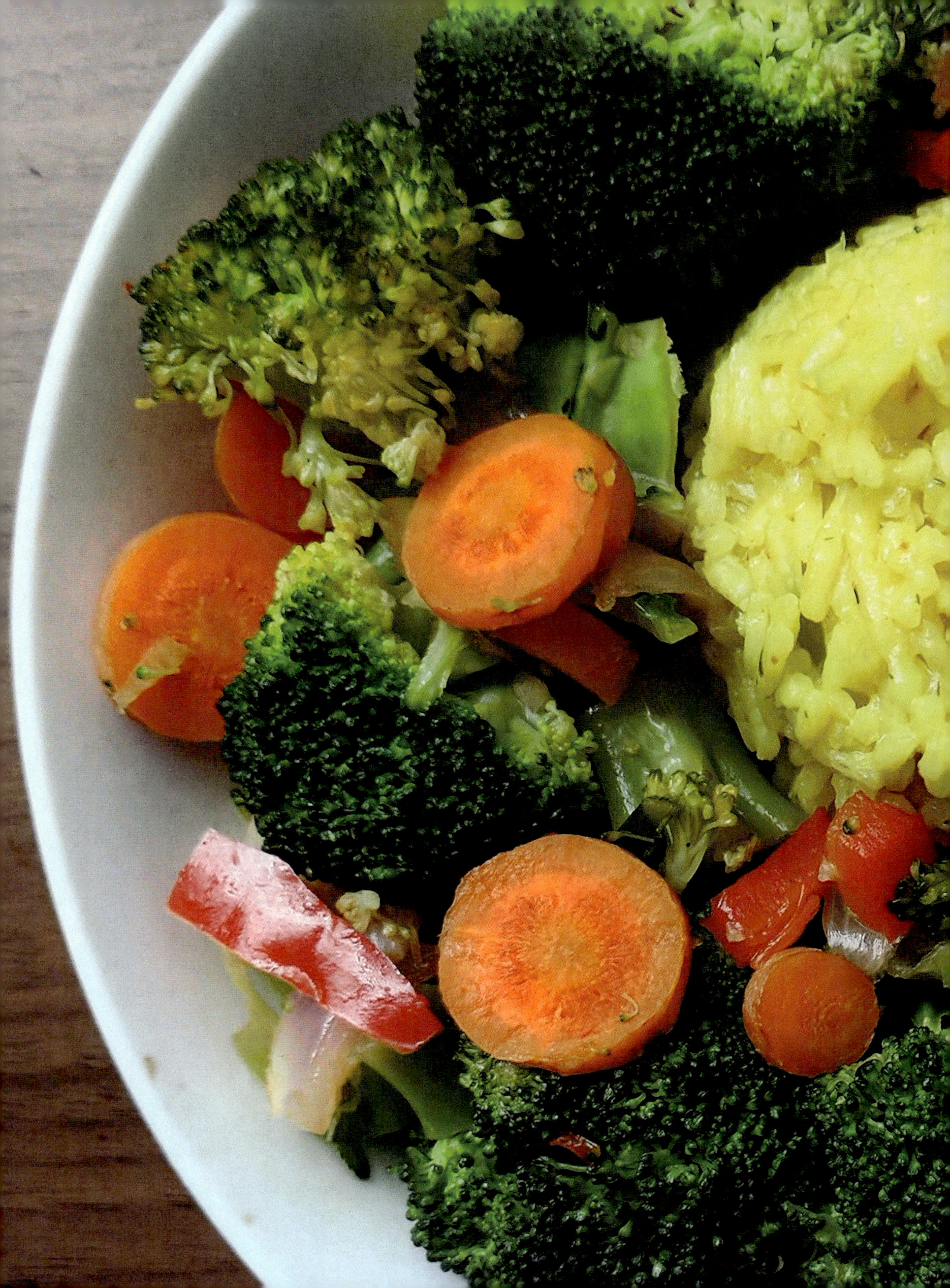

Bountiful Bowls

SUPPER

I prefer my meals in a bowl, which is why most of the meals in this book are in bowls! Simply building your meal in a bowl can make it appear more bountiful and appetizing. Here I share how I combine many of the savory sidekicks and sauces in this book to make easy and delightful meals that nourish and satisfy.

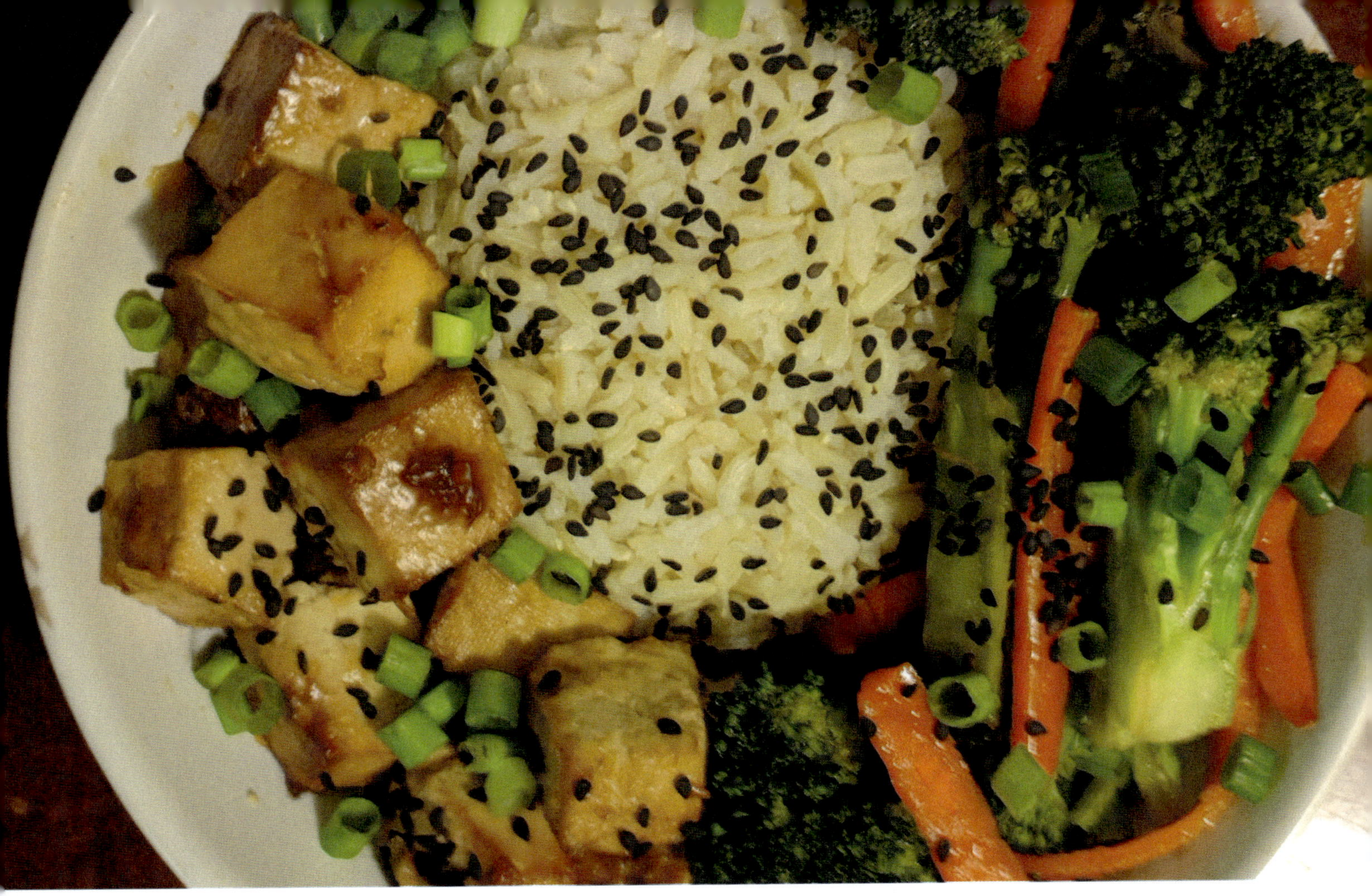

TERIYAKI TOFU BOWL

Teriyaki Tofu served with whole grain brown rice and steamed veggies and topped with green onions and toasted sesame seeds makes a satisfying savory supper.

Serves: 4

INGREDIENTS:

- Teriyaki Sauce (use whole recipe pg. 57)
- 16 oz. tofu (1 block)
- 3 cups broccoli, chopped
- 3 carrots
- 4 green onions
- 1 cup brown rice
- 2 cups water
- 2 tsp. sesame seeds

Keep Broccoli Green!

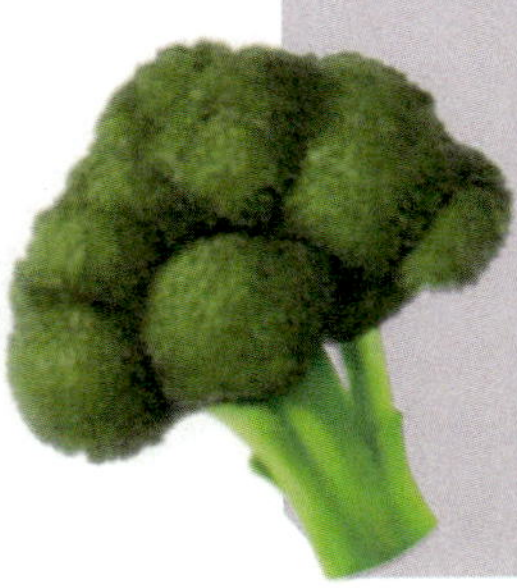

Science shows that the more broccoli is cooked, the more it loses its nutritional value. To get the most goodness out of your broccoli, it's best to minimize cook time. Lightly steaming or sautéeing broccoli so it retains it's brilliant green color and some crunch will reduce nutrient loss through cooking. Also, if you like broccoli, consider enjoying it raw from time to time to get the maximum nutrient boost that these flowers have to offer.

STEPS:

1. Prepare Basic Brown Rice, pg. 82.
2. Drain tofu and slice into cubes. Toss with Teriyaki Sauce and bake at 400°F for 30 minutes or until slightly crisp on the edge.
3. Wash broccoli, carrots, and green onions.
4. Slice carrots into thin strands. Chop broccoli into bite-sized pieces. Dice green onions into small pieces and set aside.
5. Steam carrots on stovetop for a few minutes, add broccoli, and steam for a few more minutes until broccoli turns vibrant green.
6. Use a one-cup-sized cup to scoop rice into a mound in the center of the bowl.
7. Arrange Teriyaki Tofu and steamed veggies around rice.
8. Garnish with green onions, black or tan sesame seeds, and fresh ground black pepper.

DELICIOUS WITH: Teriyaki Sauce (pg.57), Spicy Peanut Sauce (pg.57).

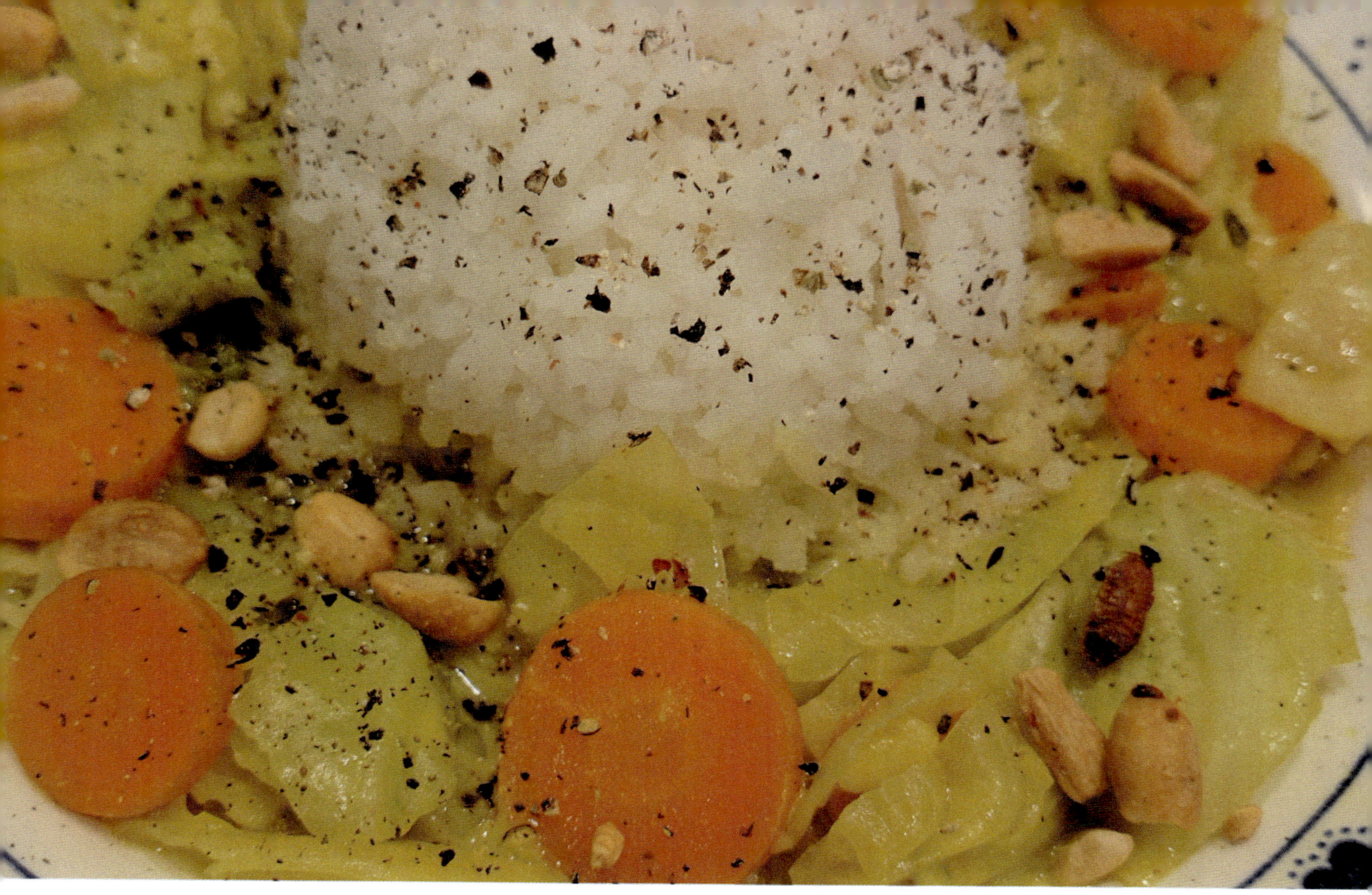

CURRY CABBAGE

Coconut cream and curry spices make this cabbage craveable.

Servings: 6

INGREDIENTS:

- 1 head cabbage
- 1 yellow onion, medium
- 2 carrots, large
- 7 garlic cloves
- 1 14 oz. can coconut cream
- 2 tbsp. fresh ginger, chopped small
- 2 tsp. turmeric
- 2 tsp. cumin
- 2 tsp. sea salt
- 1 tsp. garlic powder
- 1 tsp. thyme
- 1/4 tsp. cayenne pepper
- 2 cup + 2 tbsp. water

STEPS:

1. Chop onion, garlic, and ginger into small pieces and sauté in a large pot with 2 tbsp. water.
2. Chop cabbage into medium-sized chunks. Slice carrot into 1/2 inch rounds.
3. When onion begins to turn soft, add the carrots and cabbage to the pot.
4. Add spices, coconut cream, and water.
5. Stir to combine and cover pot with a lid.
6. Continue to cook on medium/low heat until carrots and cabbage are tender but retain a crisp crunch.

DELICIOUS WITH: Basic Brown Rice (pg.82) or Steamed Jasmine Rice (pg.82). Serve with fresh arugula or other fresh greens. Feel free to add in other vegetables like cauliflower or broccoli. Sprinkle peanuts on top for a salty crunch.

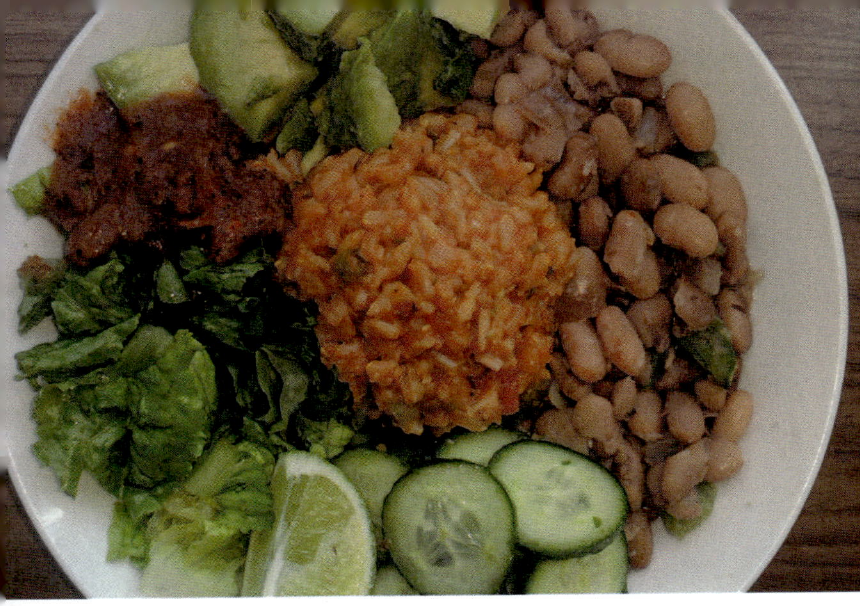

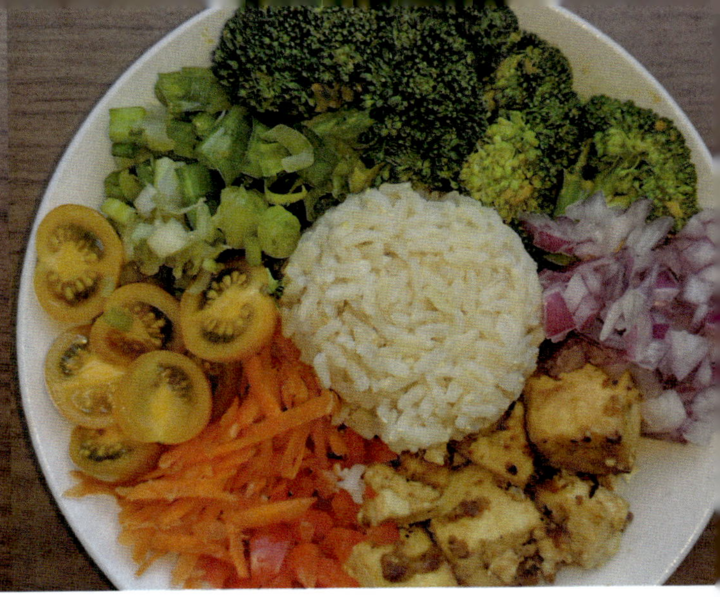

RED RICE N' BEANS BOWL

Another 100% plants meal featuring rice and beans.

Serves: 4

INGREDIENTS:

- 4 cups Red Rice (recipe page 83.)

BEANS

- 2 cans of pinto beans
- 3 green onions
- 1 tsp. onion salt

IN THE BOWL

- 2–3 cucumber
- 2 avocados
- 2 cups lettuce
- 1 lime
- salsa

STEPS:

1. Prepare Red Rice according to recipe on pg. 83.
2. Prepare four cups of pinto beans (equivalent of 2 cans).
3. Combine pinto beans, green onions, and onion salt in a saucepan and warm on low or medium heat.
4. Slice cucumber into rounds, chop lettuce into small pieces, and dice avocados into bite-sized pieces.
5. Use a one-cup-sized cup to scoop rice into a mound in the center of the bowl.
6. Arrange beans, cucumbers, lettuce, salsa, and avocado around rice.
7. Garnish with more diced green onions and/or fresh ground black pepper.
8. Enjoy!

RAINBOW RICE N' TOFU BOWL

Whole grain brown rice surrounded by a rainbow of fresh, whole-plant foods.

Serves: 4

INGREDIENTS:

- 4 cups Basic Brown Rice (recipe page 82.)
- 1 red bell pepper
- 2–3 carrots
- 1 cup yellow cherry tomatoes
- 6 green onions
- 3 cups Steamed Broccoli (recipe page 90.)
- 1/2 red onion
- 1 package of extra firm tofu, tossed with Spicy Peanut Sauce (recipe page 57.)

STEPS:

1. Prepare Basic Brown Rice, pg. 82.
2. Drain tofu and slice into cubes. Toss with 1 cup of Spicy Peanut Sauce (pg. 57) and bake at 400°F on a parchment-paper lined baking sheet, or in a shallow glass baking dish, until tofu is slightly crisp on the edge (abut 30 min).
3. Prepare Steamed Broccoli, pg. 90.
4. Shred carrots, chop bell pepper and red onion into small pieces, cut cherry tomatoes in half, and cut green onions into small pieces.
5. Use a one-cup size cup to scoop rice into a mound in the center of the bowl.
6. Arrange tofu, broccoli, bell pepper, carrots, tomatoes, and onions around rice.
7. Garnish with more diced green onions and/or fresh ground black pepper.

DELICIOUS WITH: Spicy Peanut Sauce (pg. 57).

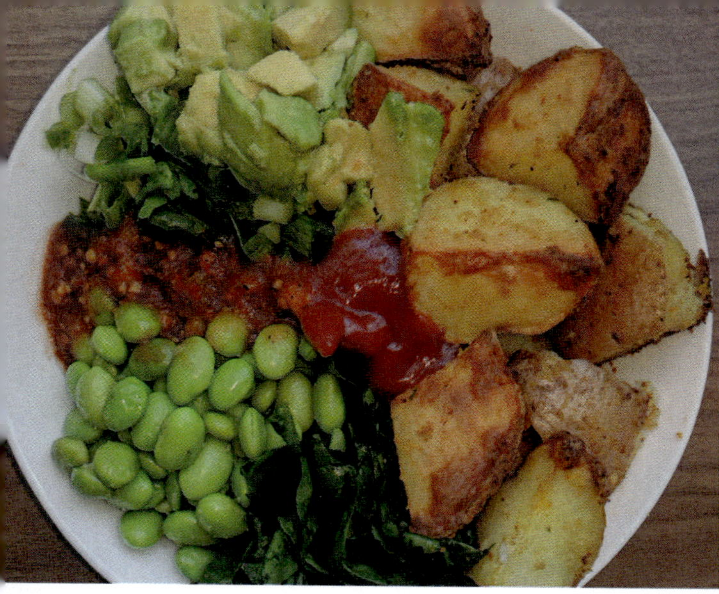

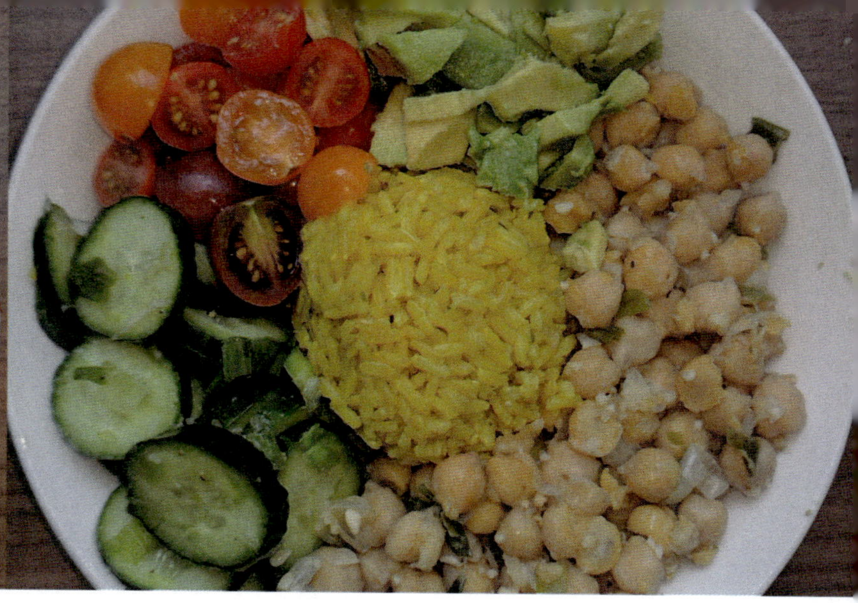

ROASTED POTATO BOWL

Another easy and satisfying plant-based meal to please the whole family.

Servings: 2 bowls/meals

INGREDIENTS:

POTATOES

- 2 large or 3–4 medium potatoes
- 3 tbsp. nutritional yeast
- 1 tbsp. garlic powder
- 1 tbsp. onion salt

SIDEKICKS

- 1 cup greens, chopped
- 1.5 cups edamame beans
- 1 avocado
- 5 green onions, diced
- 1/2 cup salsa
- organic ketchup

STEPS:

1. Wash potatoes and remove any bad spots with a sharp knife.
2. Dice potatoes into large chunks, leave skins on for nutrients.
3. Place diced potatoes into a large bowl and mix with onion salt, garlic powder, and nutritional yeast. Stir until potato chunks are evenly coated.
4. Roast potatoes in oven on 425°F until crispy browned.
5. Warm frozen edamame beans with a dash of onion salt (or use onion powder and salt or low-sodium soy sauce).
6. Serve in bowl with fresh diced avocado, green onions, chopped spinach, salsa, and ketchup.

CHICKPEAS N' RICE BOWL

Yellow rice and garbanzo beans served with a side of Marinated Cucumbers, cherry tomatoes, and avocado.

Servings: 2 bowls/meals

INGREDIENTS:

Yellow Rice (recipe pg. 83)

CHICKPEAS

- 2 cans chickpeas (aka garbanzo beans)
- 3 garlic cloves
- 4 green onions, diced
- 1 tbsp. nutritional yeast
- splash Bragg Liquid Aminos or low-sodium soy sauce

SIDEKICKS

- 1 avocado, diced
- 3 cucumbers, sliced
- 2 cups cherry tomatoes, halved

STEPS:

1. Prepare Yellow Rice according to recipe pg. 83.
2. Prepare Marinated Cucumbers according to recipe pg. 68.
3. Prepare 4 cups of garbanzo beans (~2 cans).
4. Dice green onions and garlic cloves into small pieces.
5. Combine garbanzo beans, green onions, garlic, nutritional yeast, and soy sauce in a saucepan and warm on low or medium heat.
6. Slice cherry tomatoes in half and dice avocado into bite-sized pieces.
7. Use a one-cup-sized cup to scoop rice into a mound in the center of the bowl.
8. Arrange garbanzo beans, cucumbers, tomatoes, and avocado around rice.
9. Garnish with more diced green onions and/or fresh ground black pepper.

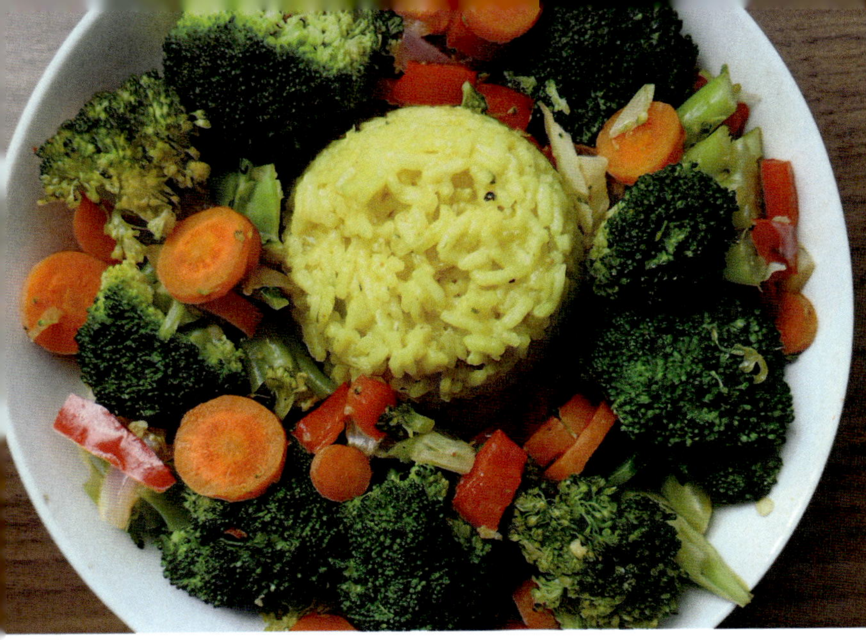

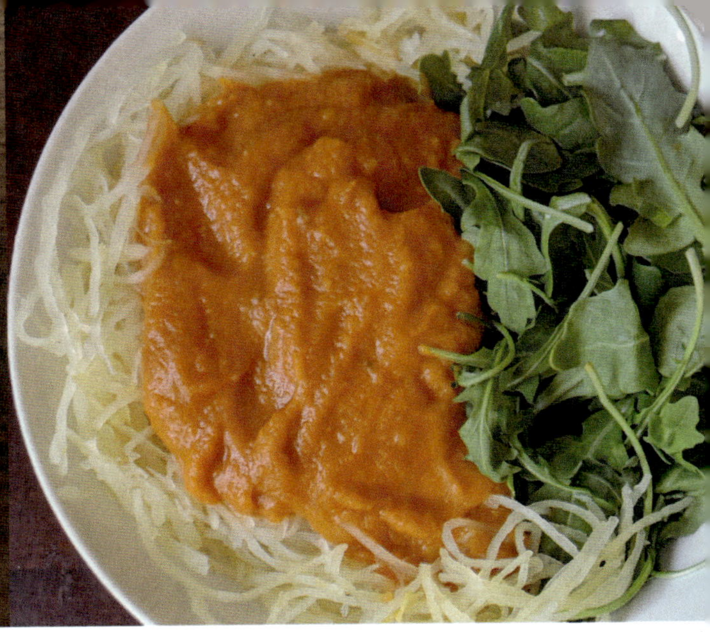

BROCCOLI BOWL

A simple, colorful, and nutritious bountiful bowl starring broccoli flowers.

Servings: 4 bowls/meals

INGREDIENTS:

- 4 cups Yellow Rice (pg. 83)
- 4 cups broccoli, chopped
- 2 carrots, large
- 1 red bell pepper
- 1/2 red onion
- 8 garlic cloves
- 1 tsp. sea salt
- 1 tsp. onion powder
- 1 tsp. water

STEPS:

1. Prepare Yellow Rice (recipe pg. 83.)
2. Wash fresh veggies.
3. Chop broccoli into bite-sized pieces.
4. Dice carrots into thin rounds.
5. Chop red onion, red bell pepper, and garlic cloves into small pieces.
6. Chop red bell pepper and onion into small pieces.
7. Sauté onion, garlic, and bell pepper in 1 tsp. water on medium heat until tender.
8. Add chopped broccoli to pan, cover with tight fitting lid, and reduce heat to low for 5 minutes.
9. Stir, return lid to pan, and turn off heat.
10. Allow broccoli to steam for another 5 minutes before serving.
11. Serve immediately so that broccoli and carrots maintain a slight crispness.

SQUASH ON SQUASH

A scrumptious bowl of squash that's purely plants and loaded with the flavors of fall.

Servings: 4 bowls/meals

INGREDIENTS:

- 1 jar of Harvest Pasta Sauce (pg. 60)
- 1 Baked Spaghetti Squash, large (pg. 88)

STEPS:

1. Prepare Harvest Pasta Sauce according to the directions on pg. 60.
2. Prepare spaghetti squash in oven according to the directions on pg. 88.
3. Scoop spaghetti squash strands out of squash shell with a big spoon being careful not to break the strands as much as possible. Fluff the squash strands with a fork so they resemble thin noodles.
4. Warm Harvest Pasta Sauce on stove.
5. Scoop squash noodles into bowl and top with sauce.
6. Serve with fresh arugula or a simple side salad. Enjoy!

I Prefer Spaghetti Squash

I cook pasta very infrequently because I'm not the biggest pasta fan. Although I can enjoy some Ch-easy Mac from time to time, pasta often leaves me feeling heavy and I much prefer the way I feel after eating spaghetti squash. I like feeling nourished and light after mealtime and for me this means prioritizing whole-plant foods on my plate.

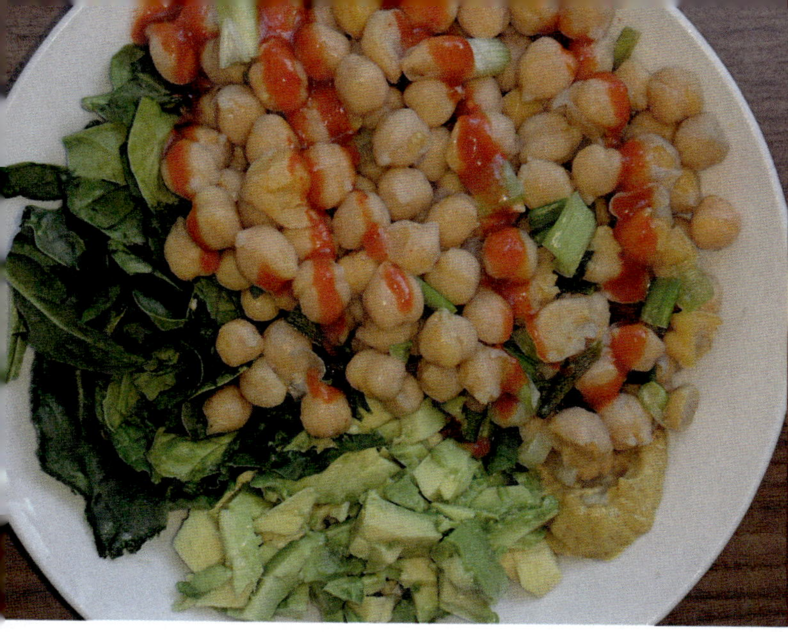

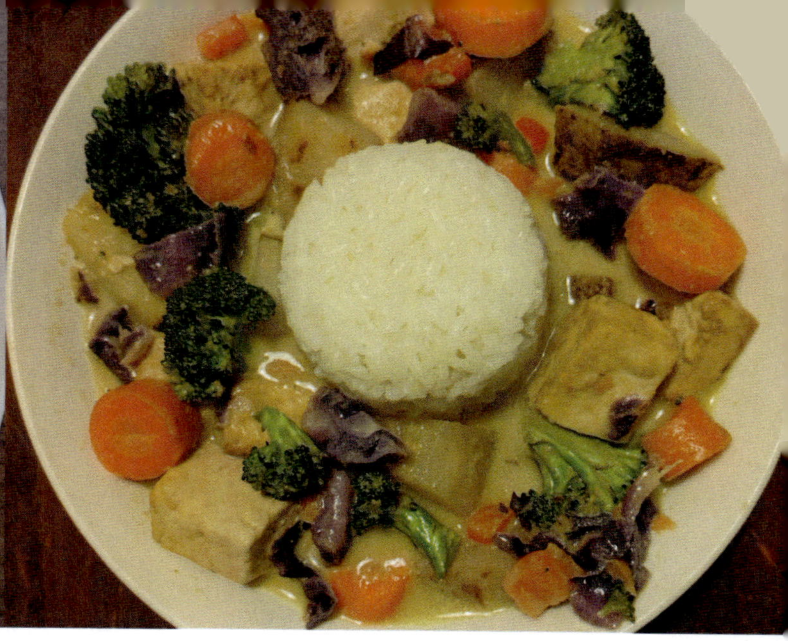

GO GARBANZOS BOWL

Savor the greatness of garbanzo beans in this nutrient-packed and satisfying meal.

Servings: 4 bowls/meals

INGREDIENTS:

- 2 cans garbanzo beans, drained
- 4 cups spinach, chopped
- 2 avocados, diced
- 4 green onions, diced
- 2 tsp. onion salt
- sriracha hot sauce (or substitute with salsa)

STEPS:

1. Wash fresh veggies.
2. Open two cans garbanzo beans, rinse, and drain liquid.
3. Warm garbanzos and onion salt on stovetop on medium heat for 3–5 minutes.
4. Add diced green onions to garbanzo beans.
5. In a bowl, combine 1 cup garbanzo beans with 1 cup chopped spinach and 1/2 diced avocado. Top with sriracha hot sauce.
6. Enjoy!

VEGETABLE CURRY BOWL

A rainbow of vegetables in sweet and spicy coconut curry sauce, served with tender baked tofu and Jasmine rice.

Servings: 4 bowls/meals

INGREDIENTS:

- 4 cups Steamed Jasmine Rice
- 1 lb tofu (16 oz.)
- 2 cups broccoli, chopped
- 2 carrots
- 1 cup red cabbage
- 1 potato, large
- 1/2 red bell pepper
- 5 garlic cloves
- 1/4 onion, medium

CURRY SAUCE:

- 1 can of coconut cream (or full-fat milk)
- 2 tsp. turmeric
- 2 tsp. garlic powder
- 2 tsp. onion powder
- 2 tsp. salt
- 2 tsp. cumin
- 1 tsp. coriander
- 1/4 tsp. cinnamon
- 1/4 tsp. ginger
- 1/4 tsp. cayenne pepper
- 1 cup water
- * optional for extra sweetness and depth: 1 tbsp. agave, juice of 1 lime, 1 tbsp. tomato paste, 1/2 fresh stalk of lemongrass or 1 tsp. dried lemongrass.

STEPS:

1. Prepare Steamed Jasmine Rice (pg. 82.) Prepare Basic Baked Tofu (pg. 92).
2. Wash fresh veggies and remove any bad spots with a sharp knife.
3. Slice carrots into thin rounds, chop broccoli, cabbage, and potato into small chunks. Dice red pepper, onion, and garlic cloves into small pieces.
4. In a pot or pan with a lid, sauté onions, red pepper, and garlic in 1 tbsp. coconut cream until they begin to turn translucent and release their aroma.
5. Add sliced carrots, potato chunks, and remaining coconut milk to the pot and cover. Allow to simmer on medium heat for 10–15 minutes stirring occasionally.
6. When potatoes and carrots start to become tender, add broccoli, cabbage, and curry sauce spices. Cover. Allow to simmer for another 5 minutes on medium heat and remove from heat.
7. Serve veggie curry immediately with Basic Baked Tofu and Steamed Jasmine Rice. Enjoy!

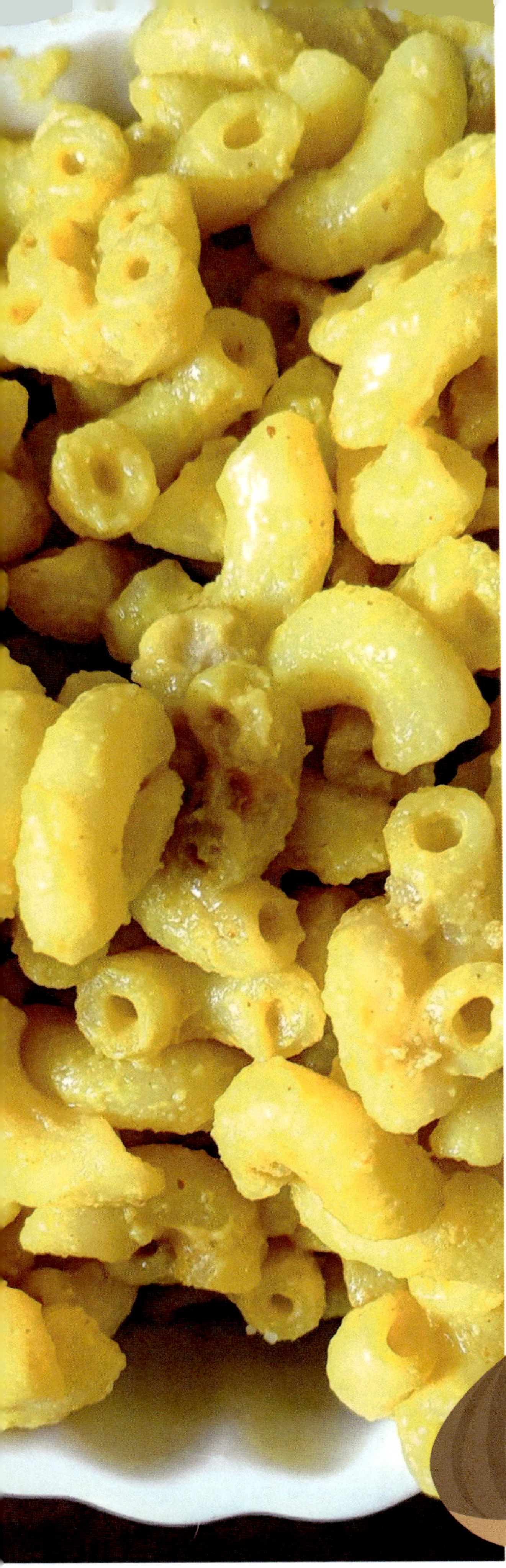

CH-EASY MAC

A creamy ch-easy pasta that's 100% plants.

INGREDIENTS:

- Regular organic macaroni, boiled and strained

..Then stir in:

- 1 cup nutritional yeast
- 1/2 cup unsweetened almond milk (or amount to create desired consistency)
- 1 tbsp. garlic powder
- 1 tbsp. sesame tahini
- 1 tbsp. yellow mustard
- 1 tbsp. soy sauce (or 1 tsp. sea salt)
- 1 tsp. turmeric
- twists of black pepper

STEPS:

1. Boil macaroni noodles according to instructions.
2. Strain macaroni and return to pot.
3. Stir in remaining ingredients until well combined.
4. Enjoy!

DELICIOUS WITH: Fresh tomato slices, diced green onions, or a sprinkle of sesame seeds. Serve with any of the following: Seven Greens Salad (pg. 66), King Kale Salad (pg. 67), Seedy Slaw (pg. 68), Three Sisters Salad (pg. 72), Rainbow Salad (pg. 73), Steamed Broccoli (pg. 90), Southern Style Collard Greens (pg.90), Peas and Carrots (pg.91), Red Pepper Corn (pg. 91).

ALTERNATE RECIPE: Try making Ch-Easy Mac with Ch-Easy Cashew Sauce, recipe page 61.

Ch-easy Sauce Made From Seeds

Cheese made from dairy is oftentimes one of the hardest things for people to let go of and probably the biggest culprit keeping many people from switching to a plant-based diet. Luckily there is an easy alternative to cheese that is just as satisfying without the downsides of dairy. Many nuts and seeds can be used to create ch-easy sauces, but my favorites are sesame seeds and cashews. The recipe above featuring tahini (ground, whole sesame seeds) is my oldest variation of Ch-easy Mac that I've been making for the last twenty years. More recently I've enjoyed making a ch-easy sauce from whole cashews (see the recipe on pg. 61). Both variations are easy to make and delicious. Use this recipe when making Ch-easy mac in just one pot. To make southern-style baked Macaroni and Ch-ease I prefer using the cashew ch-ease (pg.61). For this version, simply prepare the sauce according to instructions on pg. 61 and cook the pasta according to instructions. Then combine the sauce and pasta into a large glass baking dish and bake at 350°F for approximately 25 minutes or until the top starts to turn golden brown. This dish is a party-pleaser and favorite for the kids.

☀️CARIBBEAN RICE N' BEANS☀️

After eating numerous variations of rice and beans during my 3-month stay in Costa Rica, I decided my favorite version was hands-down the rice and beans a family on the Caribbean Coast taught me to make. This recipe is adapted from what I learned from this family, and is one of my favorite meals I have returned to again and again in the years since.

INGREDIENTS:

BEANS

- 1 lb black beans, soaked overnight
- 1 red bell pepper
- 1 yellow onion
- 7 garlic cloves
- 2 tsp. salt
- 1 tsp. cumin
- 1 tsp. coconut cream

RICE

- 3 cups Jasmine rice, dry
- 1 red bell pepper
- 1 yellow onion
- 7 garlic cloves
- 1 cup of corn
- 1 head of celery with leaves
- 1 can full-fat coconut milk or coconut cream (minus 1 tsp. for beans)
- 3 cups water

STEPS BEANS:

1. Soak beans overnight and rinse thoroughly.
2. Dice red bell pepper, onion, and garlic cloves into small pieces.
3. Sauté garlic, onion, and bell pepper in pan with 1 tsp. coconut cream until slightly tender.
4. Add beans and spices to pot and cover with plenty of water.
5. Boil beans on medium heat for 1–1.5 hours or until soft but not mushy.

STEPS RICE:

1. Dice onion, bell pepper, garlic, and celery into small pieces. Include celery leaves for best flavor.
2. Sauté diced veggies with 1 tbsp. of coconut cream in a saucepan on medium heat until tender.
3. Add dry rice to pan with corn, salt, and water.
4. Cover pan with tight fitting lid and continue to cook on low/medium heat for 15 minutes.
5. Remove pan from heat and leave covered for another 15 minutes.
6. Fluff rice with a fork and serve.

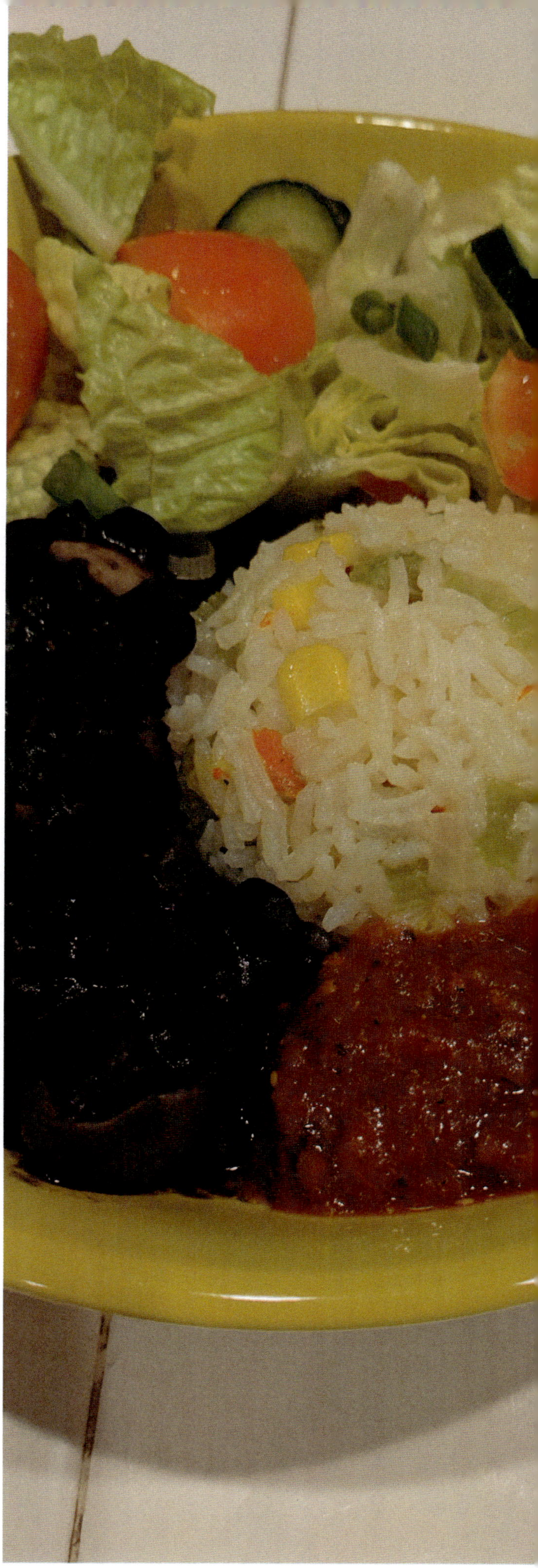

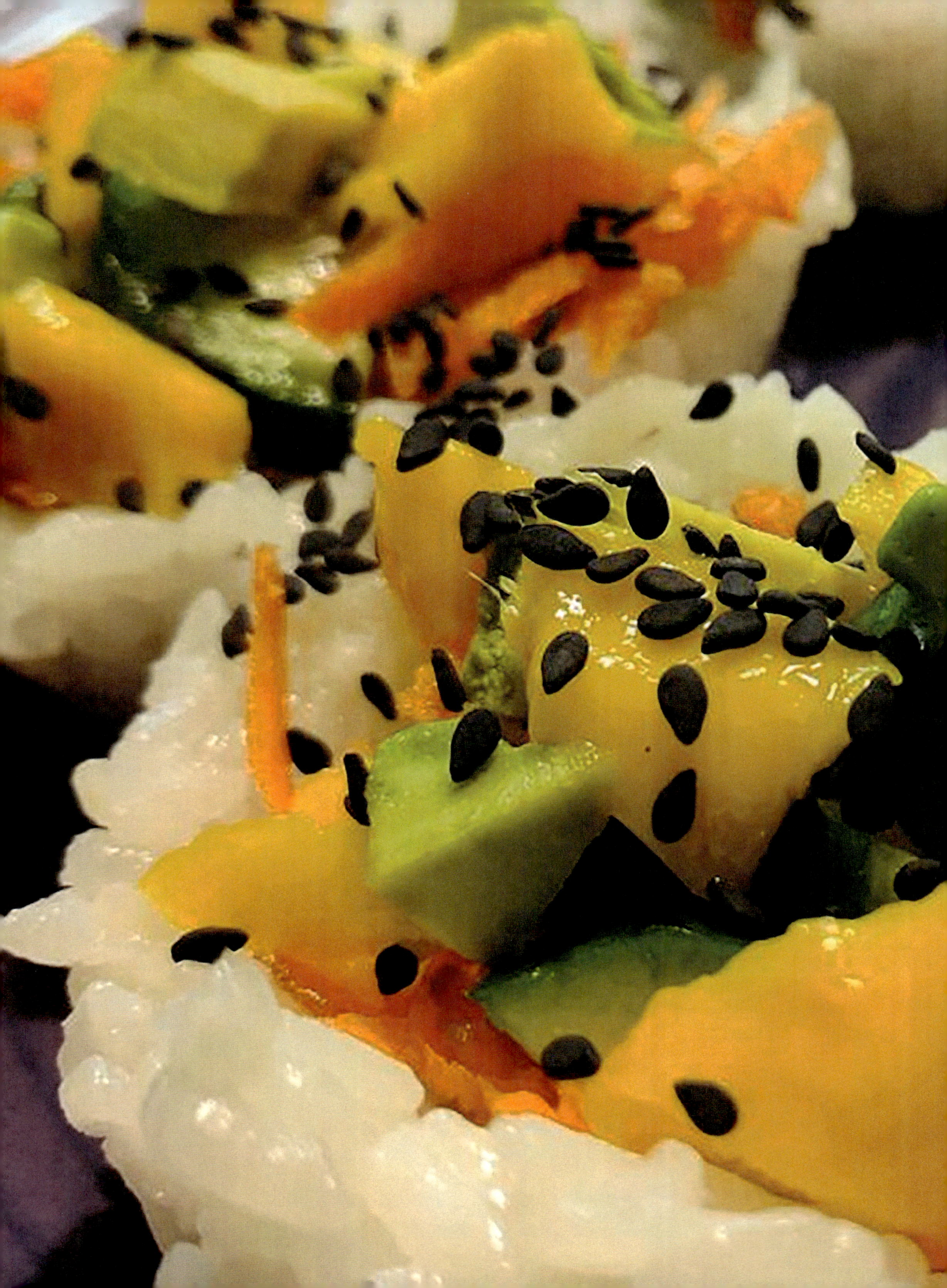

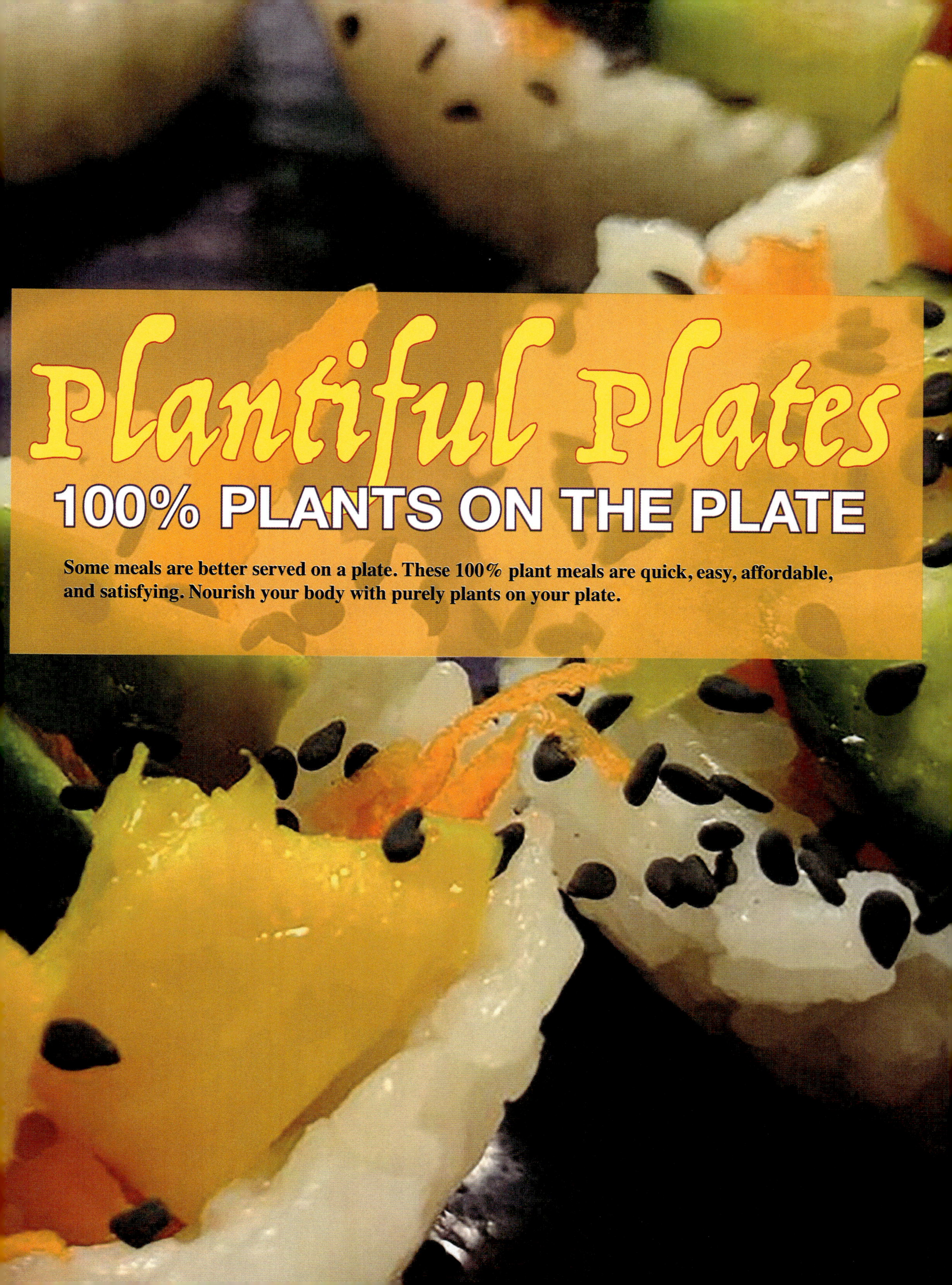

Plantiful Plates

100% PLANTS ON THE PLATE

Some meals are better served on a plate. These 100% plant meals are quick, easy, affordable, and satisfying. Nourish your body with purely plants on your plate.

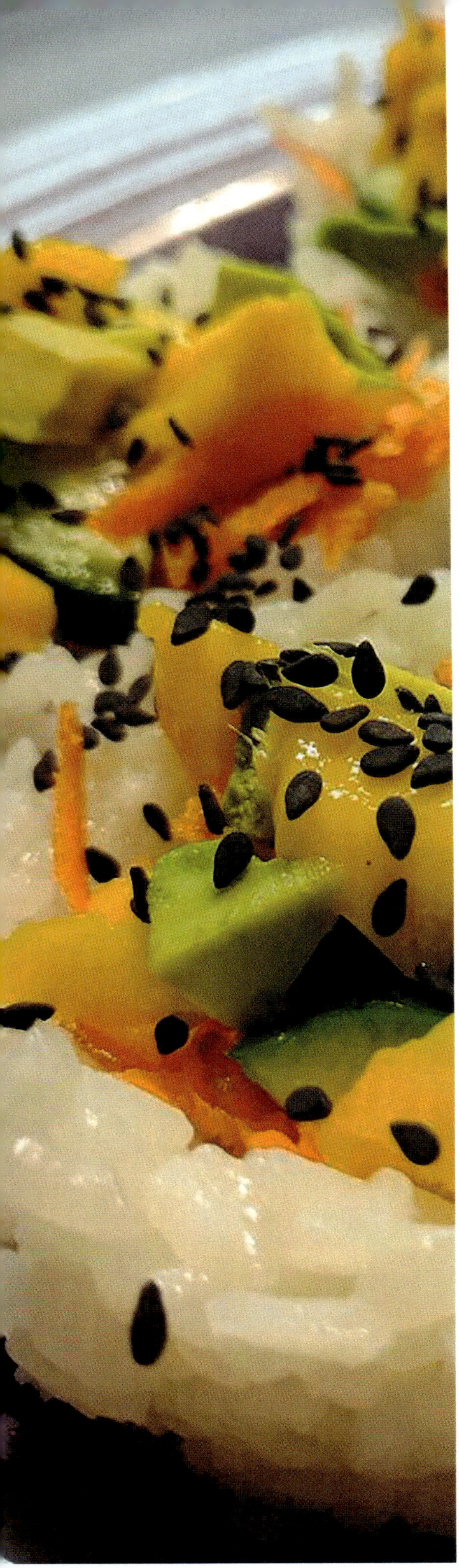

GARDEN SUSHI CUPS

Handheld sushi cups made from the garden's bounty.

INGREDIENTS:

- 12 lettuce leaves—choose large, soft, flexible leaves
- 1 avocado, diced
- 1 mango, diced
- 1 cucumber, cut in rounds and then quarters
- 1 carrot, medium, shredded
- 1 cup sushi rice, steamed
- 2 tbsp. black sesame seeds
- 1 tbsp. soy sauce (low-sodium is preferable)

STEPS:

1. Steam sushi rice according to directions on pg. 84.
2. Shred carrot. Dice mango, avocado, and cucumber.
3. Place fresh garden ingredients in small bowls for filling sushi cups.
4. Remove tough rib from lettuce leaves to end up with large flexible leaf squares.
5. Place large lettuce leaf into empty clean muffin tin and put a large spoonful of sushi rice on top.
6. Use clean fingers or gloved hands to press sushi rice into lettuce-lined cups.
7. Fill cups with carrots, cucumber, avocado, and mango.
8. Sprinkle black sesame seeds on top.
9. Gently remove the sushi cups from the mold using a spoon and put on a plate.
10. Optional: Add a dash of soy sauce to your sushi cup.

TRY IT ANOTHER WAY:

- **Substitute any of the plant fillings** for these other excellent options from the garden: radishes, green onions, edamame, purple cabbage, sprouts, and bell peppers.
- **Wrap It Up!** Try your Garden Sushi another way: roll it in the lettuce leaves to make wraps. Simply put one spoon of sushi rice in the middle of lettuce, add other sushi ingredients, and roll like a burrito. Use a toothpick to hold your wrap together if you're not eating it immediately. This is an attractive option for appetizers or a fresh lunch.
- **Traditional Seaweed Roll Style:** Try using traditional nori seaweed paper. Make a line of rice on the sushi paper, put your fruits and roots on, and roll it up. Slice your sushi roll into pieces or eat it as a roll burrito-style. You can also try cutting the sushi paper in half to make smaller sushi wraps. The advantage of nori seaweed wraps over lettuce is that they stick to the sushi rice and hold together very well. This is the best option for packing in a school lunch or picnic to go.

CUCUMBER AVOCADO TOAST

Bite into the simple and satisfying combination of creamy avocado and crunchy cucumber for breakfast. Or, enjoy this delicious and nutritious meal anytime of day.

YIELDS: 2 pieces

INGREDIENTS:

- 2 slices sprouted grain or whole wheat bread
- 1 cucumber, small
- 1/2 avocado, large
- optional: Everything But the Bagel sprinkle

STEPS:

1. Slice cucumber into thin rounds.
2. Cut avocado in half, remove pit, and slice into thin slices.
3. Warm bread in toaster or oven to desired toastiness.
4. Scoop avocado onto toast and spread evenly.
5. Top with fresh cucumber slices, a little salt and pepper, Everything But the Bagel sprinkle, or nutritional yeast.

DELICIOUS WITH: Fruit smoothie, fresh fruit, fruit salad.

Make Avocado Toast Your New Bread and Butter

"Bread and butter" has been such a staple food that in the 1700s, the three words were used to refer to a person's basic needs. In the 1800s, "bread and butter" became synonymous with a person's livelihood or income. Toasted bread with butter is such a classic breakfast menu item for Americans that most restaurants serve it as a given with breakfast and many restaurants serve some form of bread and butter as a free appetizer.

For people like me who were raised eating bread and butter, there is thankfully another equally satisfying alternative that is quite a bit healthier. You can avoid the pitfalls and health dangers of dairy by using avocado fruits for a spread instead.

Avocados are creamy and rich so make a good substitute for butter and cheese in many dishes. When it comes to avocado toast, there are many variations to try.

- Lay thick slices of avocado on toast and top with thick tomato slices, salt, and pepper.
- Smash avocado onto your toast and sprinkle with garlic powder and a dash of cayenne for heat.
- Try adding a dollop of salsa to smashed avocado before spreading on toast.
- Add shredded carrots and a sprinkle of salt and pepper on top of your smashed avocado toast.
- Thinly sliced tempeh or tempeh crumbles are delicious on top of avocado spread on toast.
- Top your avocado toast with a sprinkle of fresh herbs such as parsley, basil, or cilantro.
- Fresh arugula or diced green onions give avocado toast a nice kick.
- A sprinkle of crushed red pepper or finely minced garlic turns up the heat on your avocado toast.

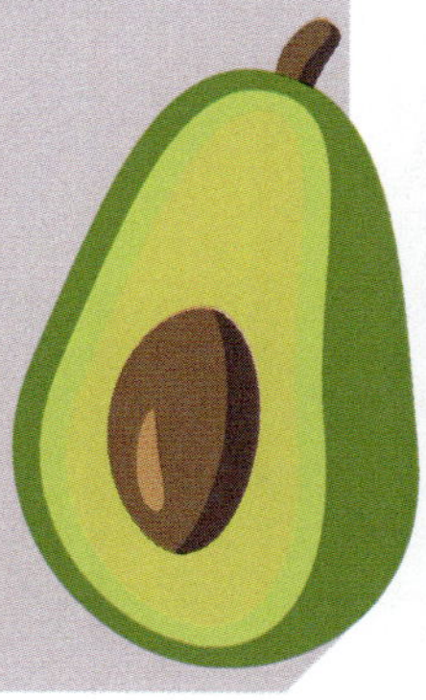

search IG #avocadotoast for more ideas

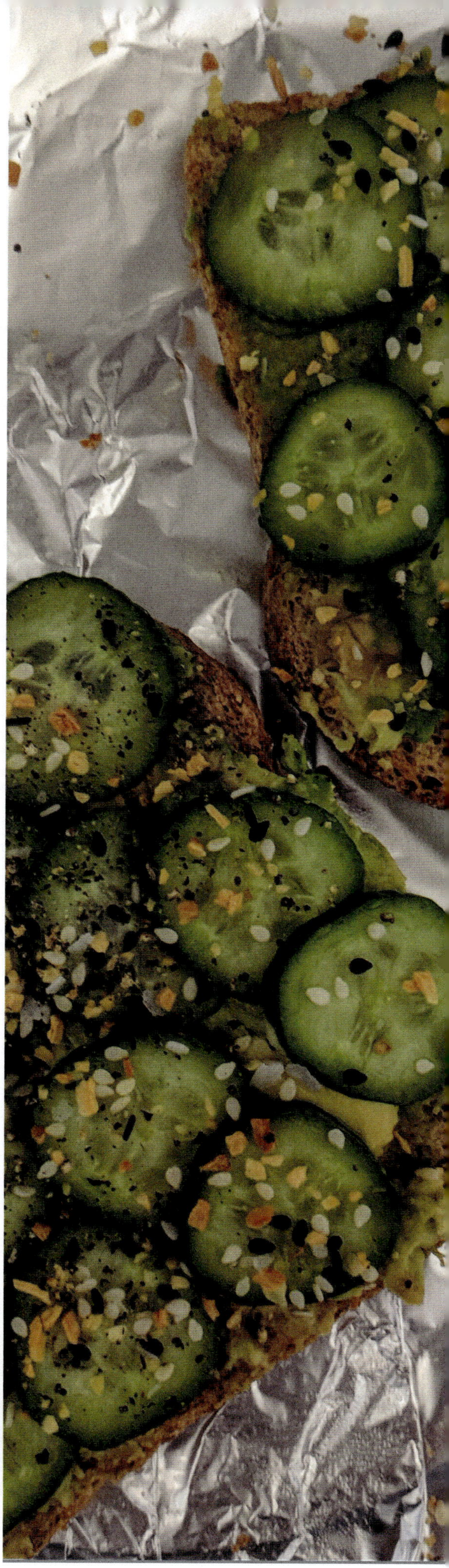

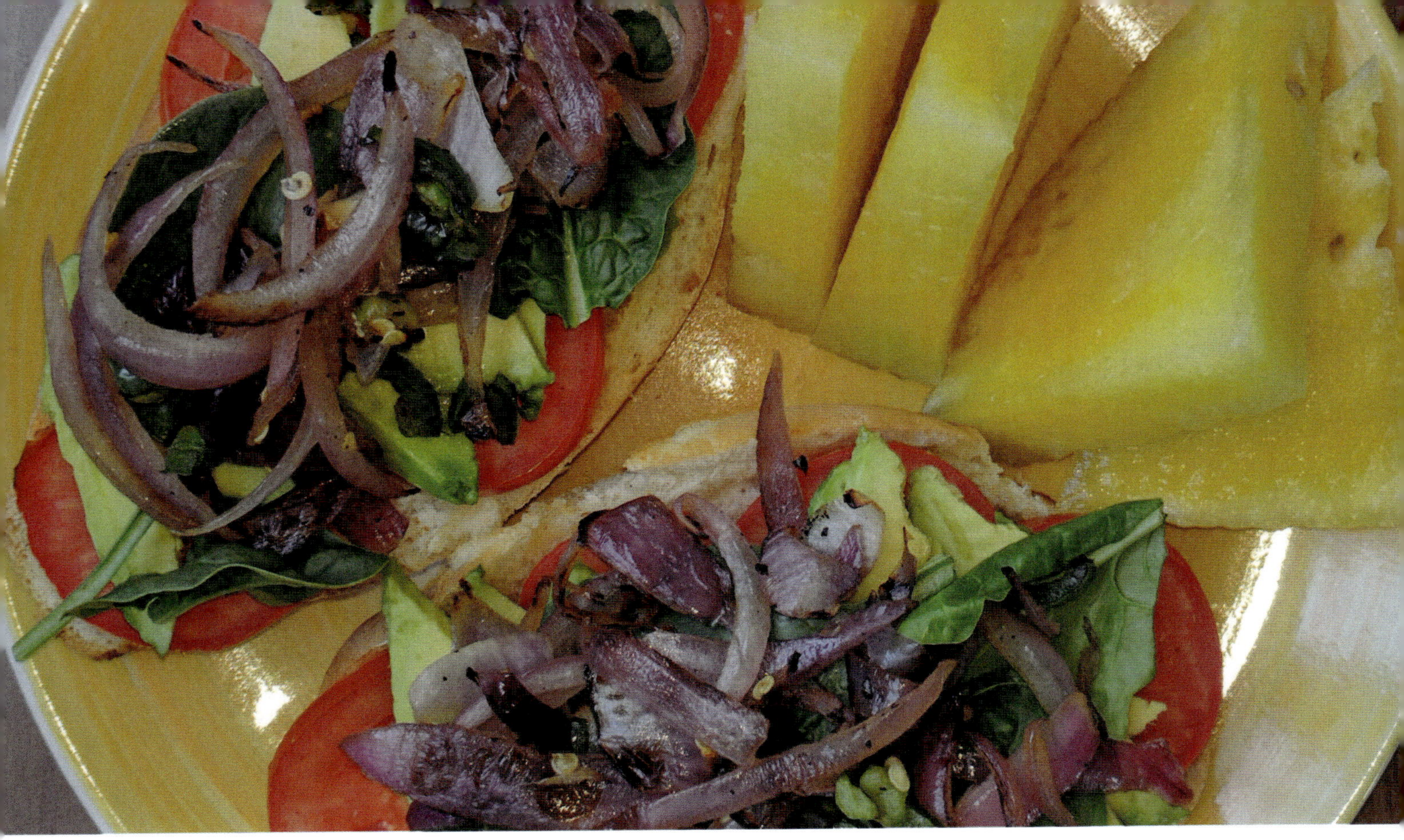

OPEN FACE PIZZA SANDWICH

An easy and fresh twist on pizza.

INGREDIENTS:

- fresh baked bread
- tomatoes
- red onion
- spinach
- avocado
- garlic salt
- pepper

Optional

- basil, fresh
- garlic, fresh, diced
- bell peppers
- mushrooms

STEPS:

1. Slice fresh bread.
   (Basic Bread pg. 86 or store bought bakery bread).
2. Sauté red onion in a teaspoon of soy sauce, water, or lime juice.
3. Slice tomato into thin rounds, dice avocado, and prepare spinach by washing and ripping into small pieces.
4. Top sliced bread with tomato slices, spinach, avocado, sautéed red onion, garlic salt, and pepper.
5. Add other optional ingredients to your liking.

DELICIOUS WITH: Simple salad, sliced pineapple, watermelon, or another seasonal fruit.

- Alternatively, top your pizza sandwich with marinara sauce or homemade pesto first before adding veggies.
- Open Face Pizza Sandwich is delectable with a sprinkle of olive tapenade.

The Key to a Perfect Pizza Is Plants

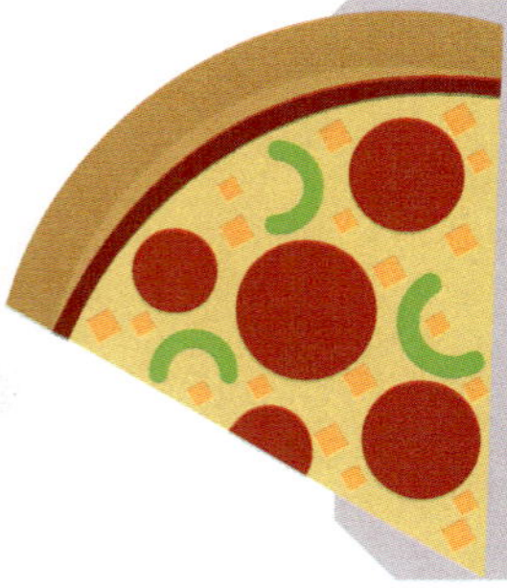

I grew up in Louisville, Kentucky, just across the Ohio River from the birthplace of Papa John Schantter, founder of the country's fourth largest pizza franchise. Papa John knew good pizza starts with the ingredients that go into it, thus the slogan, "better ingredients, better pizza," which helped grow his company into a billion-dollar enterprise. The most basic pizza ingredients have always been plants. The seeds of grasses make perfect pizza dough. Tomato fruits combine with onion and garlic roots to make the perfect sauce. What else goes on a pizza is up to your imagination. The classic red circles that top pizzas could very well be fresh tomatoes. Fresh basil, garlic, artichoke hearts, and sliced olives are just a few of the savory plant toppings that can make your pizza truly crave-worthy. And for those used to cheese-topped pizza, avocado is a nutritious and satisfying whole-plant substitute.

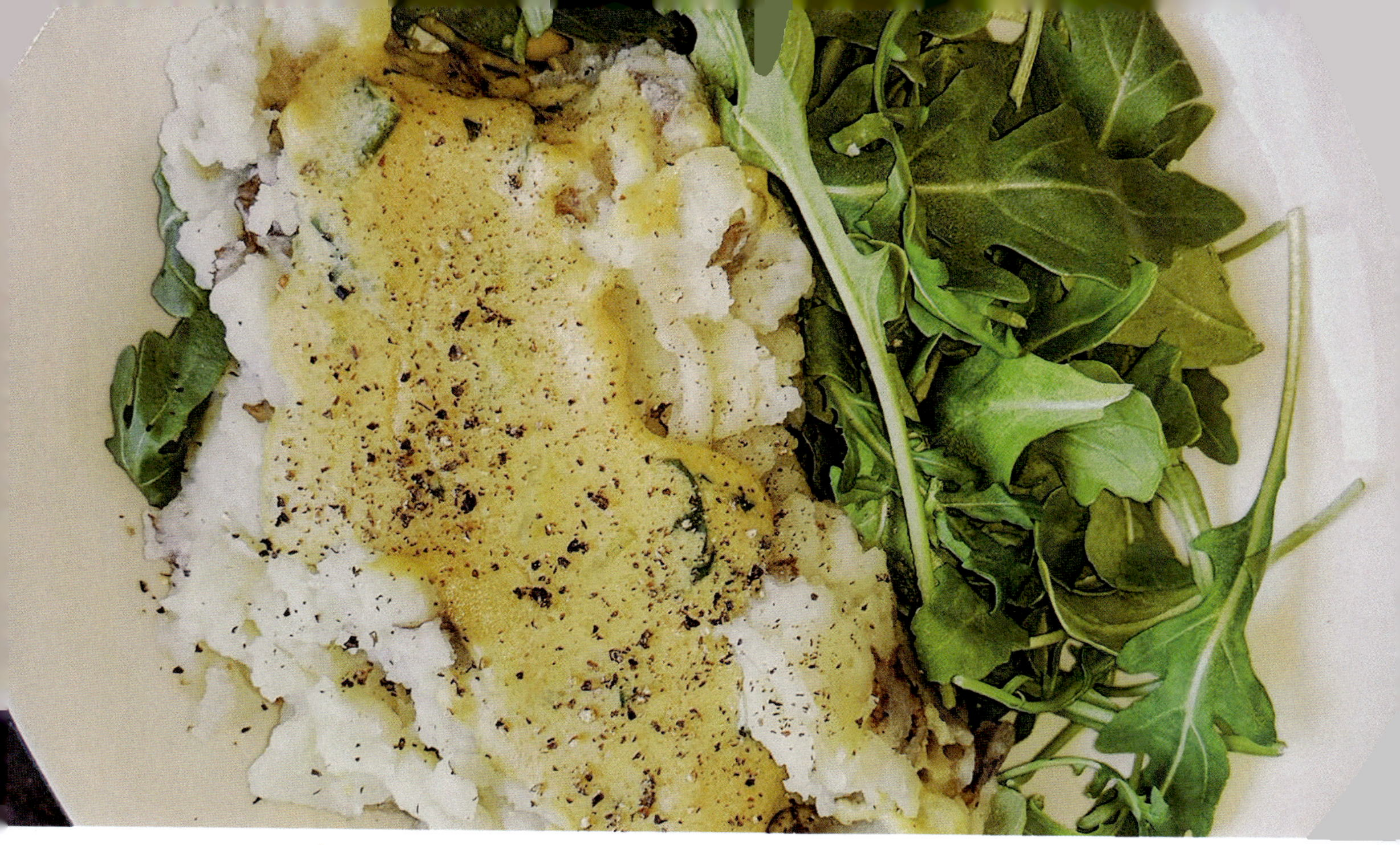

MASHED POTATOES & GRAVY

A dairy-free, 100% plants version of the classic American side dish.

INGREDIENTS:

MASHED POTATOES

- 6–7 baking potatoes, large or equivalent red or white potatoes
- 1.5 cups unsweetened almond milk.
- 1 tsp. sea salt
- generous twists of black pepper

GRAVY

See recipe for Garden Gravy, page 62 .

DELICIOUS WITH: Steamed Broccoli (pg. 90), Peas and Carrots (pg. 91), Southern-Style Collard Greens (pg. 90).

STEPS:

1. Wash potatoes and remove any blemishes. Leave skin on for nutrient value.
2. Boil potatoes until they are soft and begin to break when a fork is inserted.
3. Drain potatoes and return them to the pot.
4. Add unsweetened almond milk, salt, and pepper.
5. Blend with an electric mixer, smash with a potato masher, or stir and smash with a large fork or baking spoon. The tool you use to mash will determine the consistency of your mashed potatoes. These are good blended smooth with the electric beater and are equally as good mashed with a kitchen fork and enjoyed slightly chunky.

Make Mashed Potatoes a Regular Menu Item

Mashed potatoes seems as American as apple pie, but this simple and soul-satisfying dish originated in England, with the earliest known recipe appearing in 1747. It's quite possible they were around much earlier than that though, because this nutrient-rich root lends itself so well to being mashed and topped with a savory sauce. Mashed potatoes were my favorite Thanksgiving regular growing up, and as an adult I get to enjoy mashed potatoes much more often. In our house they can easily appear once a week, if not more. I recently attended a talk by nutrient expert and physician Dr. John McDougall who admitted that Mashed Potatoes were on the menu at least a few times a week for him and his wife. Once you try this oil-free, dairy-free recipe, you're sure to put this dish on repeat. It's hard to beat the affordability, simplicity, and satisfaction of simple Mashed Potatoes and Gravy.

For the nutrition contents of just one Russet potato, see page 23.

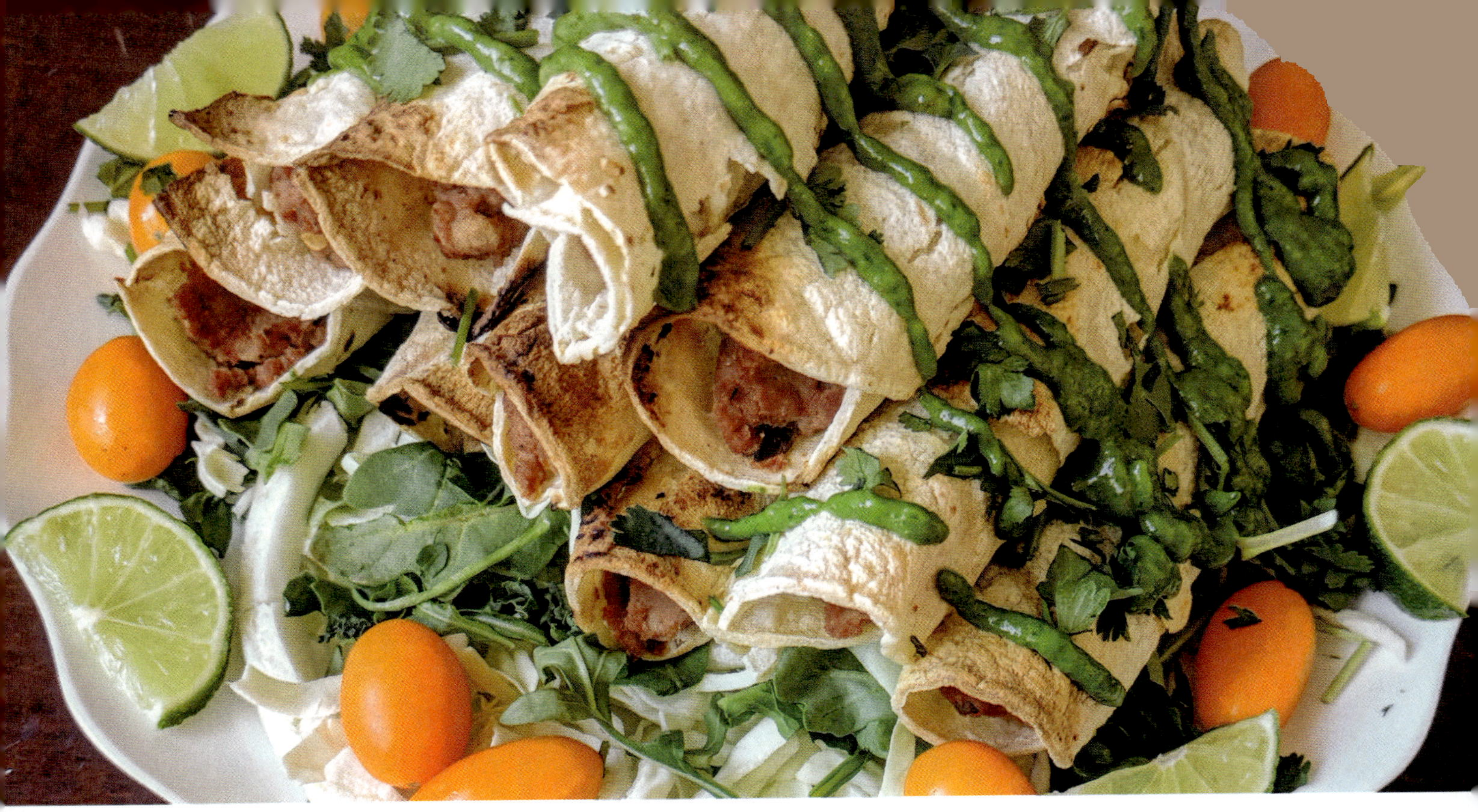

TAQUITOS

Hearty beans rolled in corn tortillas and topped with your favorite sauce or salsa.

YIELDS: 12 taquitos

BASIC TAQUITO INGREDIENTS:

- 12 corn tortillas, fresh
- 1 can refried beans (with no added oil)
- 1/4 cup salsa

Optional filling ingredients

- green chilies, diced
- onion, diced
- corn
- bell pepper, chopped
- spinach

BLACK BEAN & CAULIFLOWER TAQUITOS:

- 1 package of fresh corn tortillas
- 1 can black beans, drained
- 1 head of cauliflower, small/medium
- 1 onion, small
- 1 bunch of cilantro, small
- 2 tsp. onion salt
- 2 tsp. cumin
- 1 tsp. chipotle powder seasoning (or 1/4 tsp. cayenne)
- 1 tsp. black pepper

STEPS:

1. Warm corn tortillas on the stovetop, in steamer, or in microwave until soft and pliable.
2. For the most simple and basic taquito, place beans in mixing bowl with 1/4 cup salsa, stir until well combined, and use mixture as filling.
3. Scoop 1 heaping tablespoonful of refried bean and salsa mixture into each tortilla and spread lengthwise.
4. Optional: add chopped onion, diced green chilies, fresh spinach, corn, or diced bell pepper.
5. To make Black Bean & Cauliflower Taquitos blend all filling ingredients in a food processor.
6. Put a large spoonful of your desired filling into each tortilla and roll into a tube shape.
7. Place taquito seam-down on a baking sheet. Use a toothpick to hold shape if necessary.
8. Bake at 425°F for 15–20 minutes or until tortillas are slightly crisp and golden. Enjoy hot!

DELICIOUS WITH: Fresh salsa or hot sauce. Top with diced avocado or Garden Guacamole (pg. 63). Serve with a simple side salad or fresh tomato slices.

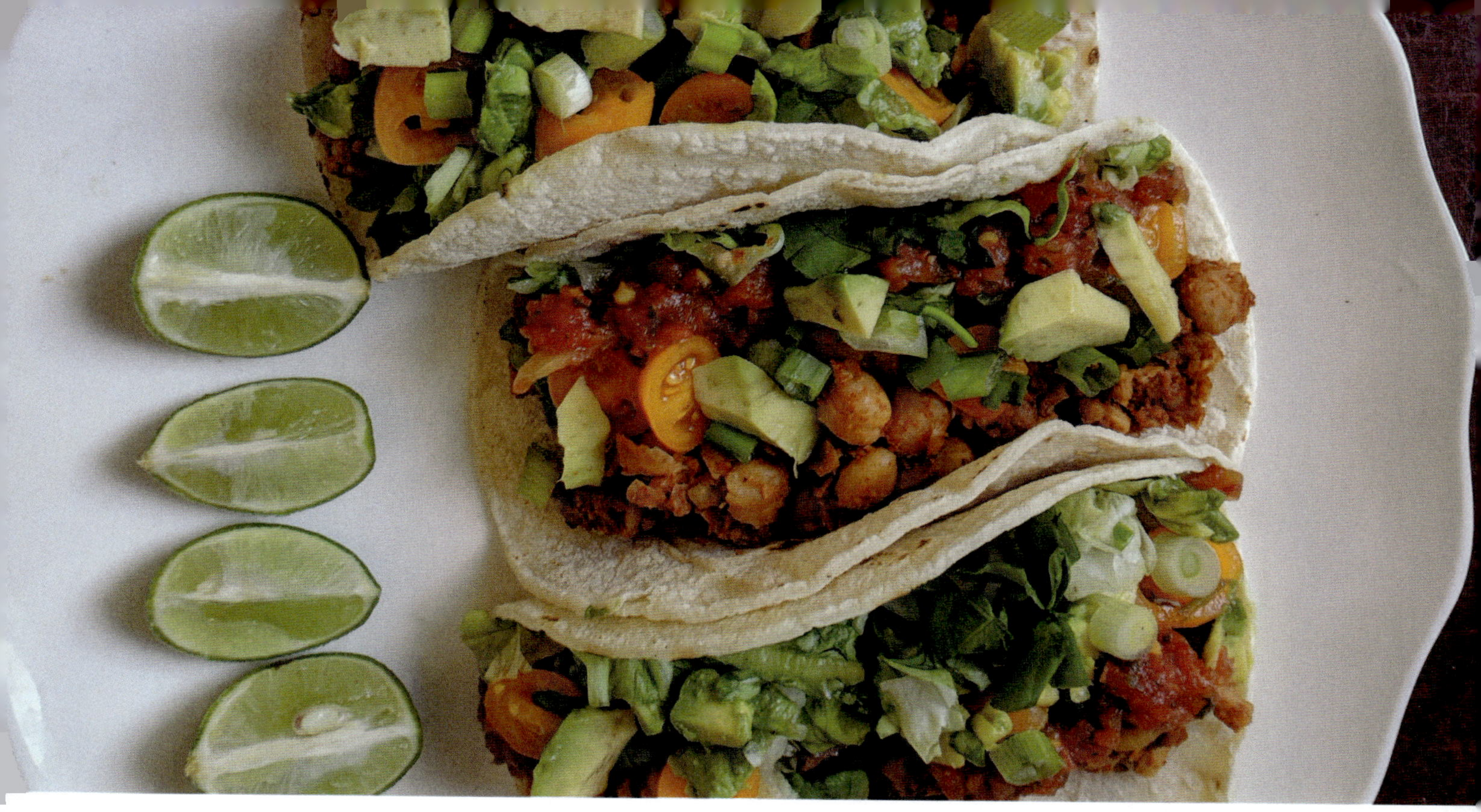

CHICKPEA TACOS

A nutritious taco stuffed with flavorful plants and a nice dose of spice to satisfy your taste buds.

YIELDS: 4 tacos

INGREDIENTS:

- 1 15 oz. can garbanzo beans
- 2 tbsp. taco seasoning (use recipe to the right, or your preferred taco seasoning mix.)
- 4 soft corn tortillas
- 1 cup of chopped lettuce, or any fresh greens
- 1/2 avocado
- handful of cherry tomatoes
- 2 green onions
- 1 lime
- 4 tbsp. salsa

STEPS:

1. Drain liquid from garbanzo beans, rinse, and pour contents into a large mixing bowl.
2. Add taco seasoning to garbanzos and mash with a fork until about half of garbanzos are smashed.
3. Warm corn tortillas on stovetop or in oven until soft.
4. Chop lettuce, dice avocado, and slice cherry tomatoes.
5. Scoop 1/4 of the garbanzo beans into each tortilla and add toppings as desired.
6. Top with salsa of your choice and add a squeeze of fresh lime.
7. Enjoy!

TACO SEASONING

YIELDS: 1/2 cup

- 1.5 tbsp. cumin
- 2 tbsp. paprika
- 2 tbsp. chili powder
- 1 tbsp. nutritional yeast
- 1 tsp. onion powder
- 1 tsp. garlic powder
- 1 tsp. salt
- 1 tsp. pepper
- 1 tsp. cornstarch

TIP: Store leftover taco seasoning in a small jar or ziploc bag and use with your next taco meal. This seasoning works with potatoes, tofu, or beans.

DELICIOUS WITH: Piña Colada Smoothie (pg. 142), Purely Pineapple (pg. 35), Strawberry Lemonade (pg. 143), orange slices.

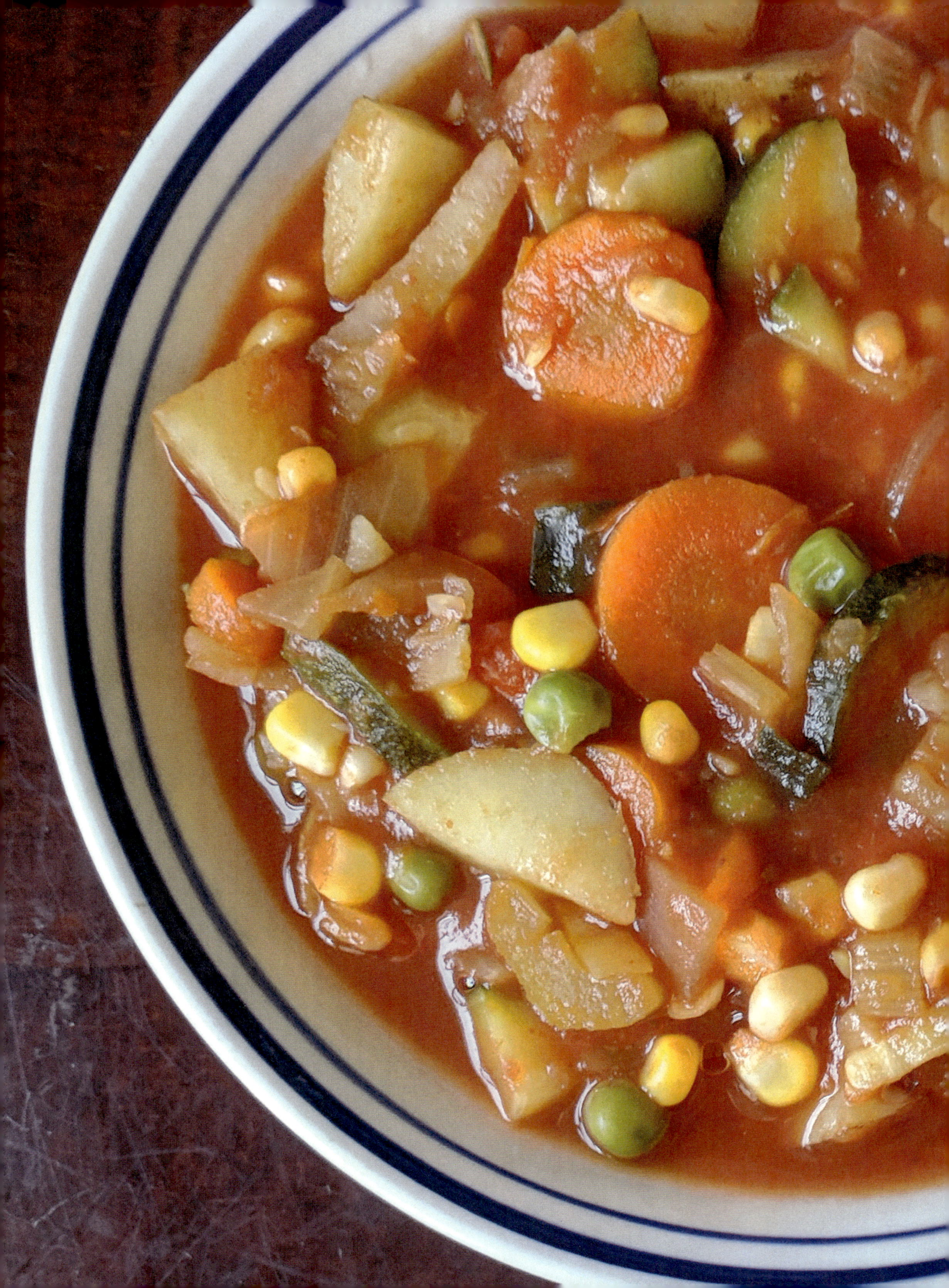

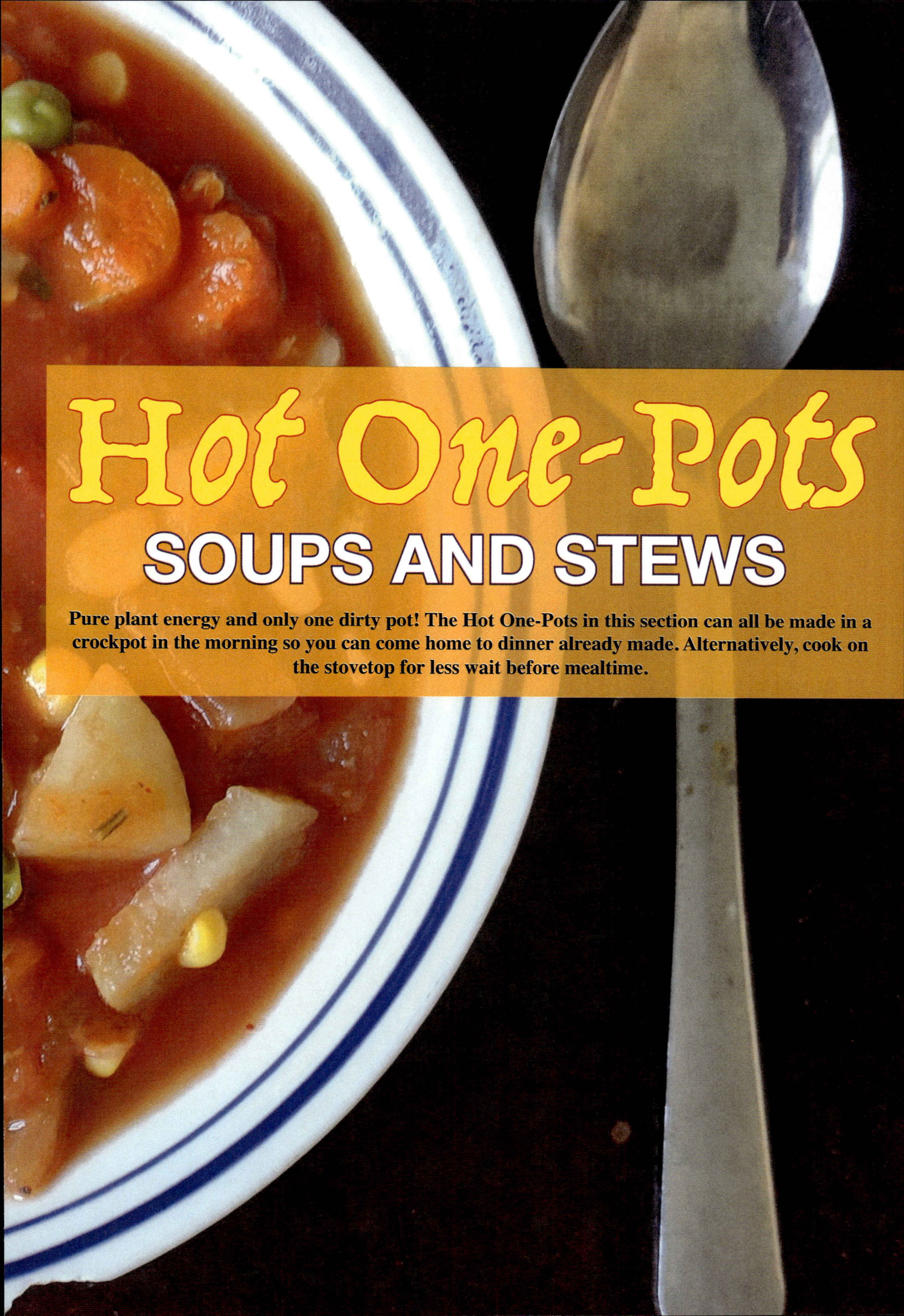

Hot One-Pots

SOUPS AND STEWS

Pure plant energy and only one dirty pot! The Hot One-Pots in this section can all be made in a crockpot in the morning so you can come home to dinner already made. Alternatively, cook on the stovetop for less wait before mealtime.

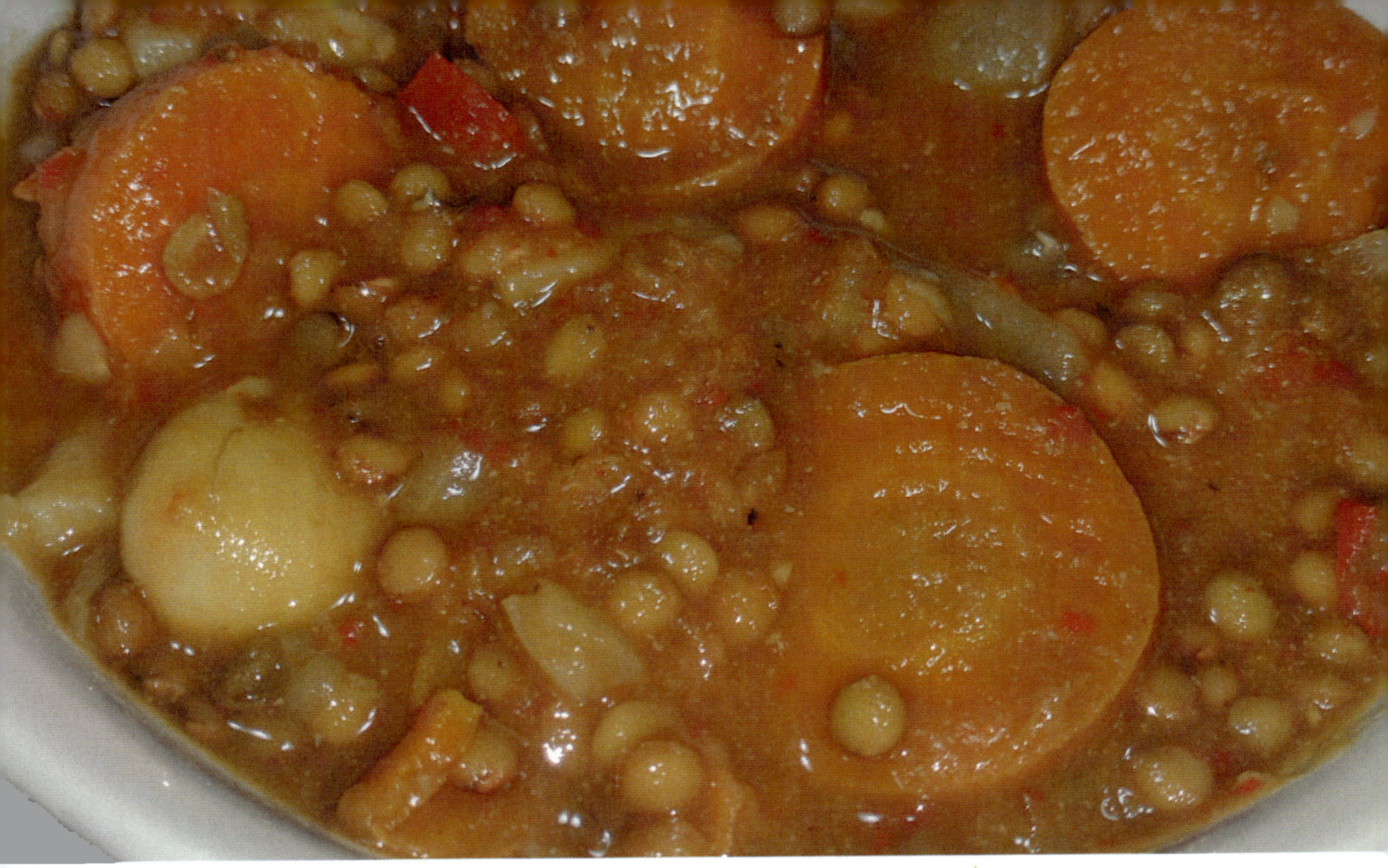

LENTIL LOVER SOUP

This hearty, nutritious and super easy soup is sure to please the entire family.

INGREDIENTS:

- 1 lb dried lentils (16 oz.)
- 1 jar marinara sauce (26 oz.)
  (I prefer organic, no salt added)
- 1 onion, large
- 3 cups potatoes
- 1 head of celery, small
- 3 carrots, large
- 16 garlic cloves
  (about 1 whole bulb of garlic, peeled)
- 1/2 cup nutritional yeast
- 2 tsp. salt
- 1 tsp. cumin
- 6 cups water
- generous twists of black pepper

STEPS:

1. Soak lentils for ~5 hours beforehand or overnight.
2. Rinse lentils.
3. Cut veggies. Dice onion and garlic into small pieces. Slice carrot into thin rounds. Chop potatoes into small chunks. Slice celery into small pieces.
4. Combine all ingredients in a crockpot.
5. Cook on high in the crockpot for 5–6 hours or until lentils are soft.
6. Share with your loved ones. Enjoy!

DELICIOUS WITH: Fresh avocado slices, a sprinkle of nutritional yeast, fresh crispy bread, or salad.

When I Lived on Lentil Soup

This recipe is my very first soup recipe I created. I adapted this from a recipe from my grandmother when I was in college. Grandma Steele sent me her hand typed recipes that were mostly vegetarian on 3 x 5 index cards. Her recipes helped teach me how to cook for myself and helped fuel my passion for creating nourishing dishes. I loved this recipe because it only cost me about $5 to make an entire pot of soup which I would eat for supper for a whole week. For much of my time in college I literally lived on lentils—very cheaply, but not suffering for any nutrition! Now it may cost slightly more to make this soup but not much—I estimate it costs $7–8 in ingredients from Trader Joe's to fill your crockpot with Lentil Lover Soup.

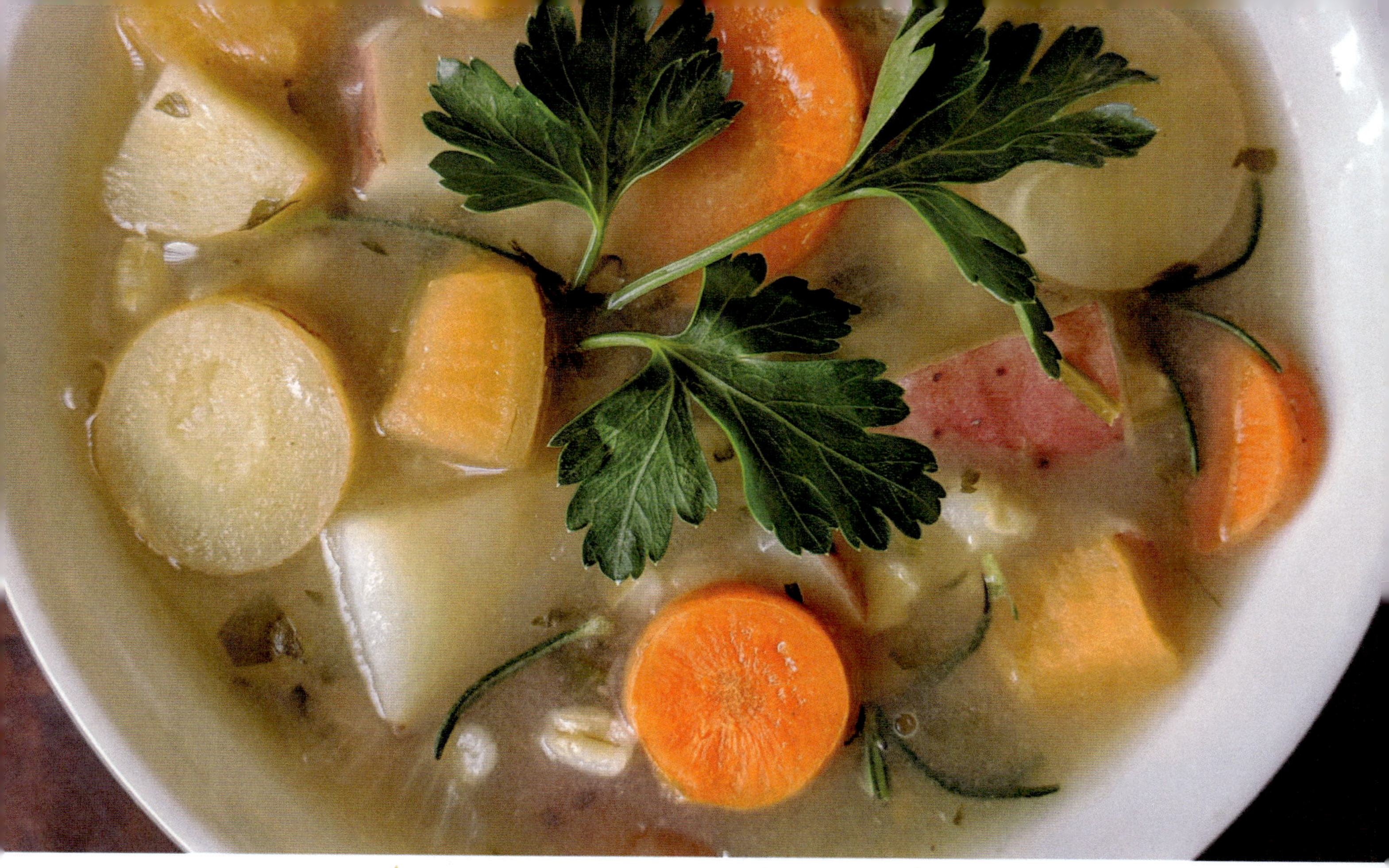

IRISH GARDEN STEW

A simple garden stew featuring traditional Irish roots and herbs.

INGREDIENTS:

- 3 potatoes
- 3 carrots
- 1 parsnip
- 2 rutabaga
- 1 onion, large (yellow or white)
- 5 garlic cloves
- 8 oz. barley
- 4 cups vegetable broth, low sodium
- 4 cups water
- 2 spring onions
- 1/2 bunch parsley
- 1 sprig rosemary
- 2 sage leaves
- 2 bay leaves
- 1.5 tbsp. corn starch
- 1 tbsp. fresh thyme leaves or 1 tsp. dry thyme
- 2 tsp. salt
- generous black pepper twists

STEPS:

1. Rinse all fresh veggies and herbs to remove dirt and debris.
2. Chop potatoes, rutabaga, carrots, and parsnips into small chunks.
3. Dice onions and garlic into small pieces.
4. Add chopped veggies to a large soup pot with fresh herbs, spices, vegetable broth and water.
5. Cook on medium/low heat for 50 minutes or until carrots, potatoes, rutabaga, and parsnips are soft and tender, but not mushy. Or cook in slow-cooker for 4–5 hours.

DELICIOUS WITH:

- Fresh parsley or chopped green onions on top.
- Serve with Green Soda Bread (pg.86).

A 100% Plants Version of Traditional Irish Stew

As my kids continue to grow so grows my desire to share our heritage—the foods, customs, and traditions of our grandparents, great-grandparents, great-great-grandparents, and onwards. I was raised as a Catholic who celebrated our Irish ancestors, and so when St. Patrick's day comes around, I like to celebrate with a traditional Irish meal. Irish Stew is a traditional food made with meat, potatoes, carrots, and spices. This recipe is a 100% plants version of the traditional recipe made with plants typical of an Irish garden.

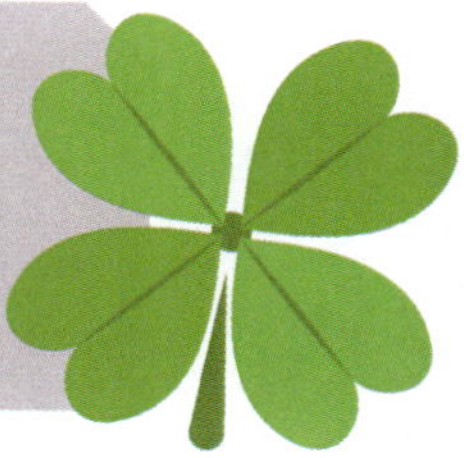

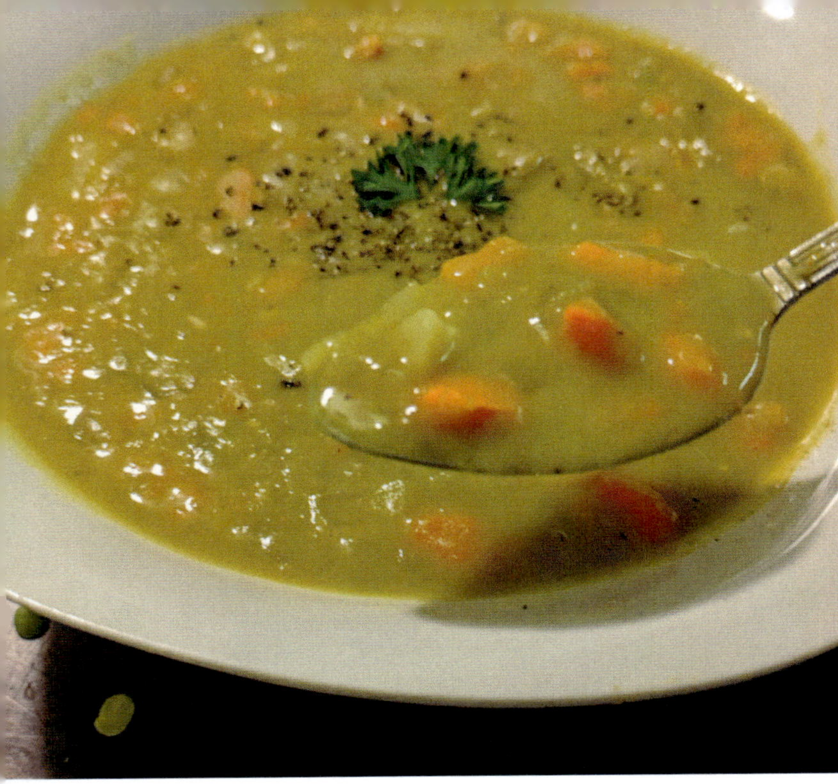

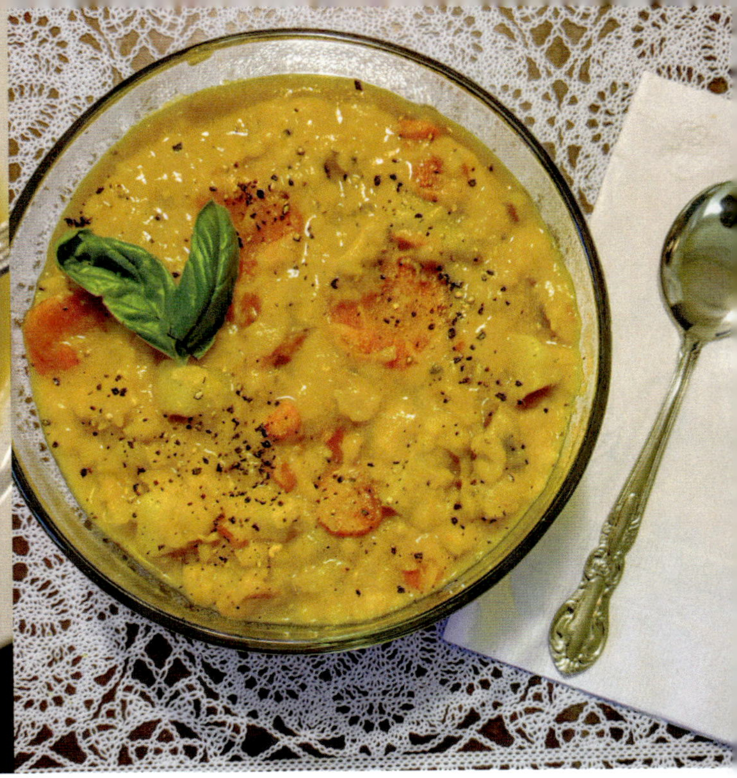

SPLIT PEA SOUP

Classic green pea soup to warm your heart and nourish your body.

INGREDIENTS:

- 1 lb green split peas (~2 cups), dried
- 5 potatoes, medium
- 1 yellow onion, large
- 4 carrots, medium
- 8 garlic cloves
- 1/2 cup nutritional yeast
- 2 tsp. salt
- 1 tsp. cumin
- 1/4 tsp. cayenne pepper
- fresh ground black pepper
- 8 cups water

STEPS:

1. Soak dry split peas overnight or for several hours to reduce cook time.[1]
2. Rinse split peas and strain excess liquid.
3. Chop onions and garlic into small pieces. Chop potatoes and carrots into small chunks.
4. Add all ingredients to crockpot or regular pot for the stovetop. Cover with water.
5. **Crockpot:** Cook on high for about 5 hours or until split peas begin to disintegrate.
   Stovetop: Bring pot to low boil and reduce heat. Cook on medium heat until peas are soft and dissolve into the soup's broth.
6. Blend half of the pots contents and return them to the pot for a slightly chunky soup. Or, blend the entire pot for a silky smooth split pea soup.

CURRIED YELLOW SPLIT PEA SOUP

Say yes to yellows with this yummy stew that will warm your heart on a cold day.

INGREDIENTS:

- 1 lb yellow split peas (~2 cups), dried
- 3 carrots
- 3–5 potatoes
- 1 can coconut cream (or full fat coconut milk)
- 1 tbsp. turmeric
- 1 tbsp. garlic powder
- 1 tsp. onion powder
- 1 tsp. salt
- fresh basil
- 6 cups water

STEPS:

1. Soak dried yellow split peas overnight or for 3–4 hours.[1]
2. Rinse split peas and add to pot or crockpot with water. (Same cooking options here as with the recipe for Split Pea Soup.)
3. Chop carrots and potatoes into small chunks and add them to the pot.
4. Add spices and coconut cream.
5. Cook on high in crockpot for about 5 hours or until yellow split peas begin to disintegrate into a thick broth for your stew.
6. Top with fresh chopped basil leaves.

1—Soaking split peas and other legumes isn't necessary, but does reduce cooking time. If you didn't presoak, simply rinse your legumes a few times before cooking or soak for a few minutes and then rinse.

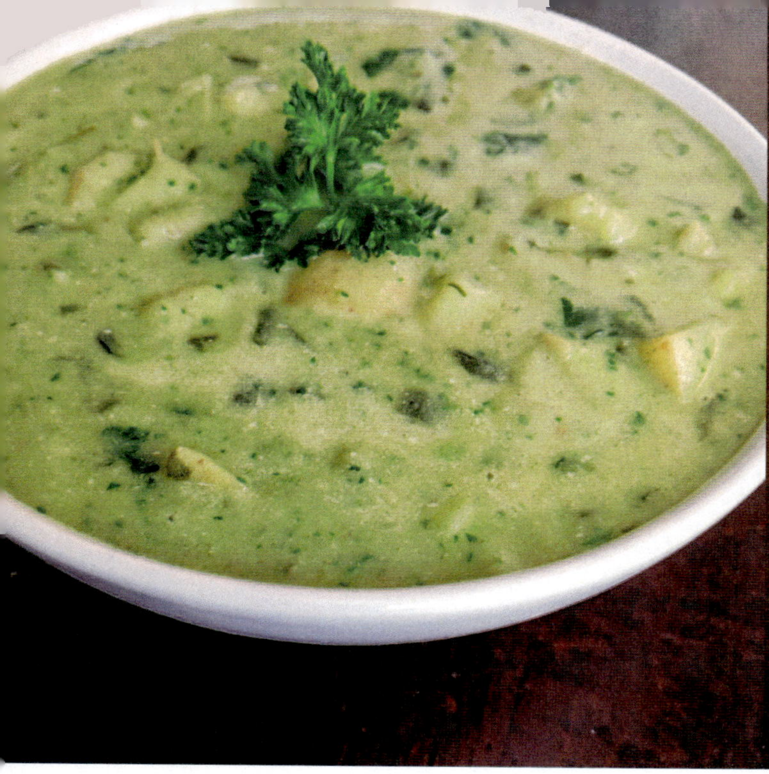

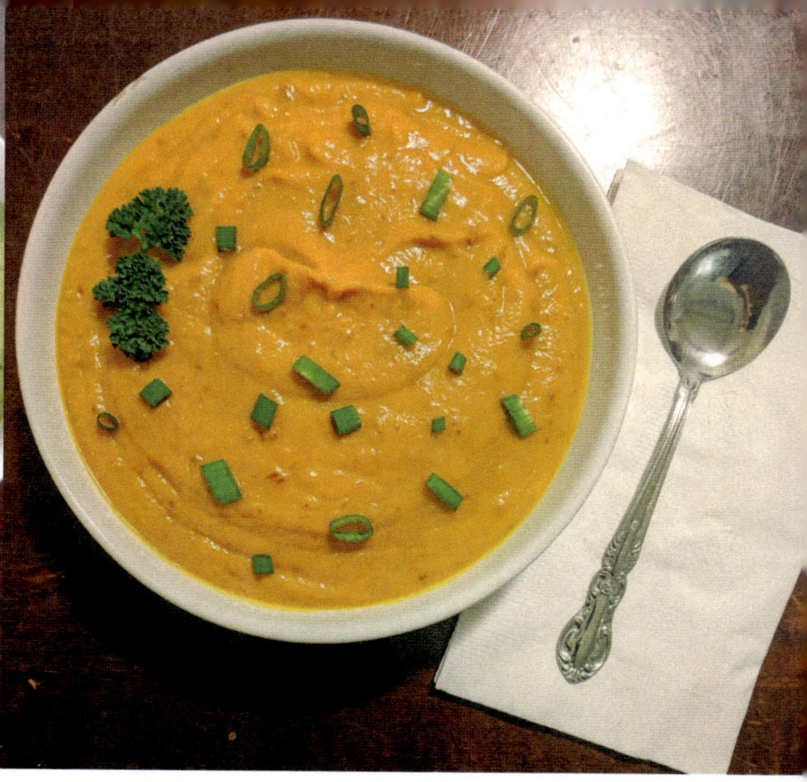

GREEN POTATO SOUP

Popeye's favorite potato soup packed with all the goodness of green.

INGREDIENTS:

- 3 lbs potatoes (~5 large potatoes)
- 1 yellow onion, large
- 2 cups spinach, packed
- 1 bunch of fresh parsley
- 1/2 cup nutritional yeast
- 1 can full-fat coconut milk
- 1 tbsp. garlic powder
- generous black pepper twists
- 7 green onions
- 5 garlic cloves
- 1 tbsp. salt
- 4 cups water

STEPS:

1. Wash fresh veggies to remove any debris.
2. Dice yellow onion and garlic into small pieces and add to large pot with a lid.
3. Add 1/3 cup coconut milk and simmer on medium heat until onion starts to release smell and become translucent.
4. Chop potato into small chunks and add to pot with water and spices.
5. Bring pot to low boil, cover, and allow to boil for about 10 minutes.
6. Chop spinach and parsley into small pieces and add to pot. (Reserve small amount of parsley for garnish).
7. When potatoes are tender remove pot from heat.
8. Blend half of the soup, or 3–4 cups, in a blender and add back to pot.

DELICIOUS WITH: Salad or Basic Bread (pg. 86). Top with fresh parsley and black pepper.

YAM CURRY SOUP

The warming spices of curry mix with sweet yams for a creamy yummy soup perfect for the cool season.

INGREDIENTS:

- 4–5 yams
- 1 can coconut milk
- 1 tbsp. ginger, or 1 tsp. powder
- 1 tbsp. garlic, minced, or 1 tsp. powder
- 2 tsp. turmeric, ground
- 1 tsp. sea salt
- 1/4 tsp. cayenne pepper
- optional: black pepper

STEPS:

1. Steam yams (with skins for full nutritional value!) in water that almost covers them and add other ingredients when nearly steamed.
2. Cool for a moment and pour contents of pot into blender[1] (this recipe fills up one blender pretty nicely).
3. Pour soup back into pot and stir.
4. Add water to achieve your desired consistency.
5. Serve topped with finely diced red onion, green onions, and/or ground black pepper.

DELICIOUS WITH: Salad, Basic Bread (pg. 86).

1—Make sure your blender can handle heat. If not, you will need to wait longer to cool soup before blending and you may want to reheat soup before serving. I've had a glass blender explode with hot soup the in past, so feel obliged to give this warning.

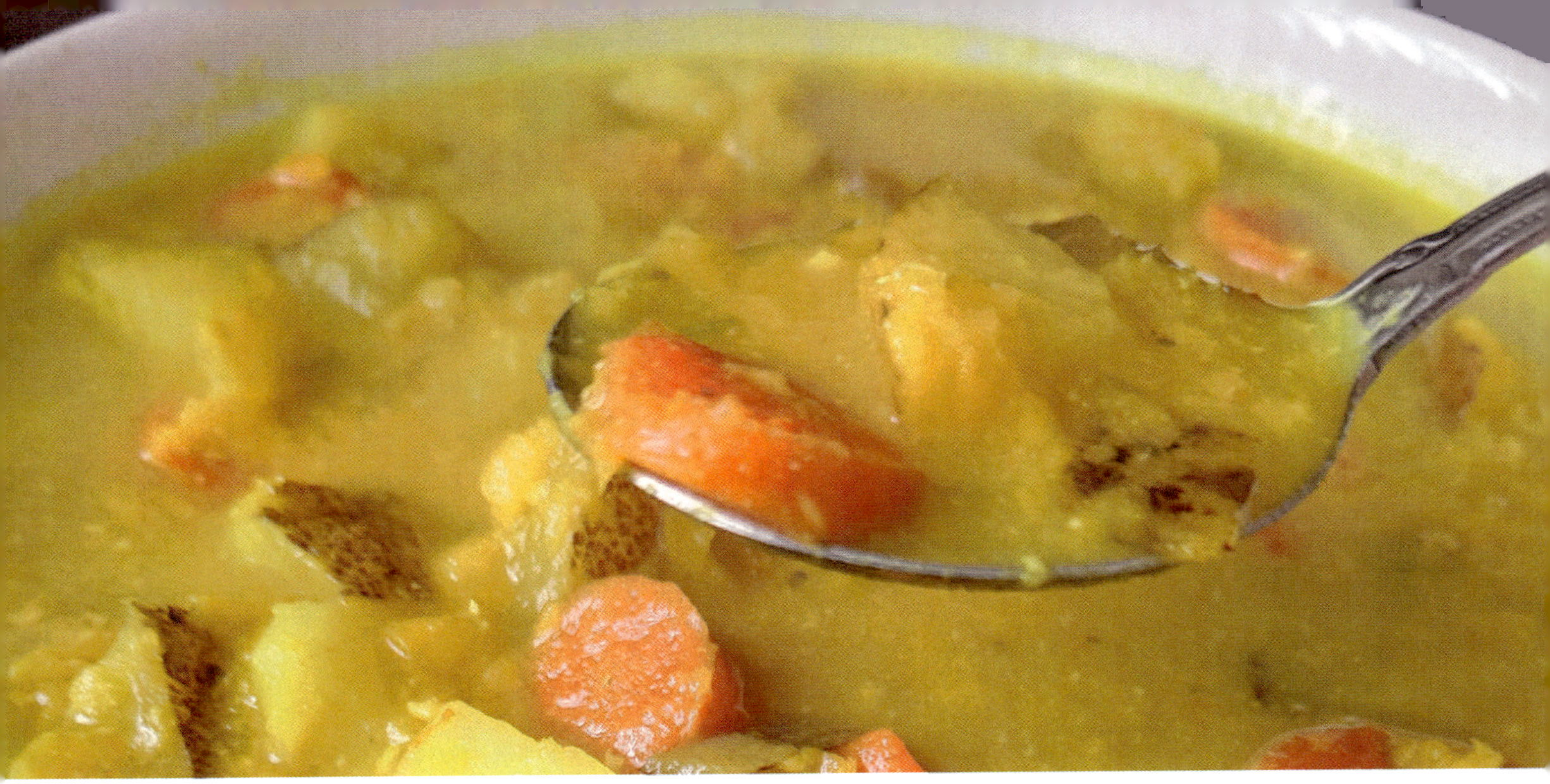

RED LENTIL COCONUT CURRY SOUP

A heart-warming and heart-healthy stew of roots in curry spices.

INGREDIENTS:

- 1 lb red lentils, dried
- 9 cups water
- 5 potatoes, medium
- 3–4 carrots
- 8 garlic cloves
- 1 can coconut cream
- 2 tbsp. turmeric
- 1 tbsp. fresh ginger (or extra 1 tsp. ginger powder)
- 2 tsp. sea salt
- 1 tsp. cumin
- 1 tsp. ginger powder
- 1/4 tsp. cayenne pepper
- 12 basil leaves
- generous black pepper twists

STEPS:

1. Soak red lentils in water beforehand for a few hours or more (if you can)[1] and then strain and rinse the soapy water off.
2. Put lentils into crockpot with fresh water and add chopped vegetables.
3. Add spices and coconut cream.
4. Cook on high, stirring occasionally, for 4–6 hours or until the red lentils are disintegrating into the soup's broth.
5. Garnish with fresh basil leaves.

DELICIOUS WITH: Salad or fresh bread.

1—Soaking lentils isn't necessary, but does reduce cooking time. If you didn't presoak, simply rinse lentils a few times before cooking. Or, soak for a few minutes and then rinse.

Make Coconut Your New Favorite Cream

Many traditional soup recipes call for heavy creamy to make a rich broth. But since science has shown that dairy is hazardous to your health, it is in your best interest to ditch the dairy. Consumption of dairy is linked to increased incidence of obesity, diabetes, cancer, and heart disease—the biggest killers of humans today. Luckily, coconut cream provides an equally rich and satisfying alternative to make soups creamy and satisfying. You will find I use coconut cream frequently in my soup recipes. Not only is coconut cream affordable and delicious, it's also full of nutrients and free of the downsides that come with dairy. Coconut cream made from whole coconut flesh can be a healthy component of a whole-foods, plant-based diet. The diet our bodies were biologically designed for has been shown to completely reverse obesity, type 2 diabetes, heart disease, and many types of cancer. Thank you coconut for being so good to us and for making our soups creamy and craveable.

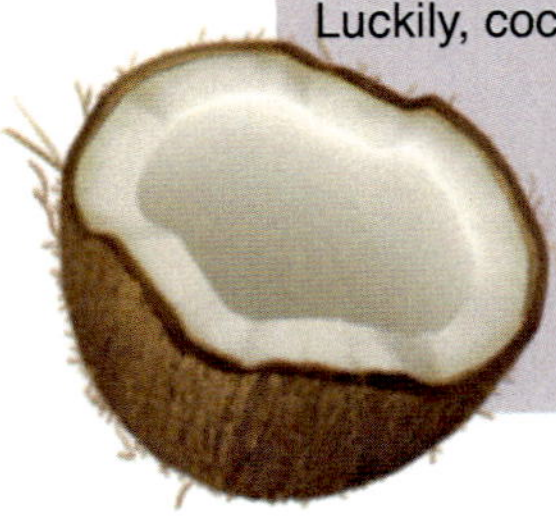

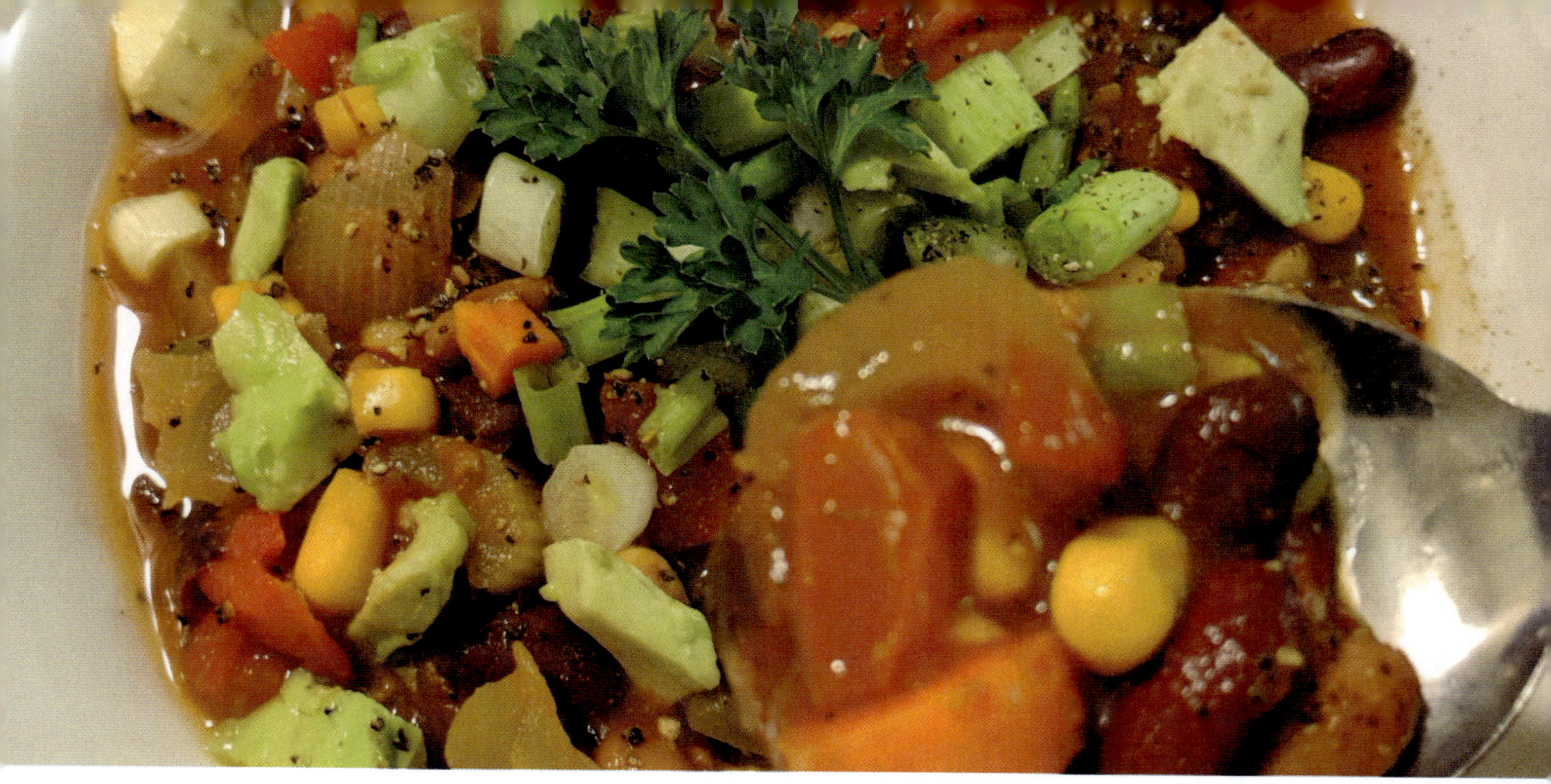

3 BEAN CHILI

A spicy chili that's purely plants and perfect for warming up a winter day.
PREP TIME: 30 minutes **BAKE TIME:** 5 hours in crockpot, 1 hr stovetop

INGREDIENTS:

- 1 can kidney beans
- 1 can pinto beans
- 1 can black beans
- 1 can diced tomatoes
- 4.6 oz. tomato paste
- 1 green bell pepper (1)
- 1 red bell pepper (1)
- 1 poblano pepper (1)
- 1 ramiro pepper (1)
- 1 jalapeño pepper (1)
- 1 onions, medium
- 2 carrots
- 2 celery stalks
- 1 cup corn
- 12 garlic cloves
- 1 tbsp. cumin
- 1 tbsp. garlic powder
- 1 tbsp. sea salt
- 5 cups water

GARNISH

- green onions
- fresh parsley
- cilantro
- lime wedge
- avocado slices

STEPS:

1. Chop all veggies and add them to crockpot.
2. Add water, beans, and spices to pot.
3. Cook on high in crockpot for 5 hours or 1 hour on the stovetop.
4. Serve chili by itself or over steamed rice or pasta.
5. Garnish with diced onion (red, green, or white), fresh parsley or cilantro, or diced avocado.

DELICIOUS WITH: Salad, cornbread, crackers, or Baked Potato (pg.89).

(1) Picking Peppers for Perfect Chili

Any type of peppers will work in this recipe. I prefer using whole fresh bell peppers and chili peppers. Most produce markets will have at least a few options of fresh, spicy peppers that add a nice flavor to chili, but if you don't have these on hand, you can substitute with chili powder and cayenne pepper. I would use 1 tbsp. of chili powder and 1/4 tsp. cayenne in place of the hot peppers. There's no substitute for fresh bell peppers, though which color they are doesn't matter too much.

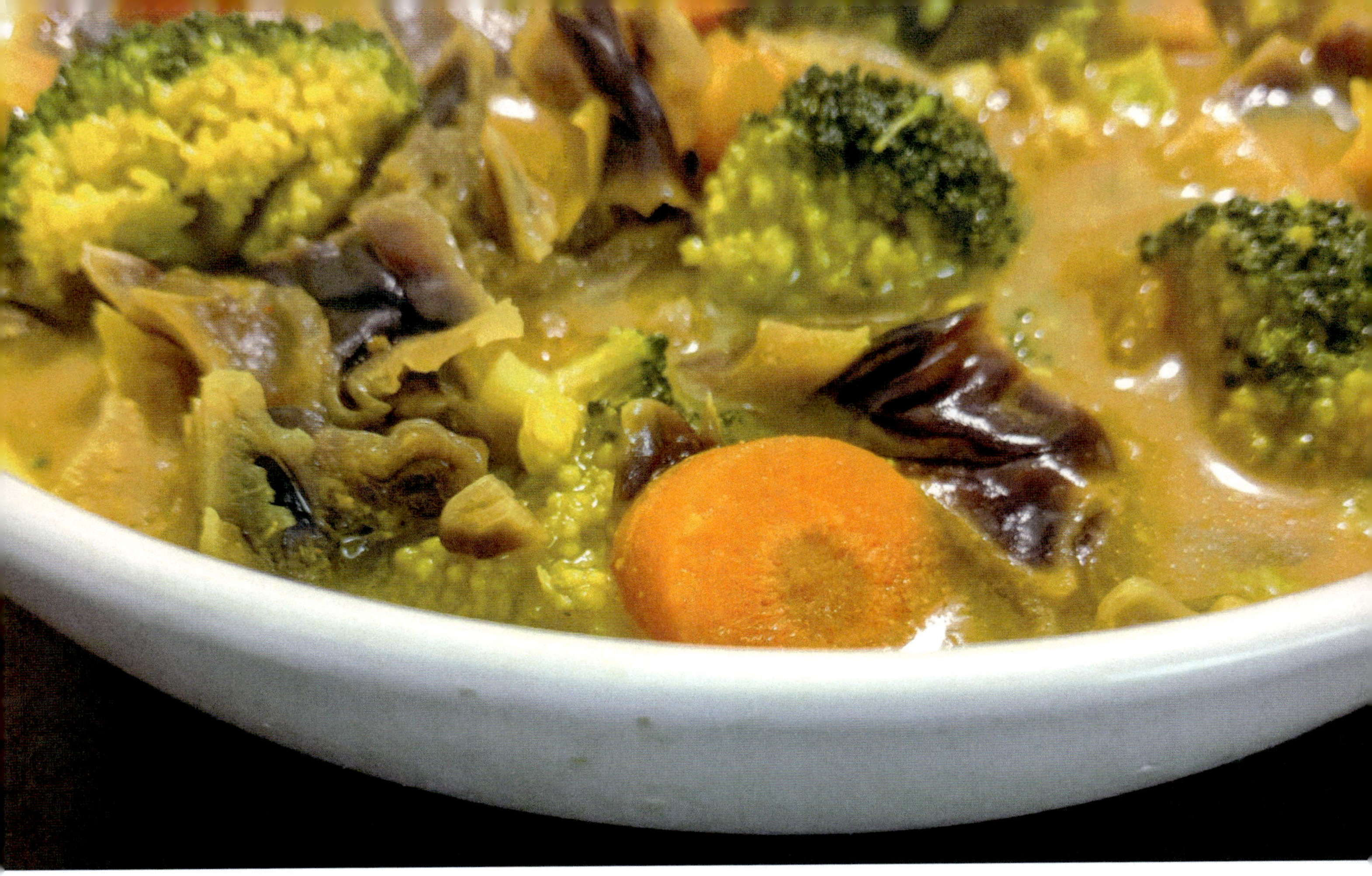

VEGETABLE CURRY SOUP

A warming pot of roots, shoots, flowers, and seeds that's comforting on a cold day.

INGREDIENTS:

- 1/4 cabbage, medium
- 2 carrots, large
- 1 onion, large, diced small
- 1 bell pepper
- 4 cups broccoli, chopped
- 12 garlic cloves
- 6 cups water
- 1 can coconut cream (or full-fat coconut milk)
- 2 tbsp. corn starch

SPICE:

- 2 tbsp. turmeric
- 1 tbsp. garlic*, fresh (or 1 tsp. garlic powder)
- 1 tbsp. onion powder
- 1 tbsp. ginger*, fresh (or 1/4 tsp. ginger powder)
- 2 tsp. salt
- 1 tsp. cayenne pepper
- 1/2 tsp. cinnamon
- 1/2 tsp. cumin
- 1/2 tsp. black pepper

* chopped small

STEPS:

1. Wash fresh veggies to remove any debris.
2. Slice carrots into thin rounds. Dice onions, bell pepper, and garlic into small pieces. Chop broccoli and cabbage into bite-sized chunks.
3. Add onion, pepper, and carrots to pot with a couple spoons of coconut cream and sauté on medium heat until they begin to release their aromas.
4. Add spices and remainder of ingredients to pot and bring to a low simmer.
5. Cover pot and allow soup to simmer on medium/low heat for 10–15 minutes or until veggies are tender, but not overdone.
6. Remove pot from heat before broccoli loses its vibrant green color.
7. Serve immediately. Share with loved ones. Enjoy!

TIP: Leftovers store in the fridge for 3–5 days, but this soup is best enjoyed right after cooking to preserve freshness and slight crunch of carrots, broccoli, and cabbage.

DELICIOUS WITH: Fresh basil leaves, fresh parsley, chopped chives, or roasted peanuts. This soup is delicious with most fresh vegetables. Consider adding eggplant, kale, collard greens, cauliflower, brussels sprouts, yellow squash, or winter squash.

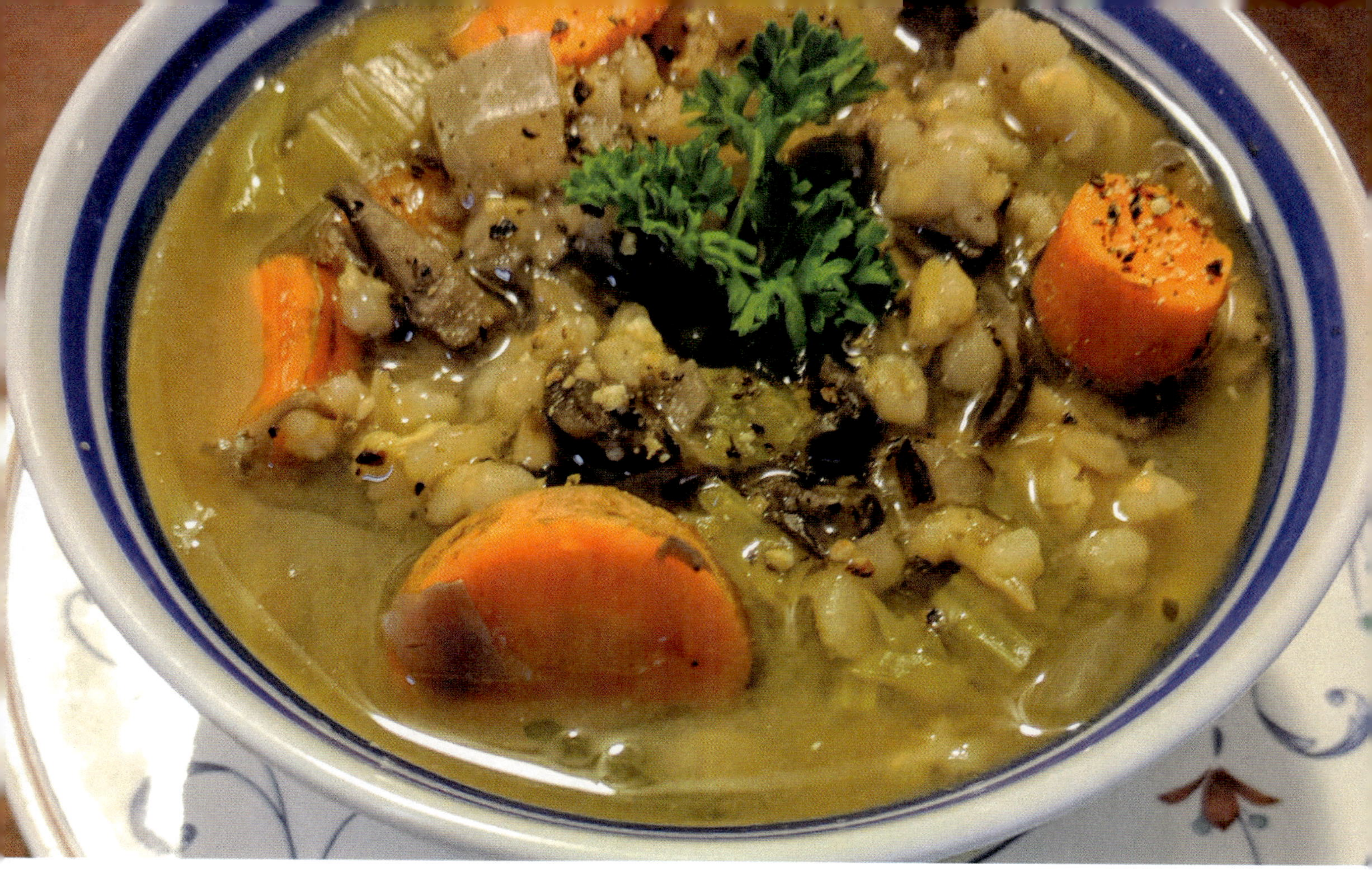

MUSHROOM BARLEY SOUP

A simple savory soup that makes an affordable, hearty and nutritious meal. I make this soup in a crockpot and let it slow cook all day so that it's stewed to perfection by supper time. Use any type of mushrooms, onions, and garlic you have on hand.

INGREDIENTS:

- 3 carrots
- 1 head of celery
- 2 cups portabella mushrooms
- 4 cups white mushrooms, sliced
- 1 cup dried barley
- 1 red onion
- 4 cups vegetable broth, low-sodium
- 7 cups water
- 1–2 tbsp. garlic powder (to taste)
- salt and black pepper sprinkles (to taste)
- nutritional yeast sprinkles (to taste)

STEPS:

1. Wash fresh veggies to remove any debris.
2. Chop mushrooms and onion into small pieces. Cut carrots into thin rounds and celery into thin pieces.
3. Add mushrooms and veggies to crockpot with veggie broth, barley, and spices.
4. Cook 3–4 hours on high or 5–6 hours on low.
5. Share with loved ones. Enjoy!

DELICIOUS WITH: Side salad, Baked Potato (pg. 89), Basic Bread (pg. 86).

Ayla's Favorite Soup: Mushroom Barley Soup

I was never a fan of mushrooms growing up, but thankfully I grew out of my dislike for them as an adult and my nine-year-old daughter already has a taste for mushrooms. Like her mom, Ayla loves meals starring mushrooms. This soup is her favorite soup I make. The inspiration came from Whole Foods Market. While it's extremely rare for me to purchase their hot soups because they are so costly ($5 for a small cup of soup), one day the Mushroom Barley Soup called out to me and Ayla and after one taste we wanted more. So, I ventured to create my own recipe at home. This super easy recipe resulted from my trial and error and it won't break the bank! While mushrooms can be pricey, I find good mushrooms frequently at the 99¢ Only store and you can definitely use the most affordable mushrooms at market for the 6 cups of mushrooms required for this recipe.

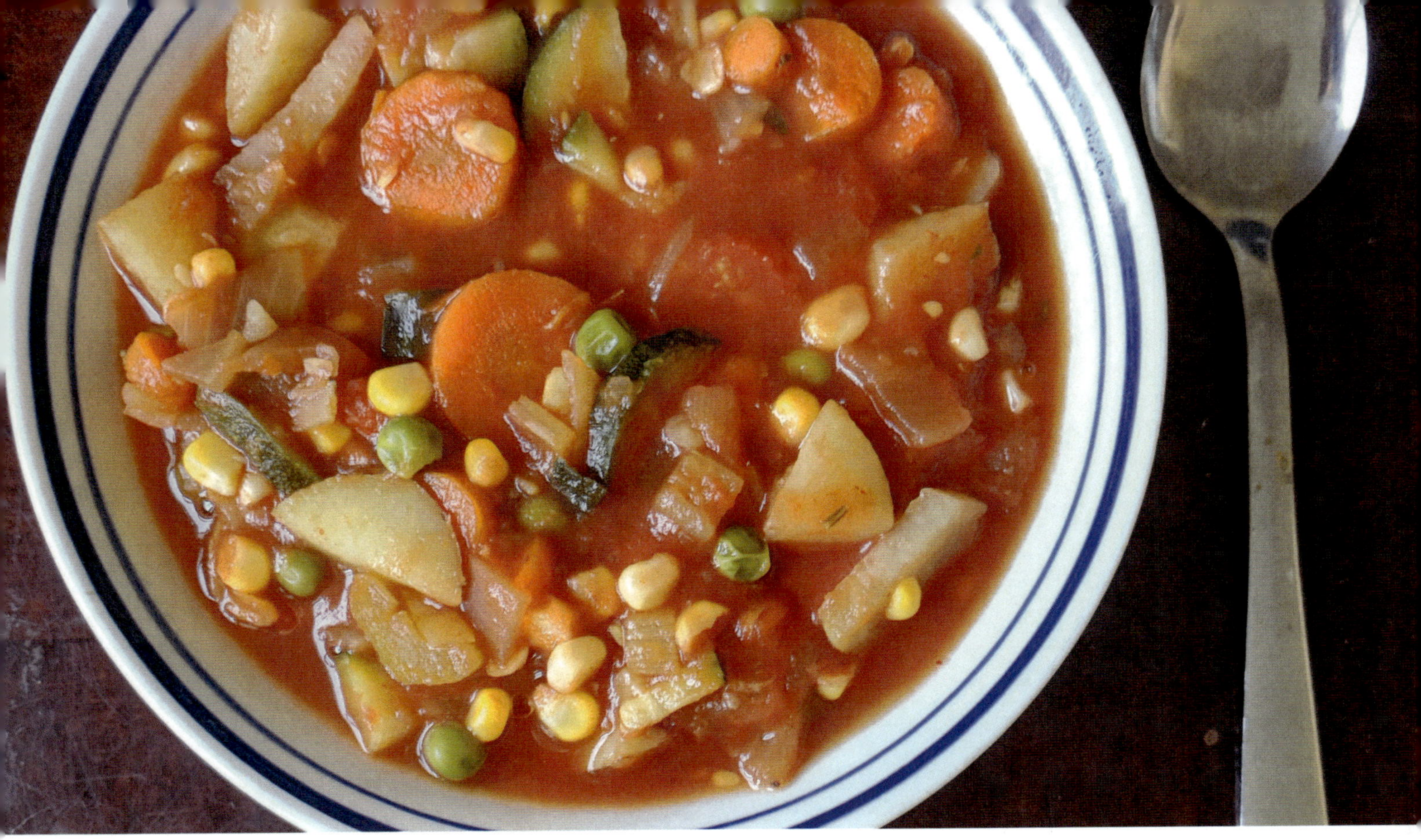

VEGETABLE SOUP

This classic American soup is warming, nourishing, and delightful to the palate.

INGREDIENTS:

- 1 can marinara sauce (low or no-sodium preferred) or 2 15 oz. cans tomato sauce.
- 5 potatoes, medium/large
- 4 carrots
- 2 zucchini
- 2 corn ears or 1 cup frozen corn
- 2 celery stalks
- 1 onion, large
- 1 cup green peas, fresh or frozen
- 4 garlic cloves (or 1 tbsp. garlic powder)
- 1 tbsp. herbs, fresh (basil, rosemary, sage, thyme, oregano) or use 1 tbsp. Italian herb seasoning
- 2 tsp. salt
- 4 cups water

DELICIOUS WITH: Basic Bread (pg. 86), Green Soda Bread (pg. 86), Cornmeal Almond Milk Biscuits (pg. 87), side salad. Try topped with diced avocado. If it sounds good to you, add a can of beans or a chopped bell pepper.

STEPS:

1. Wash fresh veggies and herbs and remove any bad spots.
2. Chop carrots into thin rounds, chop potatoes into small bite-sized chunks, dice celery into thin pieces, chop onion, garlic, and zucchini into small pieces.
3. Cut fresh herbs into small pieces.
4. Put all ingredients into a crockpot or a large pot with a lid.
5. HEAT—**Stovetop:** Simmer soup on medium heat until all veggies are tender. **Crockpot:** Cook on high for 4–5 hours until all veggies are tender.
6. Stir, serve, and enjoy!

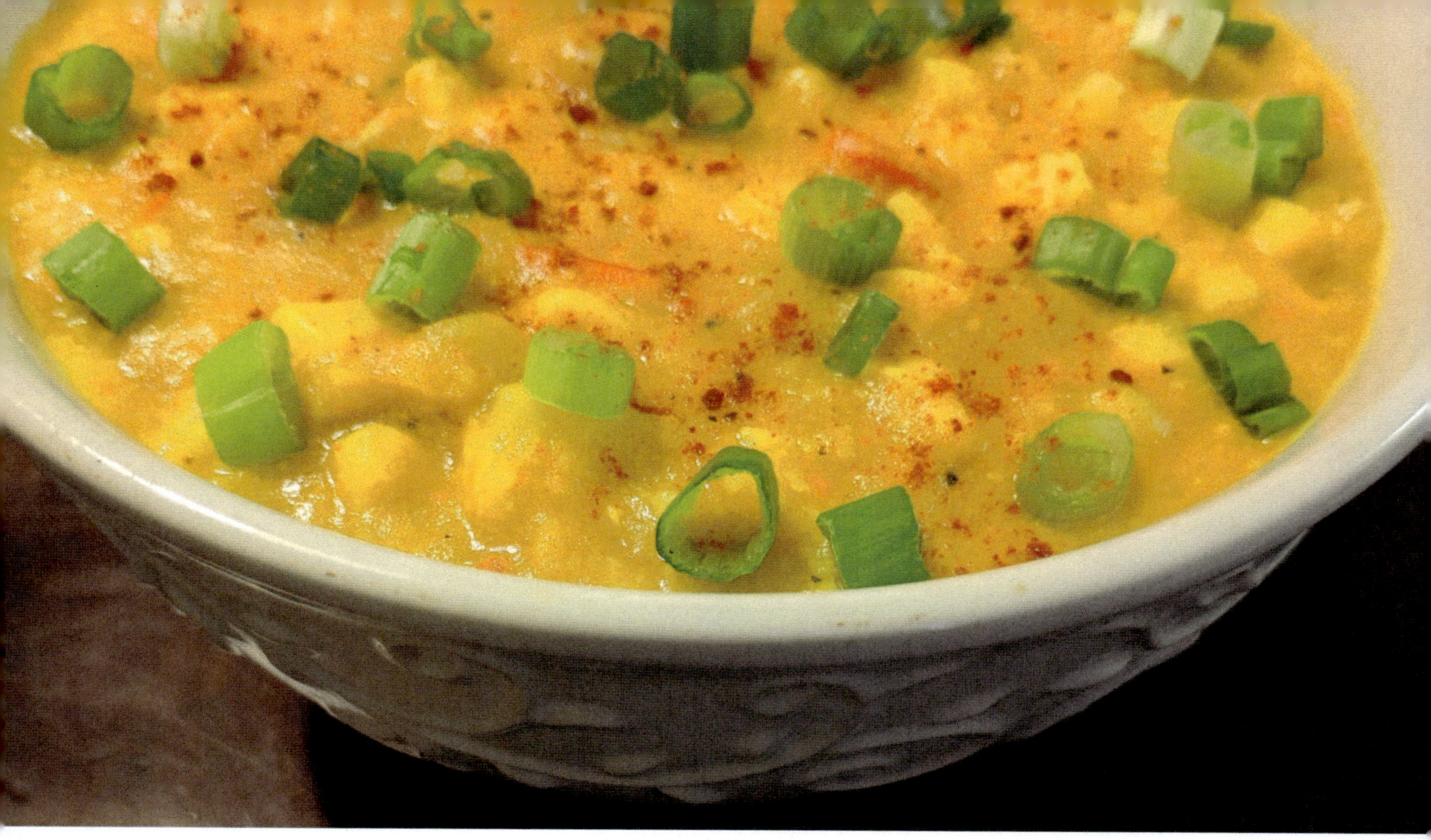

RED PEPPER N' CORN CHOWDER

A creamy golden corn chowder with a touch of spice that's particularly satisfying.

INGREDIENTS:

- 6 cups corn
- 5 potatoes, medium
- 1 can coconut milk
- 1 yellow onion, medium
- 3 carrots, small
- 1 red bell pepper
- 7 garlic cloves
- 1/3 cup of nutritional yeast
- 1 tbsp. onion powder
- 2 tsp. chipotle seasoning*
- 2 tsp. of salt
- 1 tsp. turmeric
- generous twists of black pepper
- 6–8 cups water depending on desired thickness

*Note: The chipotle powder seasoning gives it a slight kick, but if you don't have chipotle you can use cayenne pepper instead. I'd substitute 1/2 tsp. cayenne pepper for equivalent heat.

DELICIOUS WITH: Fresh green onions, fresh ground black pepper, cayenne pepper.

STEPS:

1. Chop onion, garlic, and red bell pepper into small pieces.
2. Sauté diced onion, garlic, and pepper on medium heat in a soup pot with a small amount of water or coconut milk to prevent sticking to the pot.
3. Chop carrot and potatoes into small pieces and add them to the pot after the onions begin to turn translucent and release their aroma.
4. Add corn, coconut milk, water, and spices to the pot.
5. Cook on medium heat until potatoes and carrots are soft.
6. Blend half of the soup in a blender and then mix it back into pot so that there's some chunks remaining.
7. Enjoy!

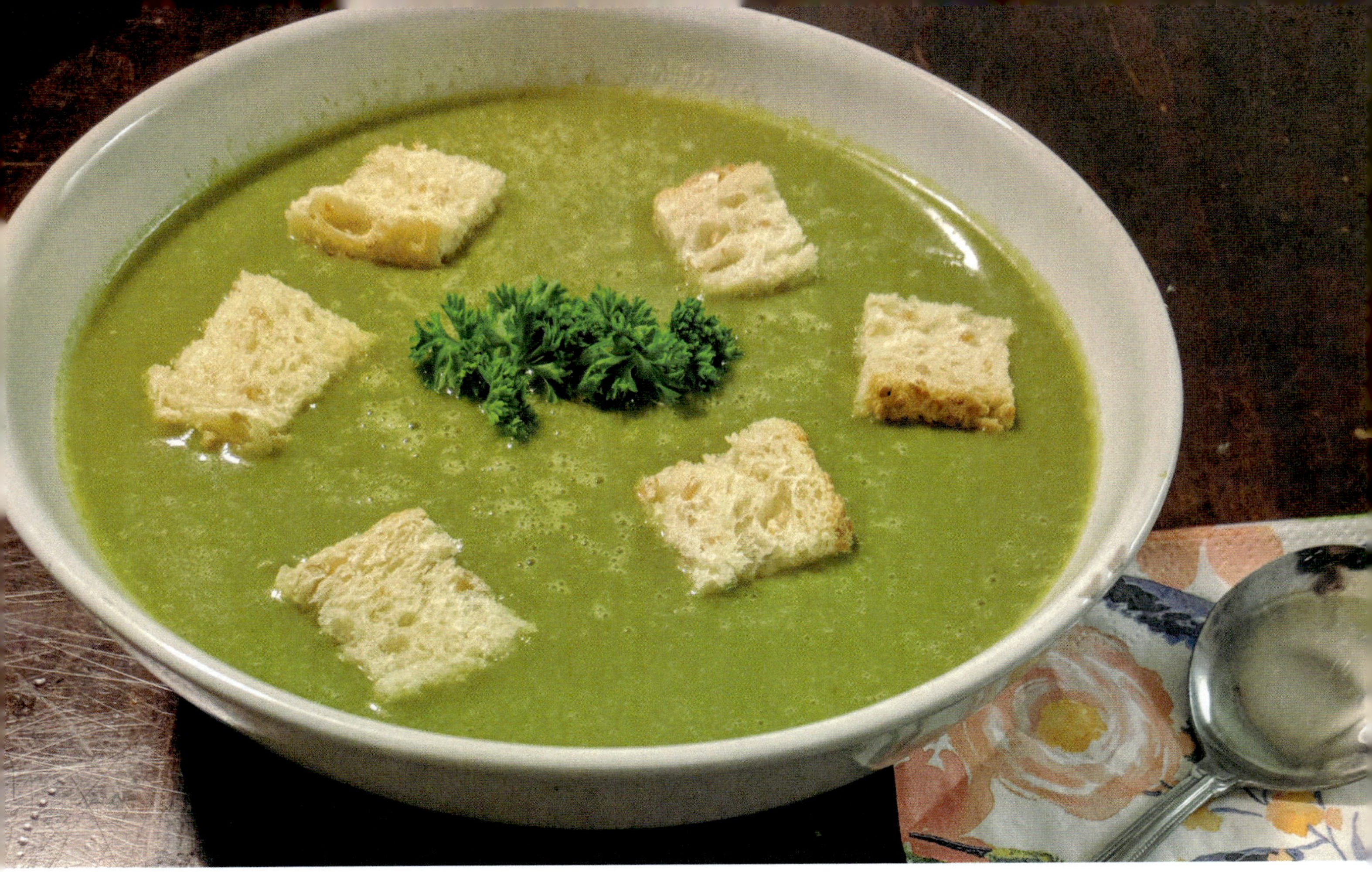

GREEN POWER SOUP

The power of green in a creamy and savory soup.

INGREDIENTS:

- 12 oz. spinach leaves
- 6 potatoes, small
- 16 garlic cloves
- 1/2 onion, large
- 1 head of celery
- 5 green onions
- 1 can coconut cream
- 7 cups water
- 4 cups vegetable broth (low sodium)
- 1/2 cup nutritional yeast
- 1 tbsp. garlic powder
- 1 tsp. sea salt
- 1/4 tsp. cayenne pepper

DELICIOUS WITH:

Side salad, Basic Bread (pg. 86), crackers.

STEPS:

1. Chop onion, celery, and garlic cloves into small pieces.
2. In a large soup pot, sauté onion, celery, and garlic with 1 tbsp. water, lime juice, or soy sauce on low until they turn tender and their aroma begins to release.
3. Wash potatoes and dice them into small pieces. Add potatoes, water, and vegetable broth to pot with onions, celery, and garlic.
4. After potatoes are nearly cooked, add spinach and spices.
5. Once potatoes are completely cooked, remove pot from heat and allow to cool for 5–10 minutes.
6. Add soup to a heat-safe blender[1] and blend until smooth.
7. Return blended soup to pot and add coconut cream.
8. Warm soup on low heat and stir in coconut cream.
9. Enjoy!

1—Make sure your blender can handle heat. If not, you will need to wait longer to cool soup before blending and you may want to reheat soup before serving. I've had a glass blender explode with hot soup the in past, so feel obliged to give this warning.

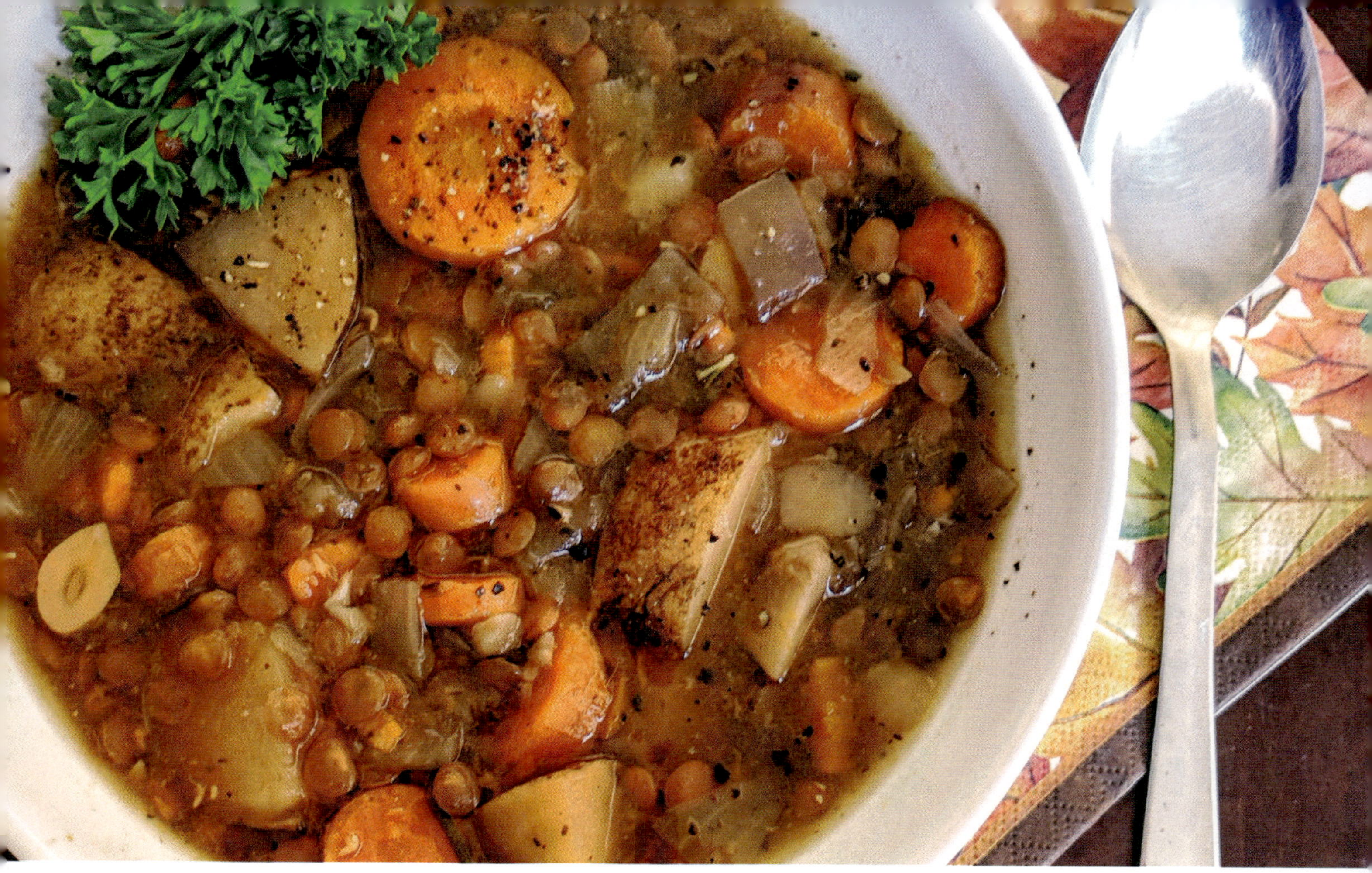

ROOT STEW

The most wonderful thing about winter may be warming up with roots.

INGREDIENTS:

- 4–5 potatoes, medium
- 4–5 carrots
- 1 yellow onion, large, diced small
- 1 cup lentils (green/brown)
- 5 garlic cloves, fresh, diced (or substitute with dried)
- 1 tbsp. Italian herbs, chopped. Fresh is best but dried will work. Choose fresh herbs you have on hand or use a prepared Italian seasoning. These herbs work well:
    - thyme
    - rosemary
    - oregano
    - basil
- 2 tsp. salt
- 7 cups water
- generous twists of ground black pepper

STEPS:

1. Wash fresh vegetables.
2. Use a sharp knife to remove any bad spots from veggies.
3. Chop potatoes and carrots into large chunks.
4. Dice onion and garlic into small pieces.
5. HEAT—**Crockpot:** Add all ingredients to crockpot and cook on high for 5 hours. **Stovetop:** Add all ingredients to large covered pot. Cook on medium heat for about 30 minutes or longer until potatoes and carrots are soft and lentils are partly dissolved into the soup's broth.
6. Stir, serve, and enjoy!

DELICIOUS WITH: Basic Bread (pg. 86), Cornmeal Almond Milk Biscuits (pg. 87), Green Soda Bread (pg. 86). Top with diced avocado, diced green onions, or a sprig of fresh parsley.

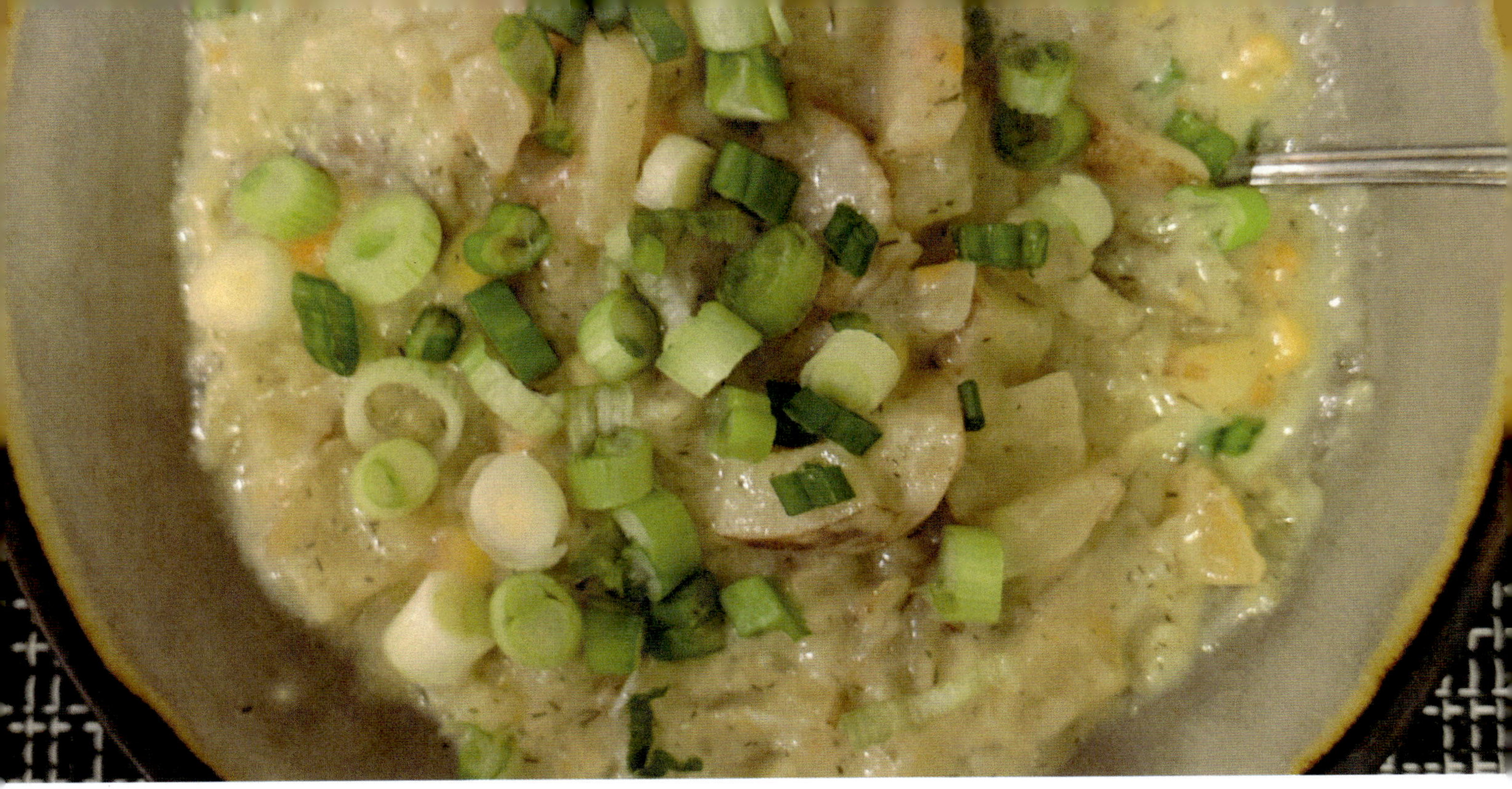

POTATO CHOWDER

Classic comforting chunky potato soup made from 100% whole plants.

INGREDIENTS:

- 3 lbs potatoes
- 1 carrot
- 1 yellow onion
- 1 cup corn
- 1/2 green bell pepper
- 12 garlic cloves
- 4 cups plain almond milk[1]
- 5 tbsp. nutritional yeast
- 3 tbsp. corn starch
- 1 tbsp. dill
- 1 tbsp. garlic powder
- 1 tsp. pepper
- 1 tsp. salt
- 1 cup water

STEPS:

1. Wash potatoes, carrots, onion, and bell pepper.
2. Dice onion, garlic, carrot, and green bell pepper into small pieces.
3. Sauté onion, garlic, pepper, and carrot with 1 tsp. water in soup pan until onions are translucent.
4. Remove any bad spots from potatoes and chop into small (1/2 inch–1/4 inch) squares.
5. Place potato squares into a large colander and rinse with cold water to remove any remaining dirt.
6. Add potatoes and remaining ingredients to pot with veggies.
7. Simmer on medium heat until potatoes are tender enough to puntcure easily with a fork. Remove pot from heat and allow to sit covered for another 5–10 minutes.
8. Serve topped with diced green onions and black pepper. Enjoy!

1 Or, for a creamier soup, try using a 13.5 oz can of coconut cream or full-fat coconut milk + 4 cups of water.

Making Potatoes the Star of Supper

Potato is the star of many dishes in our home and many recipes found in this book. I really can't sing the praises of potatoes enough. It's really a shame so many people today have been scared away from this affordable, delicious, and nutrient packed food which has been a staple for our ancestors for countless generations. Potatoes are one of the cheapest foods a person today could subsist on and, if considering the nutrients they deliver (see pg. 23), one would be hard pressed to find better nutritional value per dollar. One winter my kids and I lived off-grid at a place where potatoes had been grown and we were one of the only people harvesting from a couple raised beds of potatoes. The potatoes fed us all winter long and comprised the bulk of our diet that winter. My appreciation for this super tuber grew then as I saw how easy it was to simply dig up the potatoes I needed for supper each day. I wrapped them in tinfoil and cooked them in the ashes of our fire and this sustained us through the winter. The only thing I would add to that supper was perhaps a winter squash baked the same way, a small amount of avocado, and basic salt and pepper. The recipe above is quite fancy in comparison. Still, I want to share for anyone who is struggling to afford food, that potatoes make a filling and nutritious staple food to rely on.

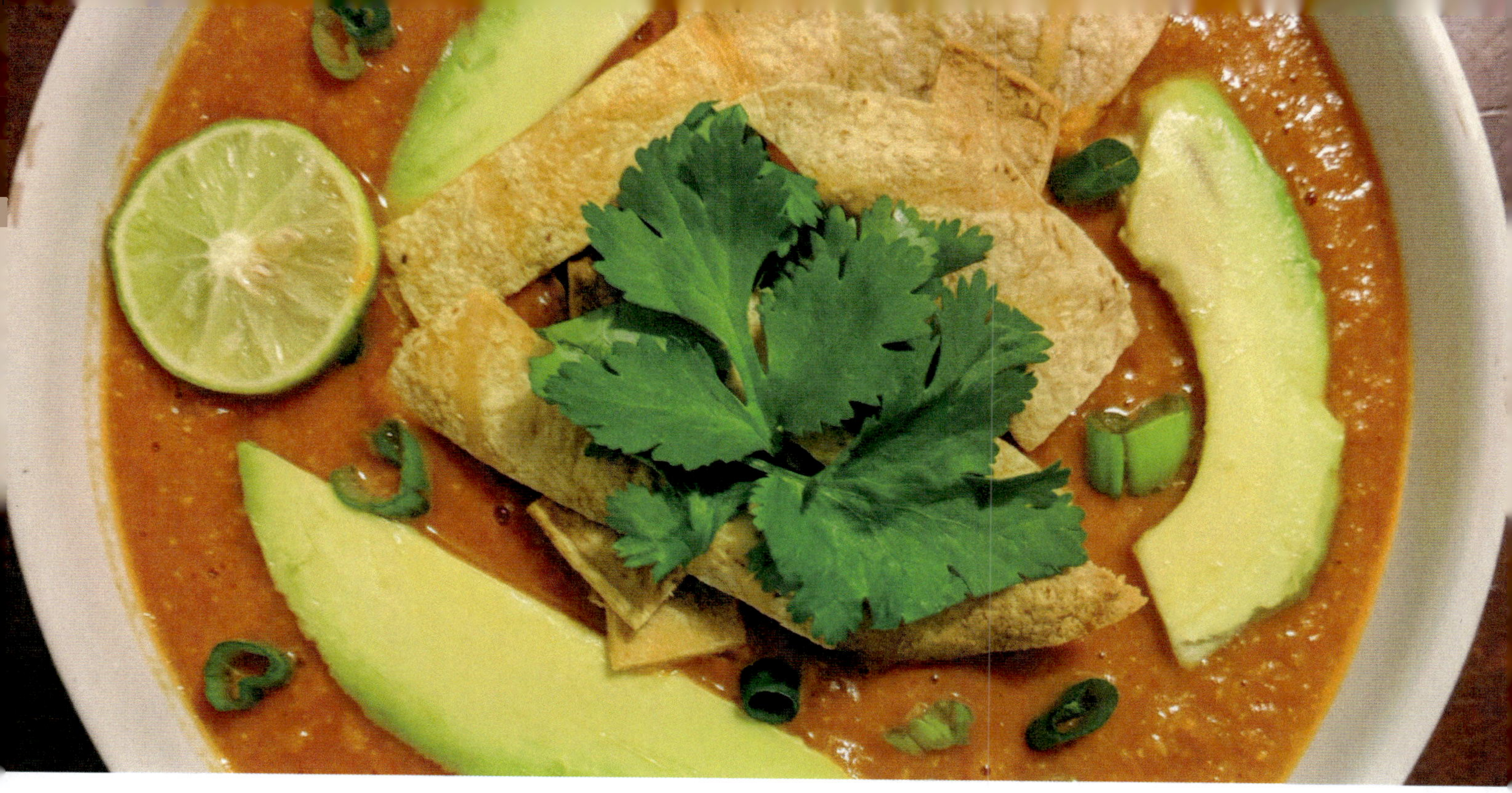

TORTILLA SOUP

A spicy and satisfying soup topped with avocado slices and tortillas.

INGREDIENTS:

- 3 cup white corn (~1lb)
- 1 yellow onion
- 1 red bell pepper
- 1 zucchini, medium
- 2 tomatoes, medium
- 5 garlic cloves
- 2 cans tomato sauce
- 6 oz. tomato paste
- 4 cups vegetable broth
- 2 tbsp. cumin
- 1/2 tbsp. chipotle powder
- 1 tsp. garlic powder
- 1 cup almond milk
- 1/2 cup nutritional yeast

GARNISH:

- cilantro
- lime
- avocado
- tortilla strips, toasted

✓ See important tip about adding heat in caption to the right.

STEPS:

1. Dice onion, bell pepper, and green onions into small pieces. Sauté in 1/4 cup of vegetable broth on stovetop until onions are slightly tender and translucent.
2. Move onion and peppers into blender and add 1 cup of corn, zucchini, and remainder of broth.
3. Blend on high until well mixed.
4. Pour mixture back into pot and add spices, almond milk, nutritional yeast, and remaining cup of corn.
5. Cook soup slowly on low heat for 30–40 minutes to incorporate all flavors.
6. Garnish with homemade tortilla chips, avocado slices, and chopped green onions.

✓ Adjust to Your Desired Level of Spice

Tortilla soup is one of my very favorite soups and I have experimented with several different ways of spicing this soup just right. Feel free to adjust the spice in this recipe to match your desired level of heat. It's easy to kick up the heat by adding canned chipotle peppers in adobo sauce or more chipotle powder. The recipe above is a mild amount of spice that is friendly for my kids. When I add 1/2 tbsp. more chipotle powder, I enjoy the heat, but my kids say it's too spicy. I first made this soup using a couple chipotle peppers from the can and 2 tsp. of chipotle powder and I really enjoyed the strong chipotle heat, but the kids rejected it. Since I prefer the chipotle kick of this soup, I want to make sure you aren't left wanting more. If you're cooking just for adults or you like spice, go ahead and turn up the heat. Find canned chipotle peppers in adobo sauce in the Hispanic or ethnic food section of your local grocery or find them online at: https://healingwithplants.us/store/shop-food-products/.

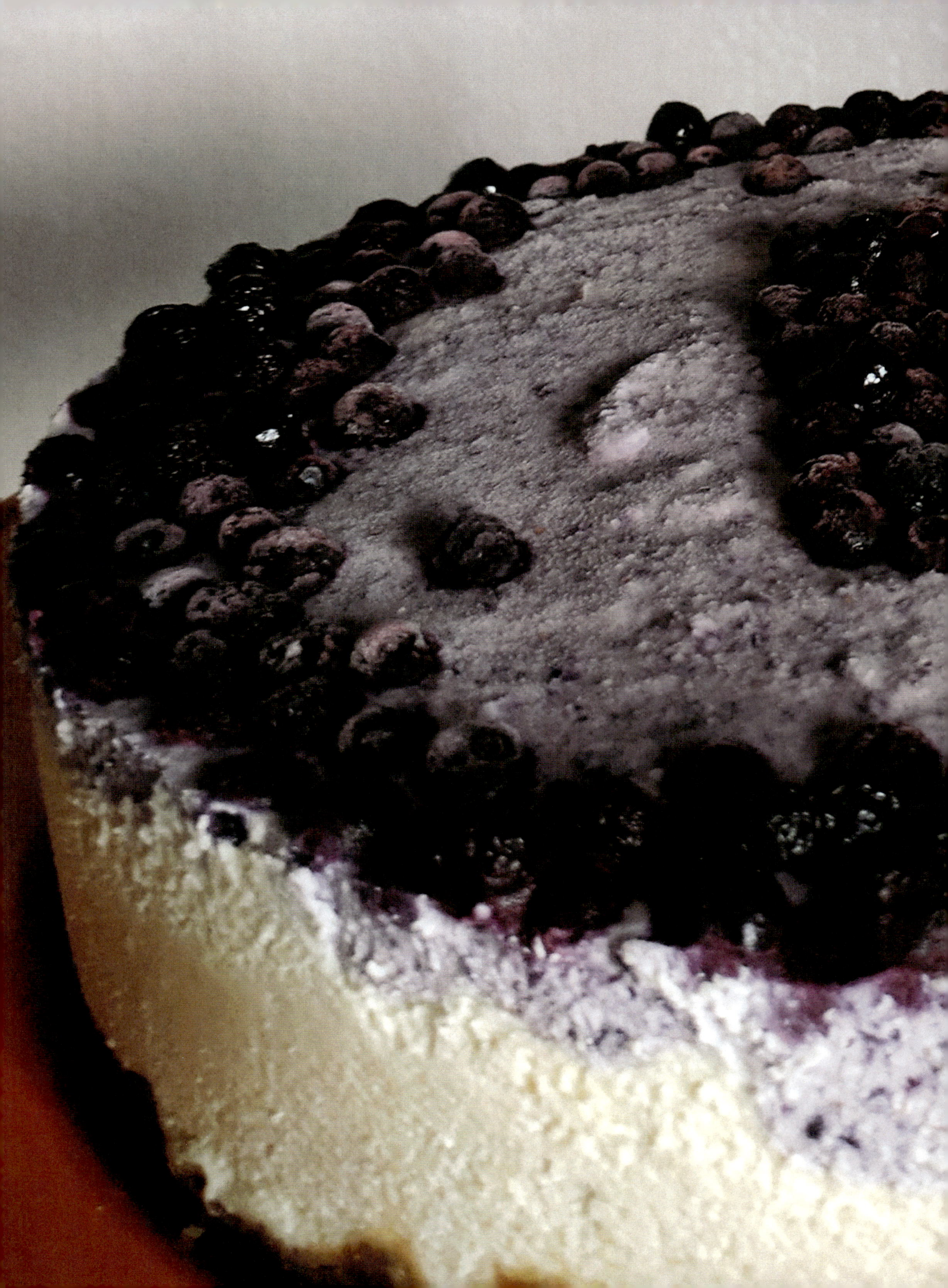

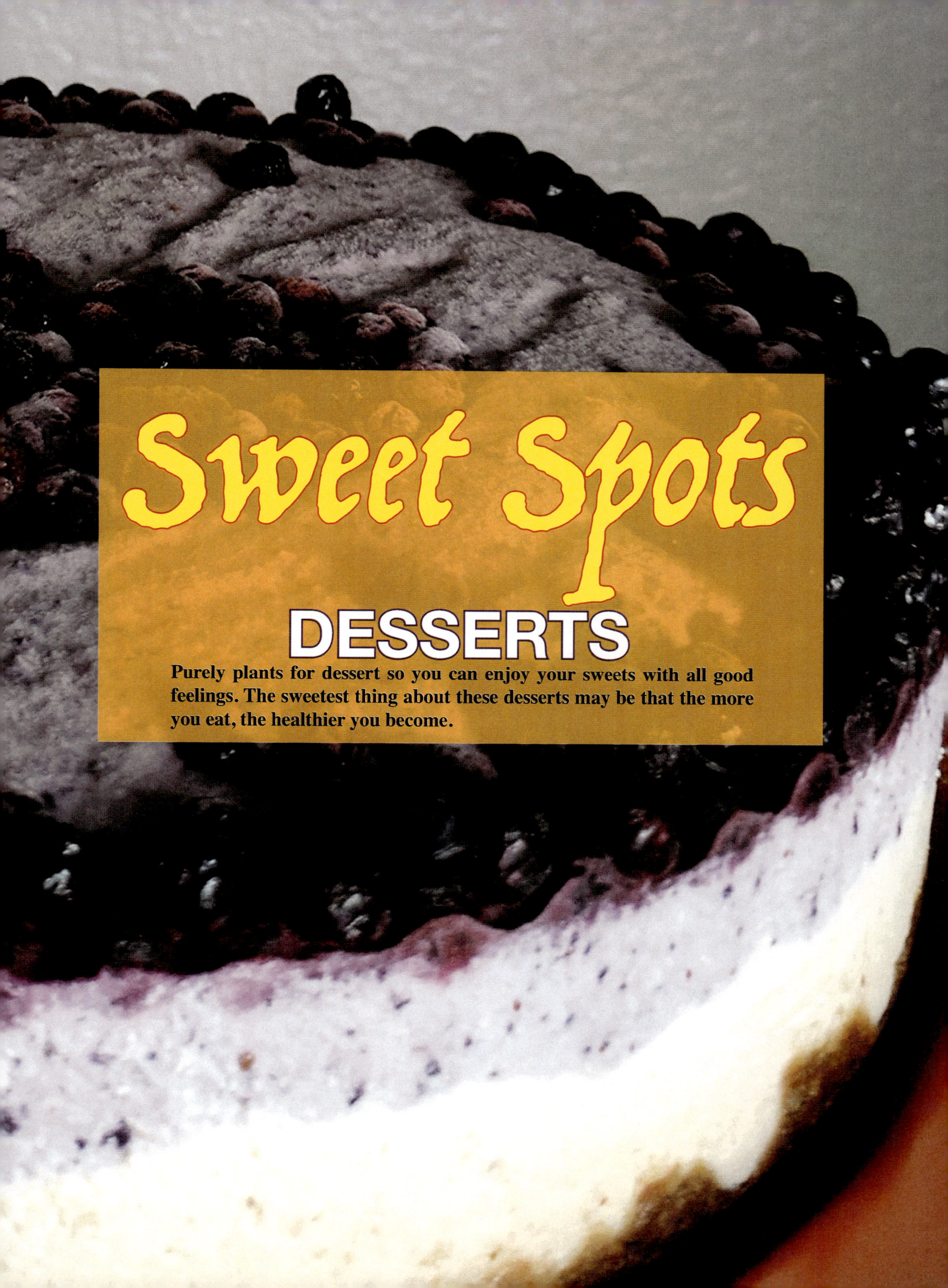

Sweet Spots

DESSERTS

Purely plants for dessert so you can enjoy your sweets with all good feelings. The sweetest thing about these desserts may be that the more you eat, the healthier you become.

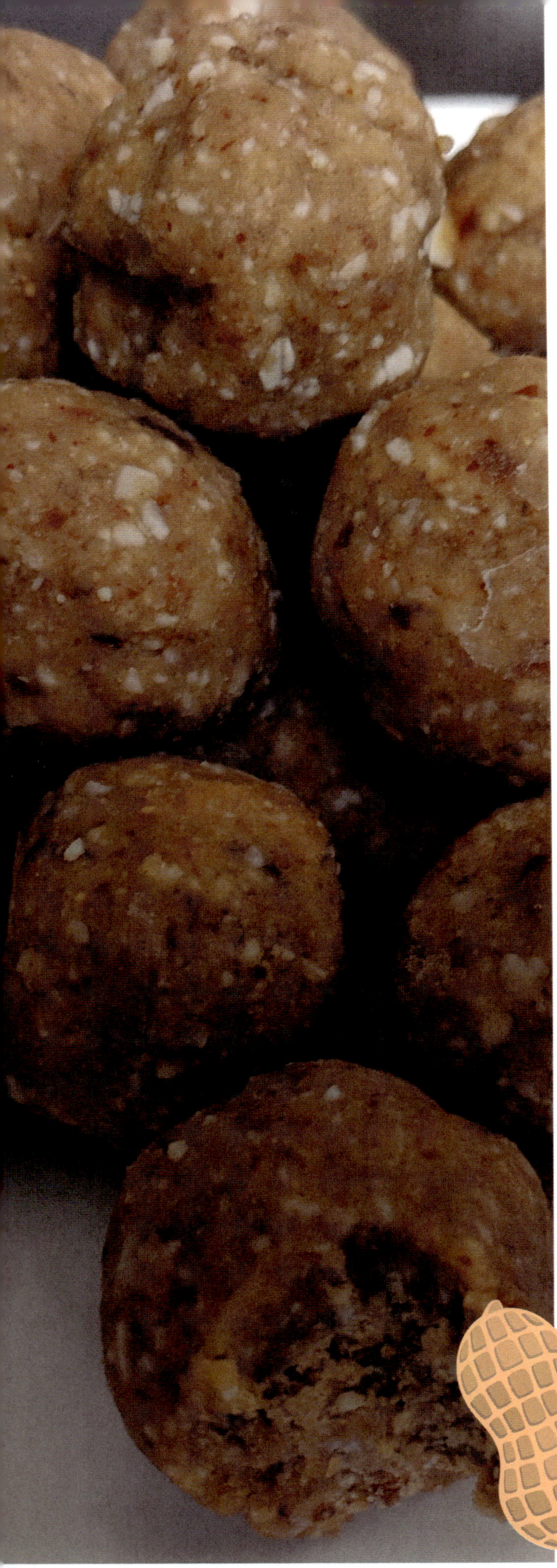

PEANUT BUTTER BALLS

These rich and creamy peanut butter balls are made with three simple ingredients and are perfect when you need quick energy on the go, or for an any-time healthy snack.

INGREDIENTS:

- 1 cup peanut butter (just peanuts)
- 2 cups coconut flakes
- 12 medjool dates, pitted

STEPS:

1. Remove pits from dates.
2. Put peanut butter, coconut flakes, and dates into a food processor and blend.
3. Stop and push contents down into blade in order to blend thoroughly. The mixture should turn into one lump of rather firm dough.
4. Scoop mixture from food processor into a bowl.
5. Roll mixture into bite-sized balls. I aim for three-bites sized or about 1 tbsp. of mixture per ball.
6. Enjoy! Store balls in freezer in a Tupperware container and enjoy as a healthy snack or dessert.

DELICIOUS WITH: Try dipping these into melted chocolate if you desire an even more decadent sweet treat.

The Story of Peanut Butter Balls

Growing up my mother's grandma—known affectionately by all who knew her as G-ma—was an important part of my life. She was the one who watched me after school while my parents worked. G-ma was my caretaker whenever I was sick and couldn't go to school, and often if my parents went out on dates or traveled, we were with G-ma. Every year around Christmas, G-ma made peanut butter balls dipped in chocolate. She called them Buckeyes because they resembled the seeds of the Ohio Buckeye tree, which are so named by Native Americans for their resemblance to the eye of a buck deer.

G-ma's peanut butter balls were made with butter and powdered sugar which replicated for some years before my desire to create a healthier version of her recipe took hold. After some experimentation, I discovered that dried coconut flakes substitute for the stiffening effect of the powdered sugar, while dates gave the balls the perfect amount of sweetness using whole fruits—no powdered sugar needed.

Now my kids have come to expect Buckeyes at Christmas, but we enjoy plain old peanut butter balls as a less-rich treat other times of the year. These balls store great in the freezer or fridge, and 1–2 can be just right for a little treat or quick energy boost. They can also be dipped in dark chocolate to become just like G-Ma's Buckeyes for a more indulgent ball of 100% plants bliss.

CHOCOLATE SUNFLOWER BALLS

These bliss balls combine four raw, whole-plant food ingredients into a delicious, chocolaty, nutrient-packed snack, perfect for a small dessert or on-the-go snack.

YIELDS: 40 balls

INGREDIENTS:

- 3 cups raw sunflower seed kernels (or ~16 oz.)
- 1/2 cup cacao powder
- 2 cups medjool dates, pitted (or ~16 oz.)
- 1 tbsp. raw sunflower seed butter*

STEPS:

1. Add raw sunflower seeds to high-powered food processor and begin to blend.
2. Add dates and cacao powder to food processor and continue to combine.
3. Add raw sunflower seed butter and finish combining in food processor.
4. Remove blade from food processor and roll mixture into tightly-packed balls about 1–2 inches in diameter.
5. Share with your loved ones. Enjoy!
6. Store Chocolate Sunflower Balls in the fridge or freezer.

TIP: Sunflower seed butter is purely sunflower seeds ground into a thick paste, just like peanut butter. You can substitute peanut butter or almond butter if you don't have this ingredient on hand.

The Story of Sunflower Balls

I began experimenting making homemade energy bars the first time I took a long distance bike ride when I was 22 years old. I wanted bars that were healthier than what I saw at the super market and I didn't want to pay $1 or more per bar. Plus, it was fun to make homemade energy bars to share with my biking companions. My energy bars were made purely of plants with no artificial or hyper-processed ingredients. My bars were purely made of nuts, seeds, and dried fruits.

Over the years since, my energy bars turned into balls as I found the shape easy to make and easy to eat in a few bites, oftentimes all that I needed for a little energy boost. Energy balls are easy to pack, easy to store in the freezer, and packed with whole-plant nutrition. I have enjoyed experimenting with different combinations and sharing these with friends over the years. Now I prefer the name Bliss Balls for these treats.

Sunflower seeds have been my favorite ingredient for these balls much of the time because they are the most affordable of the raw seeds. I also enjoy using almonds, pecans, and walnuts, but these seeds are considerably pricier. So for someone who's been on a tight budget, sunflower seeds have often been the only seed I could afford.

Besides being affordable, I like that sunflower seed balls are actually a traditional American food. In *Buffalo Bird Woman's Garden*, Gilbert Livingston Wilson interviews Buffalo Bird Woman of the Hidatsa indian tribe, who practiced traditional Hidatsa agriculture. She describes how sunflower seeds were a staple crop along with corn, beans, and squash. Sunflowers were the first crop to be planted and the last to be harvested each year, and the kernels were used to make a dense ball which men would carry with them as they were out on their day's journey. These Chocolate Sunflower Balls can be used much the same way as the ones made by the Hidatsa in centuries past.

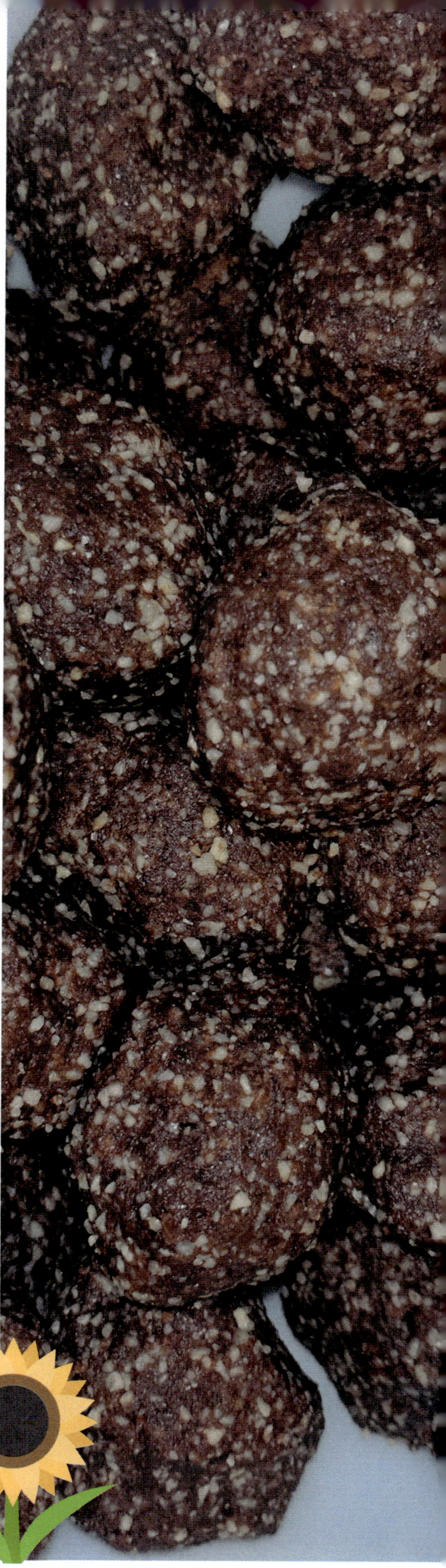

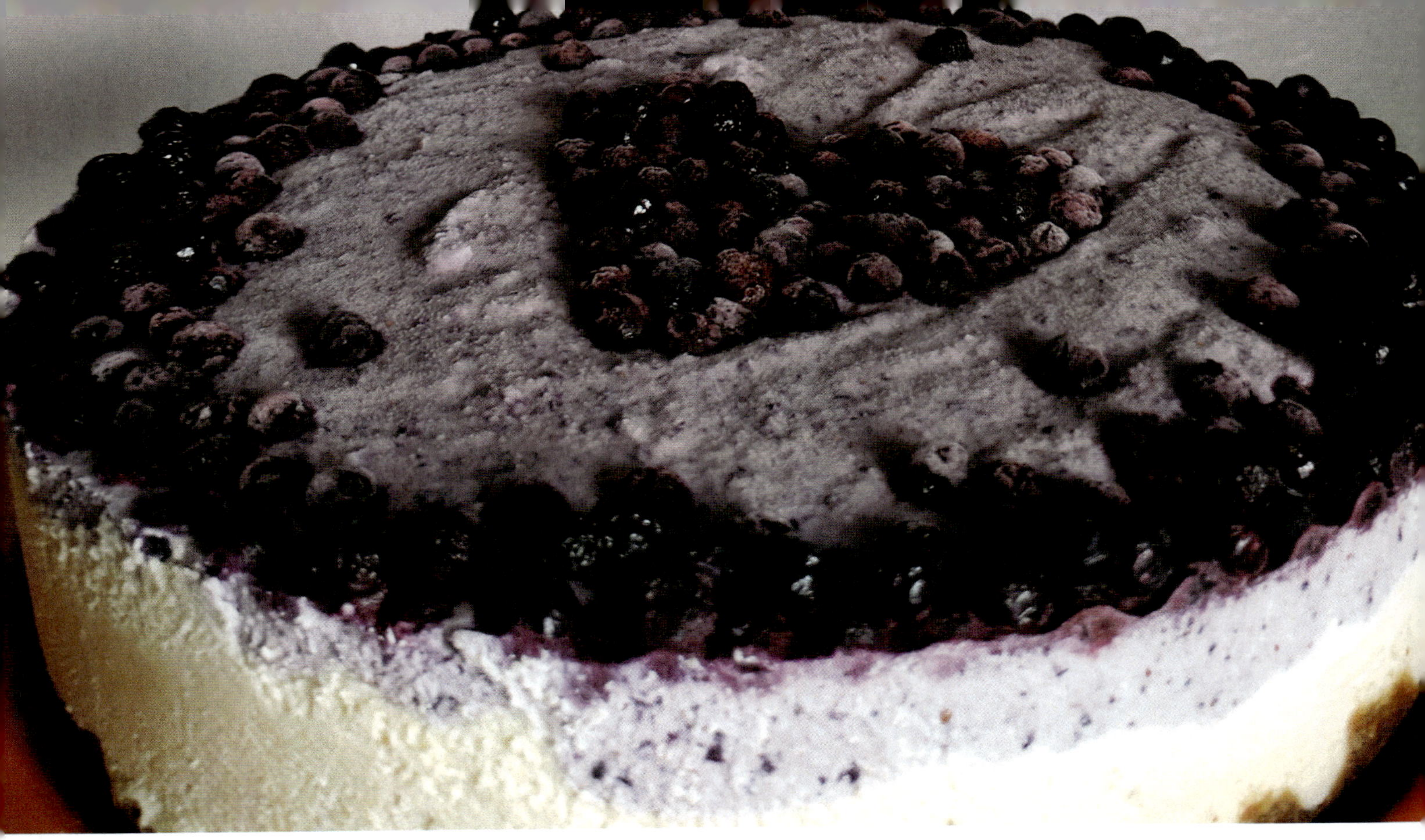

☀BLUEBERRY BLISS CH-EASE-CAKE☀

Blueberries star in this rich and creamy cake that any ch-ease-cake fan will fall in love with.

For this ch-ease cake, I modified the recipe by Minimalist Baker to end up with a nice, thick, layered cheesecake that slices beautifully.

INGREDIENTS:

CRUST:

- 1 cup medjool dates, pitted, packed
- 1.5 cups walnuts

FILLING:

- 5 cups cashews, raw, soaked
- 1 lemon, large (or 2 small), squeezed
- 1 cup maple syrup
- 1 can coconut cream (or full-fat coconut milk with hard cream on top)

STEPS:

1. Soak cashews overnight in fridge.
2. Rinse liquid off cashews.
3. Blend ingredients for crust in food processor and press into bottom of springform pan.
4. Clean food processor, then blend ingredients for filling.
5. Pour all but 2 cups of filling into the pan on top of crust.
6. Add 1 cup of frozen blueberries to the remaining 2 cups of filling and blend.
7. Pour blueberry mixture on top of ch-ease layer.
8. Top cake with fresh or fozen blueberries.
9. Freeze cake until firm and serve.

✅ **TIP:** If your ch-ease cake is fully frozen, thaw for 10–15 minutes before serving. If cake is frozen, to help make a neat slice, warm knife with hot water before slicing.

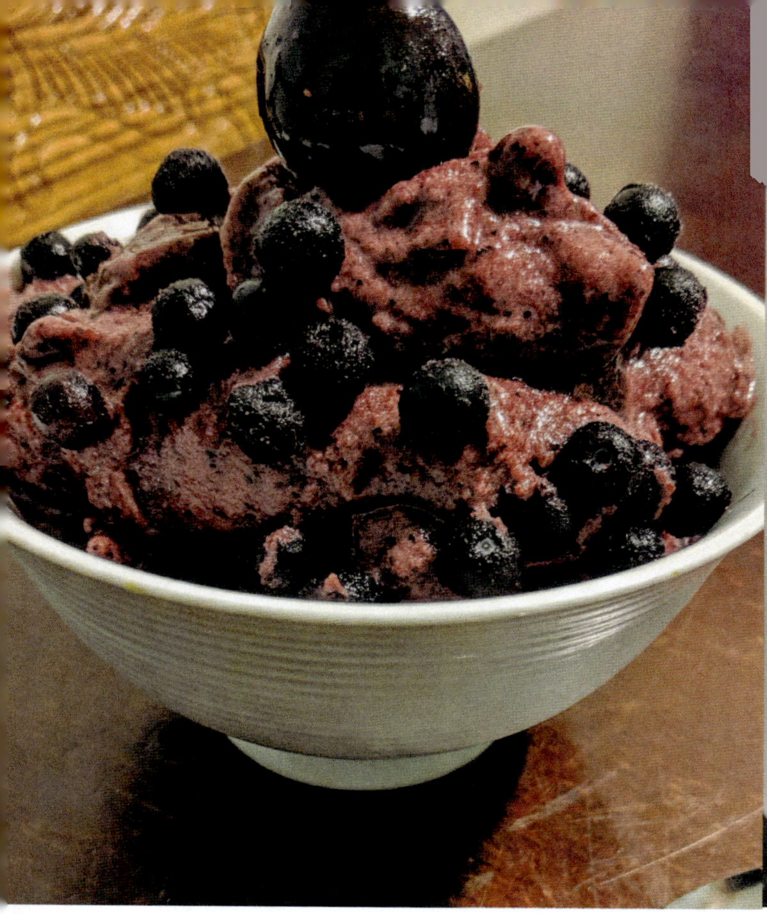

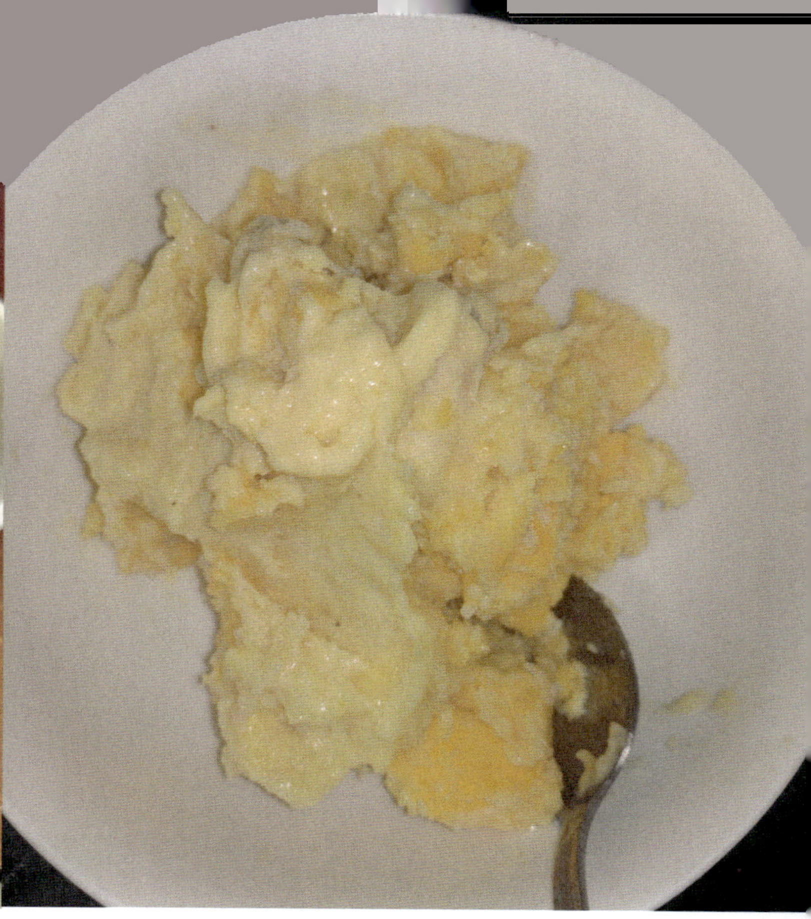

BERRY CHERRY NICE-CREAM

Nice-cream—so-called because it's nice to your body, animals, and the planet—is delicious served in a cup or bowl with fresh fruit and nuts on top.

Serves: 4

INGREDIENTS:

- 2 cups cherries, frozen
- 2 cups blueberries, frozen
- 4 bananas, frozen
- 2.5 cups vanilla almond milk

STEPS:

1. Peel bananas and freeze ahead of time.
2. Wash and freeze cherries and blueberries ahead of time or buy frozen.
3. Combine frozen fruits and almond milk in blender or food processor. Blend on high.
4. Pause to stir and push down chunks.
5. When mixture is smooth, spoon from blender into serving bowls or cups.
6. Top with desired topping.
7. Enjoy immediately soft-serve style, or put nice-cream bowl(s) in freezer to firm up for up for 5–10 minutes before serving.

DELICIOUS WITH: Fresh blueberries, fresh cherries, or a sprinkle of chopped almonds.

MANGO NICE-CREAM

*A light and sweet nice-cream treat made purely from fruits.**

Serves: 2

INGREDIENTS:

- 2 bananas, frozen
- 2 cups mango chunks, frozen
- 1 cup vanilla coconut milk

STEPS:

1. Peel bananas and freeze ahead of time.
2. Freeze chunks of diced mango or purchase frozen mango from the market.
3. Combine frozen fruits and almond milk in a blender or food processor. Blend on high.
4. Open the blender to push chunks of frozen fruit down into blades.
5. When mixture is smooth, transfer it from blender into serving bowls or cups.
6. Top nice-cream with desired topping.
7. Enjoy immediately or return finished nice-cream to freezer to firm up for 5–10 minutes before serving.

DELICIOUS WITH: Top with shredded dried coconut, fresh diced mango, or dried mango fruit chopped into small pieces.

**Botanically, coconut is considered a seed and a fruit at once.*

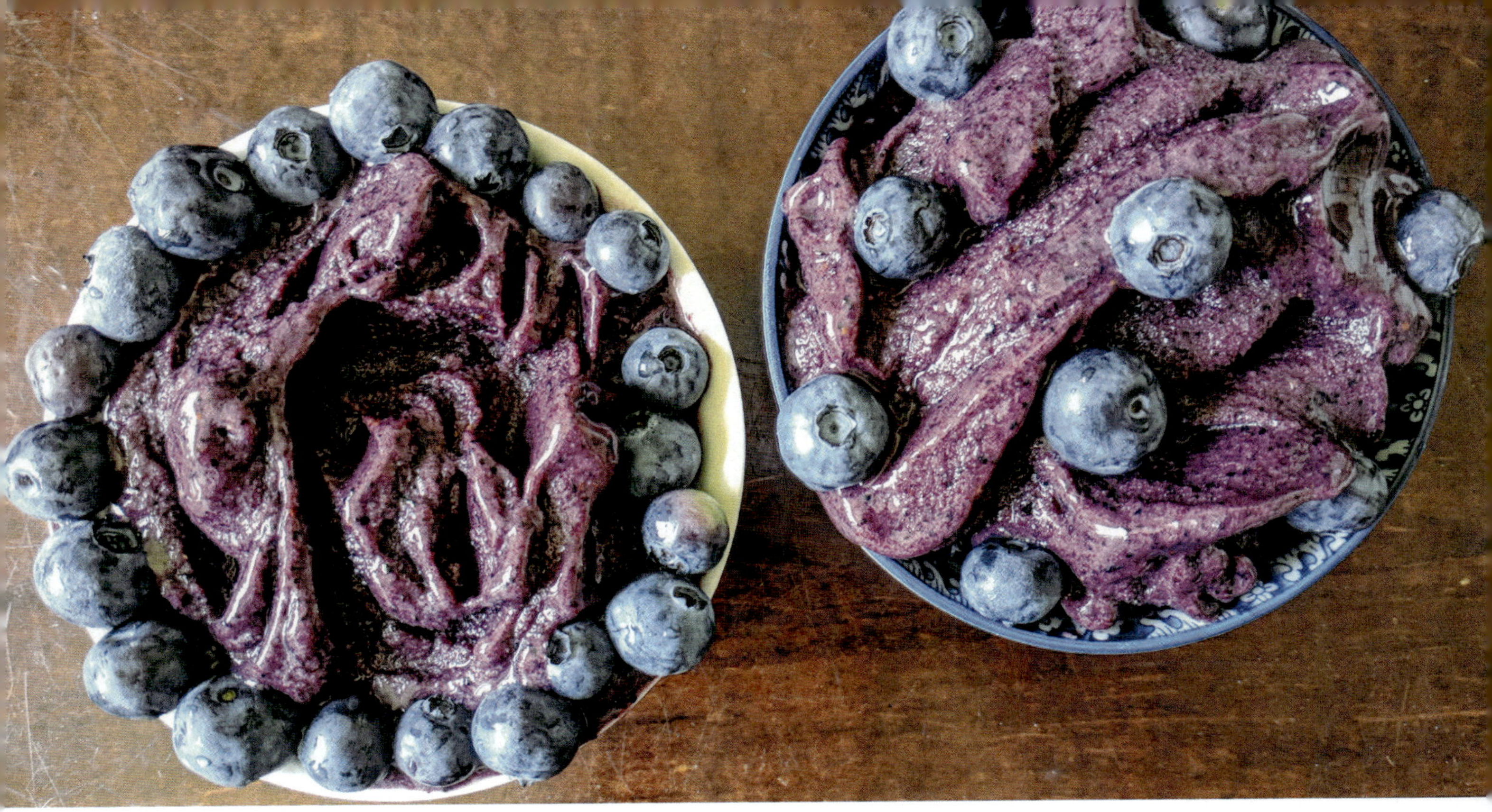

BLUEBERRY NICE-CREAM

A large bowl of blueberry nice-cream made from purely fruits and seeds makes an excellent filling, hydrating, and nutritious breakfast that's especially good for the brain.

INGREDIENTS:

- 2 cups blueberries, frozen
- 2 bananas, frozen
- 1 cup vanilla coconut milk

STEPS:

1. Peel bananas and freeze them ahead of time.
2. Use frozen blueberries or freeze fresh blueberries ahead of time.
3. Combine frozen fruits and coconut milk in blender or food processor.
4. Blend on high.
5. Open the blender to push down chunks of frozen fruit into the blades.
6. When mixture is smooth, transfer it from the blender into serving bowls or cups.
7. Top with desired toppings such as fresh or frozen blueberries, dried coconut flakes, or fresh banana slices.
8. Enjoy immediately or return finished nice-cream to freezer to firm up for 5–10 minutes before serving.

DELICIOUS WITH: Top with fresh or frozen blueberries, dried coconut flakes, chopped nuts, or fresh banana slices.

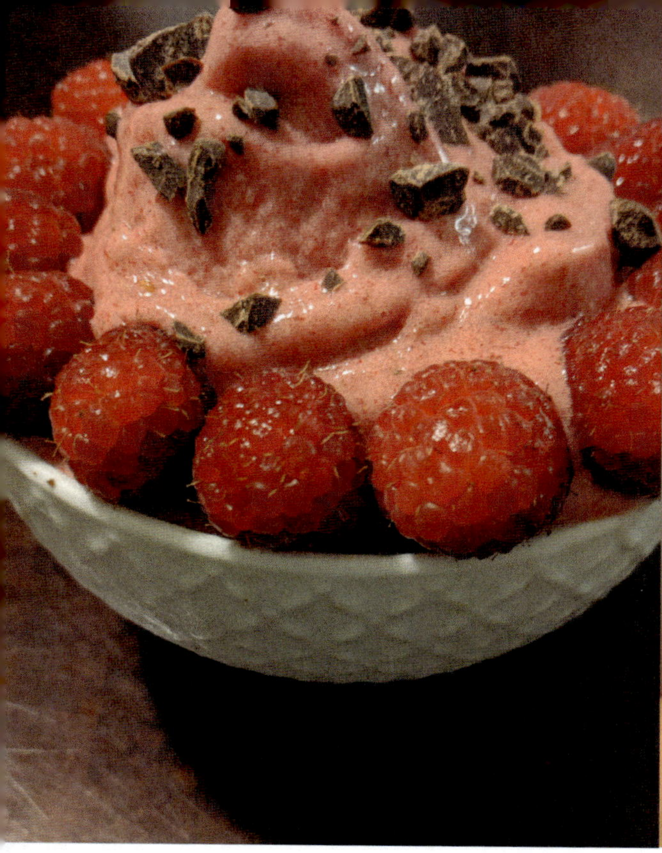

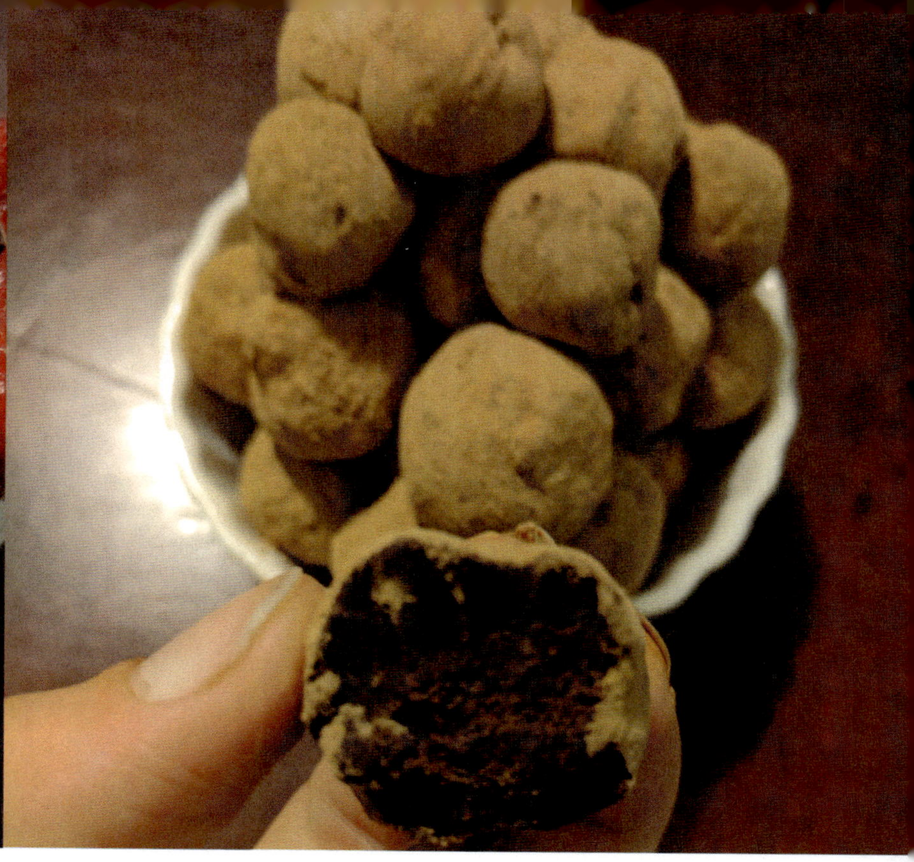

RASPBERRY NICE-CREAM

Sweet, cold, and creamy with the right touch of raspberry tang. This dessert is a healthy alternative to traditional ice-cream that's nutritious and sure to satisfy your sweet tooth.

INGREDIENTS:

- 3 cups raspberries, frozen
- 3 bananas, frozen
- 1 cup vanilla almond milk

STEPS:

1. Peel and freeze bananas and wash and freeze raspberries ahead of time.
2. Combine ingredients into a food processor or blender.
3. Blend until well combined. Stop blender and push down contents with a spoon to incorporate as needed.
4. Scoop nice-cream into a metal bowl and place in freezer for 10–20 minutes to harden. Enjoy!

DELICIOUS WITH: Top with fresh raspberries, blueberries, chopped nuts, dark chocolate flakes, or cocoa powder.

CHOCOLATE ALMOND TRUFFLES

A velvety-rich chocolate indulgence with an almond note. This dessert is mostly made of seeds.

YIELDs: 30 truffles

INGREDIENTS:

- 11.5 oz. dark chocolate (I like 65%)
- 1/2 cup coconut cream (or full-fat coconut milk from can)
- 1/4 cup cocoa powder
- 1 tbsp. almond butter
- 1 tsp. almond extract

STEPS:

1. Measure all ingredients except cocoa powder into a metal bowl.
2. Place metal bowl inside or on top of saucepan with 1—2 inches of water.
3. Warm saucepan on low heat to slowly melt chocolate. Stir contents consistently just until chocolate is melted and mixture is velvety smooth.
4. Remove from heat and allow to cool for 10 minutes. Stir pot. Place pot in the freezer for 5 minutes.
5. Spoon chocolate into dollops on a stick-proof pan and place pan in the freezer for 5 minutes.
6. Remove pan from freezer and roll the dollops into balls using clean dry hands.
7. Place chocolate balls into a large metal bowl with cocoa powder. Shake the bowl to evenly coat chocolates in powder. Serve immediately.
8. Store leftover truffles in freezer for later.

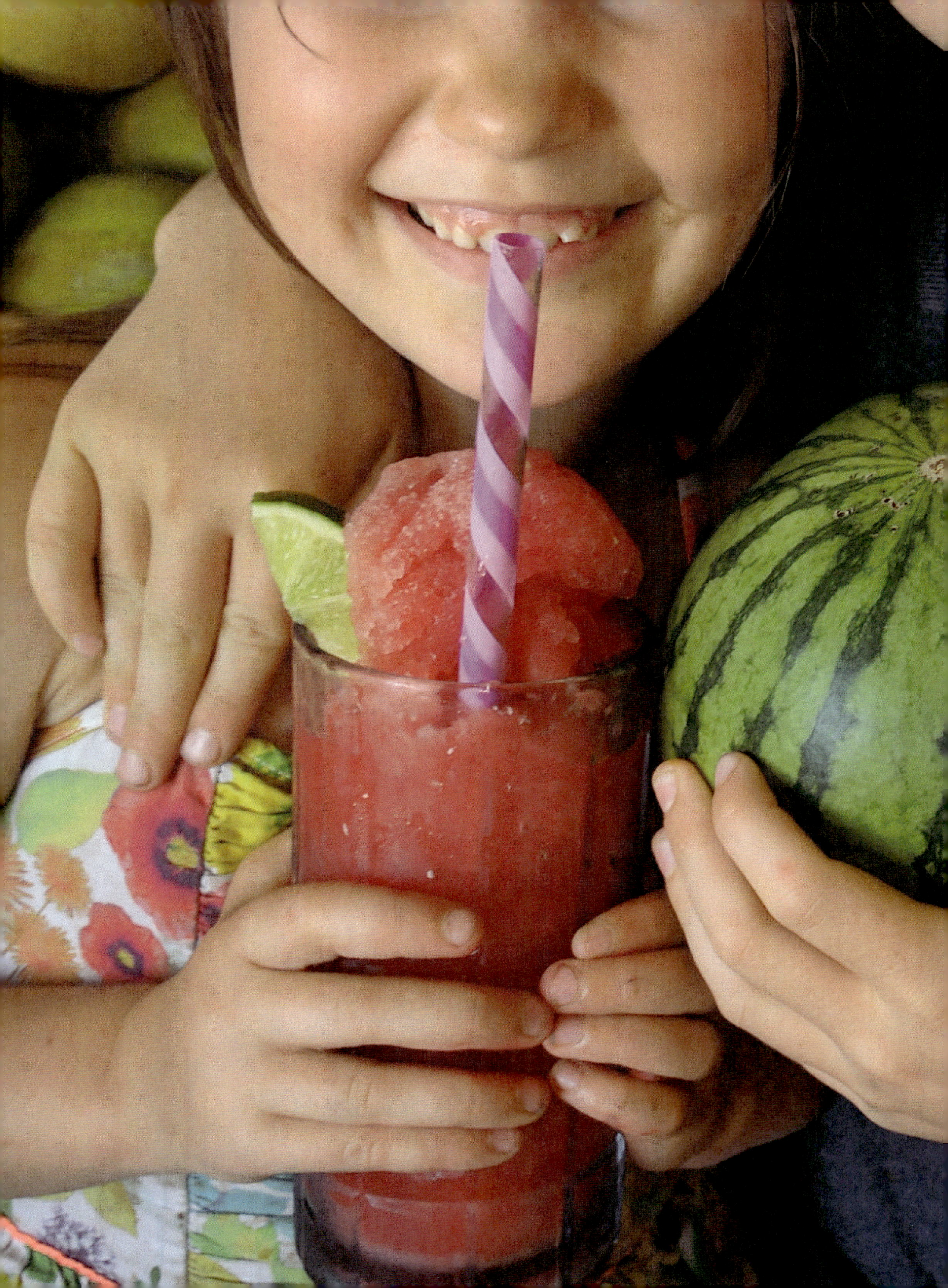

Drink to Your Health

BEVERAGES

Make drinking more delicious and nutritious with these healthy drink recipes made from 100% whole plants. Many of the recipes in this section will call for almond milk or coconut milk, but feel free to substitute for your favorite plant milk or what you have on hand. Almond, cashew, coconut, hemp, rice, oat, peanut, macadamia nut, and soy milks are all good options for making nourishing beverages.

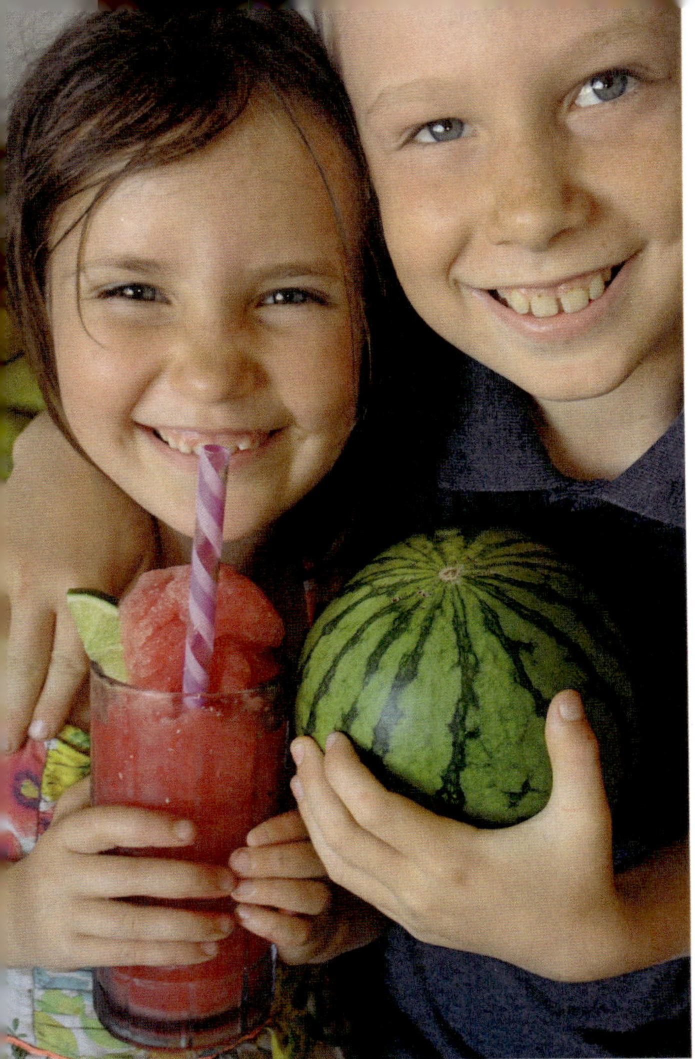

WATERMELON ICEE

A frosty treat made from one nutritious sweet fruit.

SERVINGS: 4 1-cup servings

INGREDIENTS:

- 4 cups watermelon, chopped, frozen

STEPS:

1. Chop ripe watermelon into a bowl and remove large seeds.
2. Freeze watermelon chunks until solid.
3. Blend frozen watermelon chunks on high until icee consistency is achieved.
4. Serve in your cup or bowl of choice.
5. Enjoy!

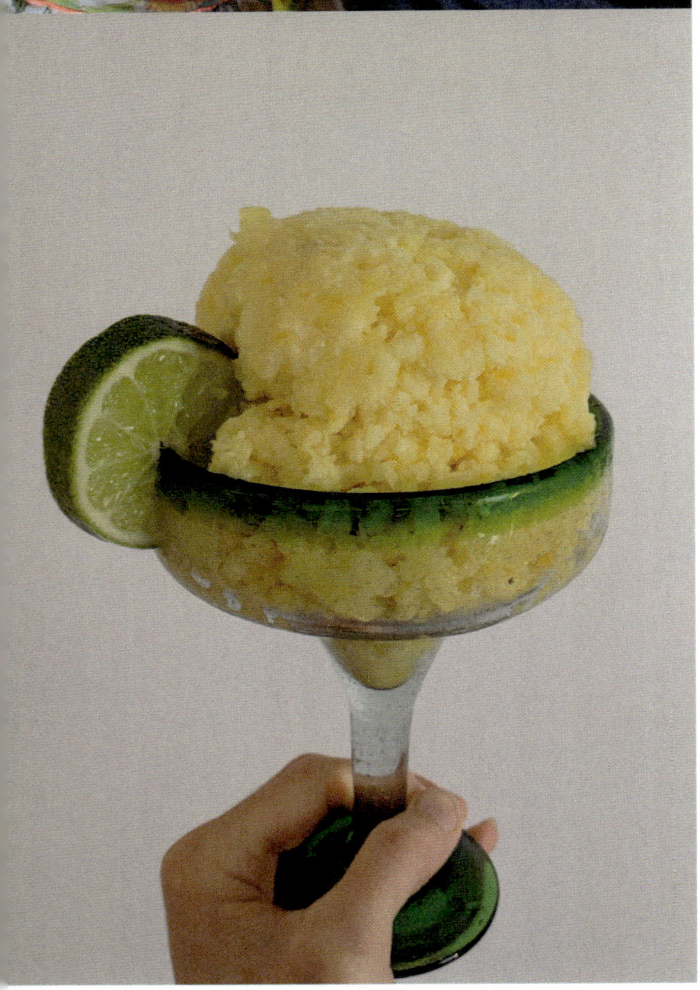

PINEAPPLE LIME CRUSH

The tanginess of pineapple and lime will tantalize the taste buds.

SERVINGS: 2 ~1.5–2-cup servings

INGREDIENTS:

- 1 pineapple
- 1 lime

STEPS:

1. Cut off pineapple top and bottom. Remove outside pineapple skin layer.
2. Chop pineapple into chunks. Discard its tough core, skin, top, and bottom.
3. Freeze pineapple chunks in a bowl or tupperware.
4. Place frozen pineapple chunks into the blender.
5. Cut lime in half and squeeze juice of both halves into the blender using a citrus squeezer so that no seeds get into the blender. If you don't have a citrus squeezer, use a strainer to catch the seeds.
6. Blend on high until well combined. You may need to pause your blender and push the pineapple chunks down into the blades.
7. Scoop blended pineapple and lime into your favorite serving cup or dish.
8. Garnish with a fresh lime slice.
9. Enjoy!

MANGO LIME CRUSH

A sweet and sour frosty beverage starring mango and lime.
SERVINGS: 2 2-cup servings

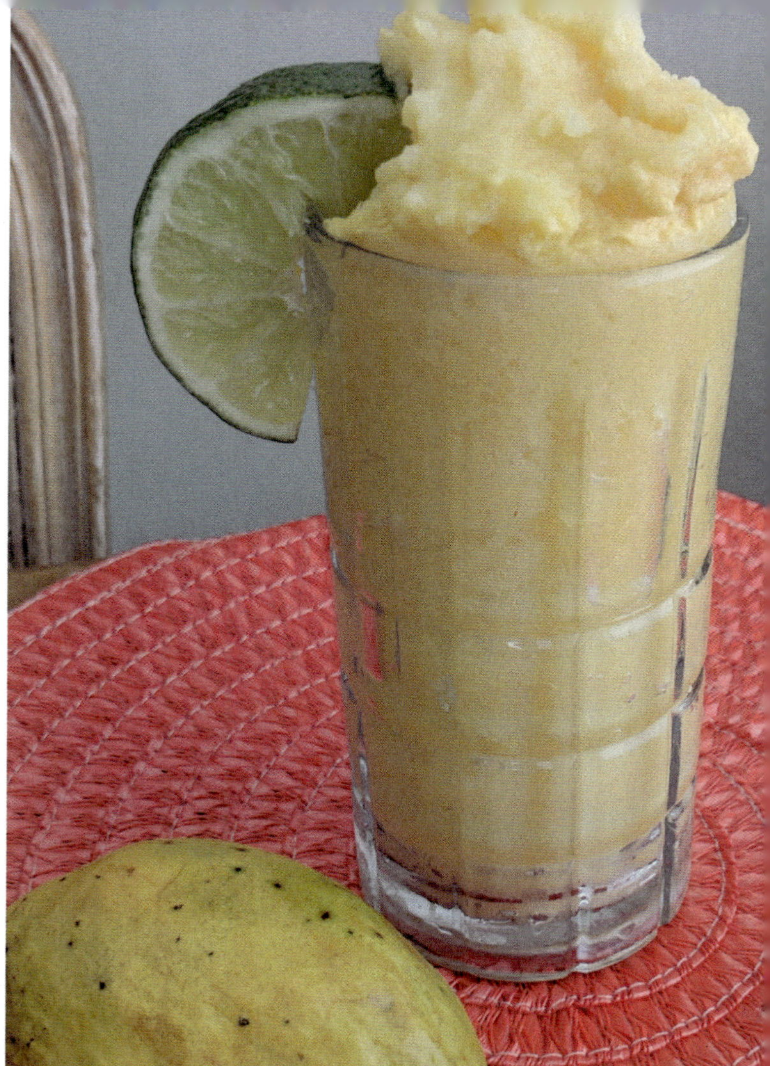

INGREDIENTS:

- 2 cups mango chunks, frozen
- 1 lime
- 1 cup coconut milk
- 1 cup coconut water
- 1/2 cup ice

STEPS:

1. Add mango chunks, coconut milk, coconut water, and ice to blender.
2. Squeeze juice of one lime into blender.
3. Blend on high until well combined and ice is thoroughly crushed.
4. Pour into two tall glasses and garnish with a lime wedge.

GRAPE ICEE

An all natural snow-cone that is simply grapes and simply nutritious.
SERVINGS: 4 1-cup servings

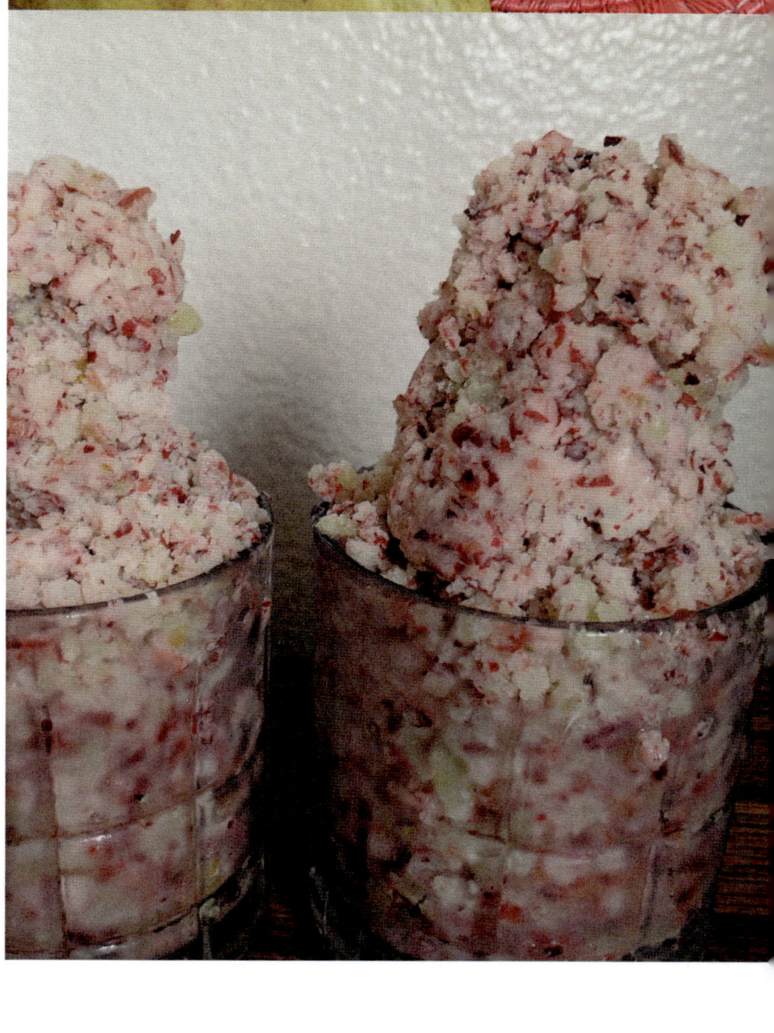

INGREDIENTS:

- 4 cups grapes, chopped, frozen

STEPS:

1. Remove grapes from stems and rinse in a colander.
2. Freeze grapes in a bowl or tupperware until solid.
3. Blend frozen grape chunks on high until icee consistency is achieved.
4. Serve in your cup or bowl of choice.
5. Enjoy!

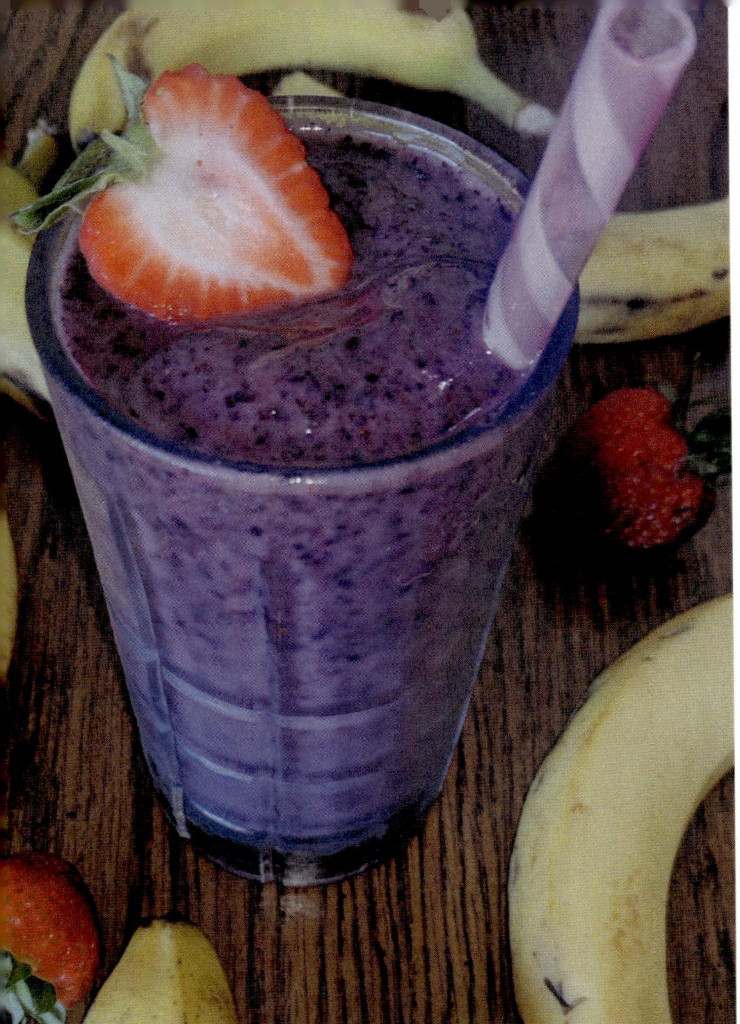

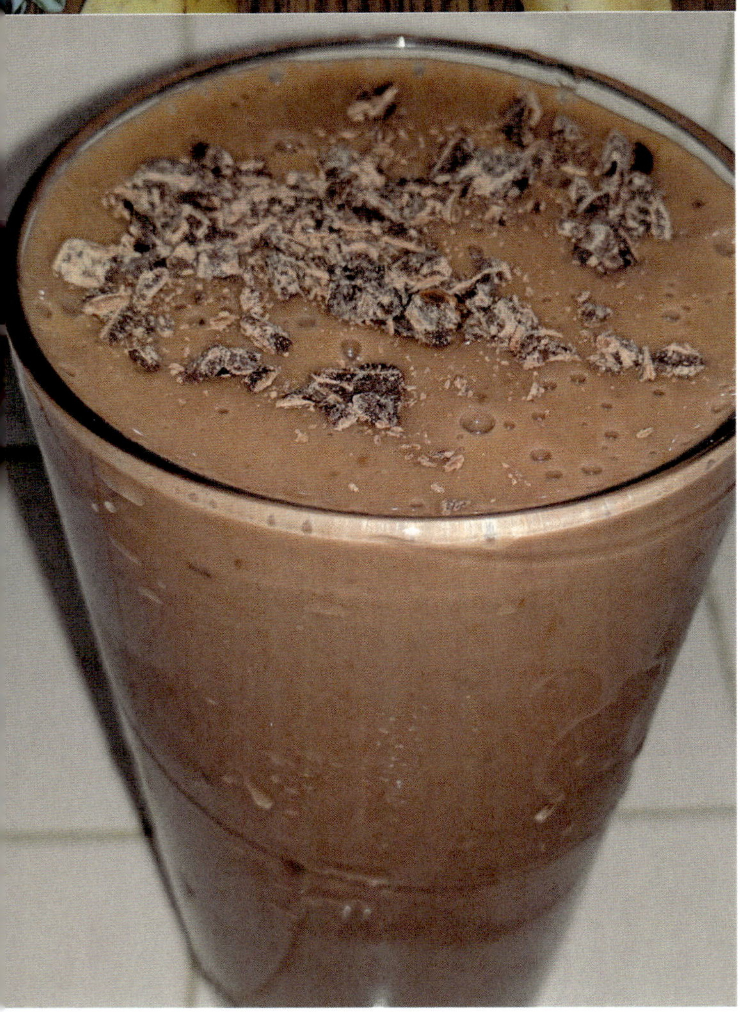

BLUEBERRY BLISSARD

Blueberries blend with bananas for cool treat with a brain-boosting benefit.

SERVINGS: 4 1-cup servings

INGREDIENTS:

- 2 cups blueberries, frozen
- 2 bananas, frozen
- 2 cups vanilla almond milk

STEPS:

1. Freeze bananas and blueberries ahead of time.
2. Combine fruits and almond milk in a blender and blend until well combined.
3. Top with your favorite garnish or topping.
4. Enjoy!

DELICIOUS WITH: Garnish with a lime wedge, fresh berries, or fresh mint leaves.

CHOCOLATE SHAKE

A chocolate shake made from nothing but fruits and seeds! This cool, creamy drink is dairy-free, cholesterol free, and full of good sun-fired energy and nutrition.

INGREDIENTS:

- 3 bananas, peeled, frozen
- 2 tbsp. cocoa powder
- 2 cups vanilla almond milk
- optional: 1 cup ice

Toppings

- chocolate shavings
- shredded coconut flakes
- banana slices
- chopped nuts

STEPS:

1. Peel and freeze bananas ahead of time.
2. Combine frozen bananas, cocoa powder, and almond milk in the blender.
3. Blend on high until smooth.
4. Pour shake into glasses and garnish with your favorite toppings.

☀MANGO SMOOTHIE☀

This simple smoothie blends bananas, almond milk, and mangoes for merriment in your mouth.

INGREDIENTS:

- 3 bananas, peeled, frozen
- 3 cups mangoes, diced, frozen
- 2 cups vanilla almond milk

Toppings

- 1 mango, fresh, diced
- 1/4 cup dried coconut flakes
- lime wedge

STEPS:

1. Peel and freeze bananas ahead of time.
2. Dice and freeze mangoes ahead of time.
3. Combine frozen mangoes, frozen bananas, and almond milk in the blender.
4. Blend on high until smooth. Open and push down fruit into the blades or add more almond milk if it is having trouble mixing.
5. Pour smoothie into three tall glasses or your super-sized mug and garnish with your favorite toppings.

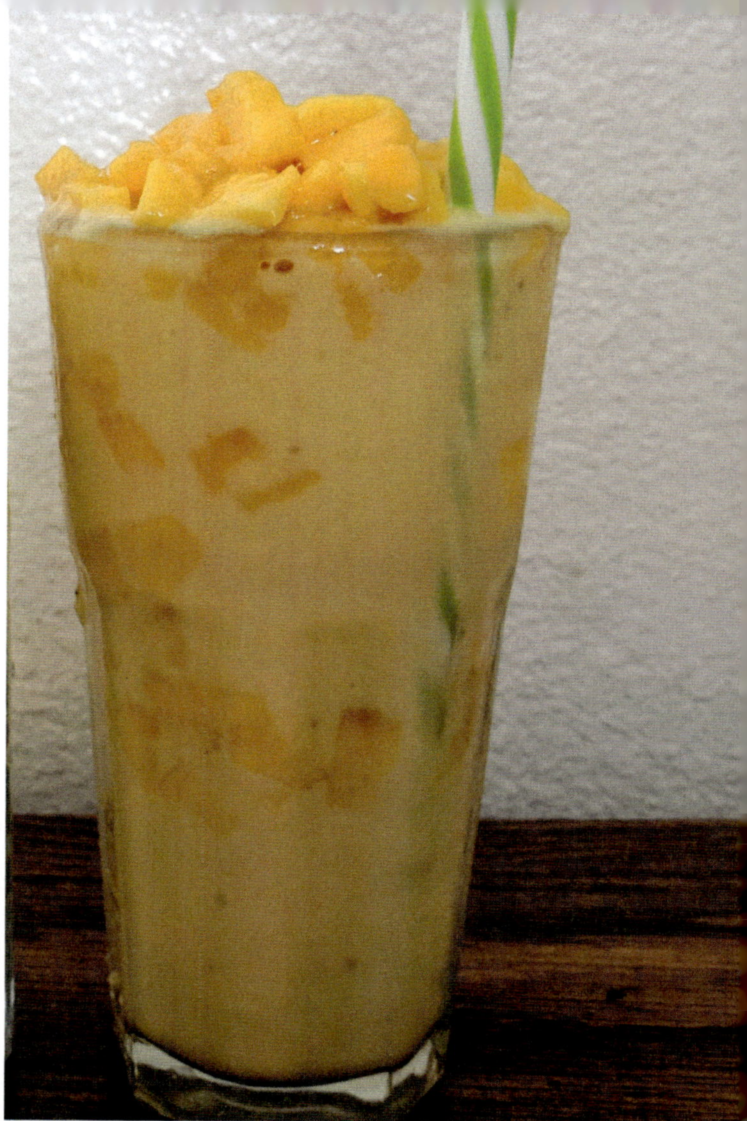

☀PEPPERMINT SMOOTHIE☀

Cool peppermint and creamy banana combine to delight in this refreshing drink.

SERVINGS: 2 1.5-cup servings

INGREDIENTS:

- 4 large bananas, frozen
- 2 cups coconut milk
- 1 cup mint leaves, fresh

STEPS

1. Peel and freeze bananas ahead of time.
2. Rinse fresh mint leaves.
3. Put ingredients into a blender and blend them together until well combined.
4. Pour smoothie in two tall glasses.
5. Garnish with fresh mint leaves. Enjoy!

DELICIOUS WITH: Garnish with fresh mint leaves.

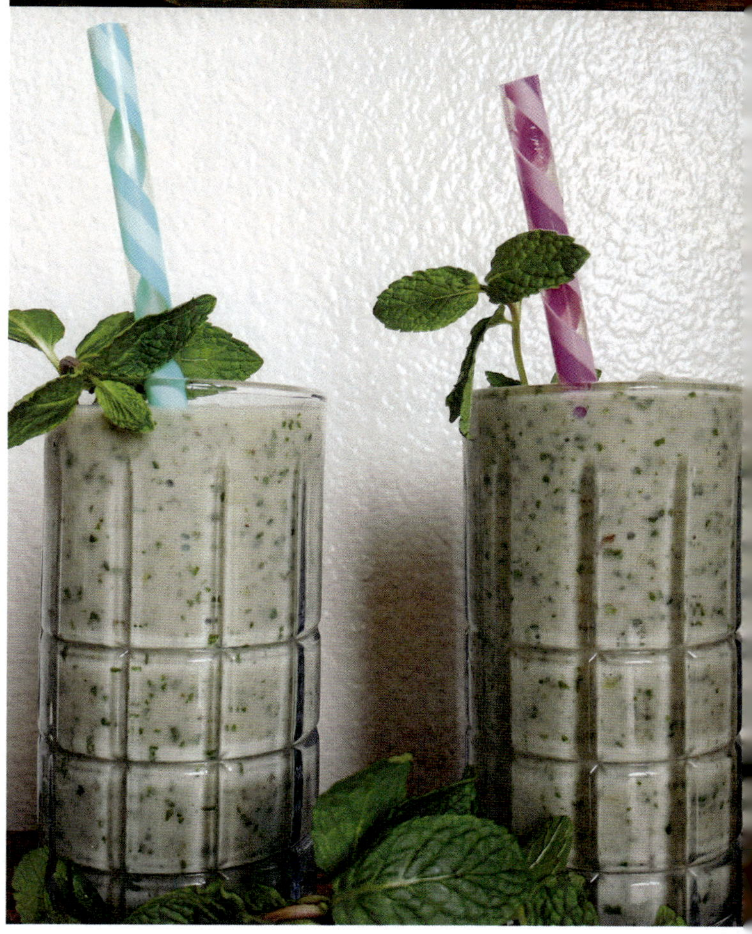

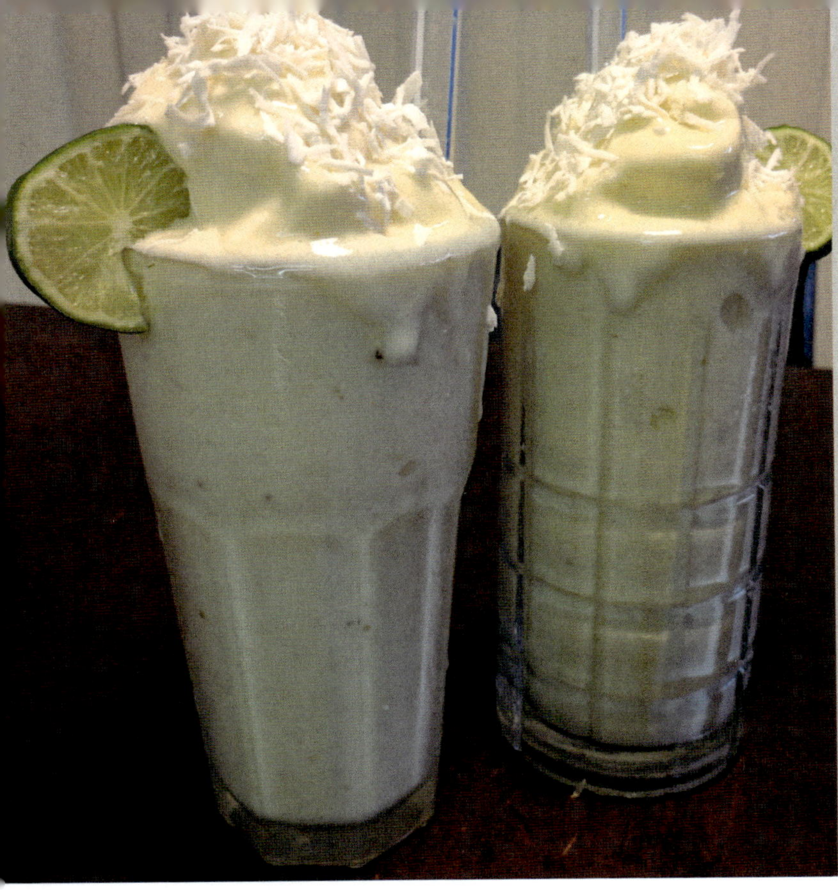

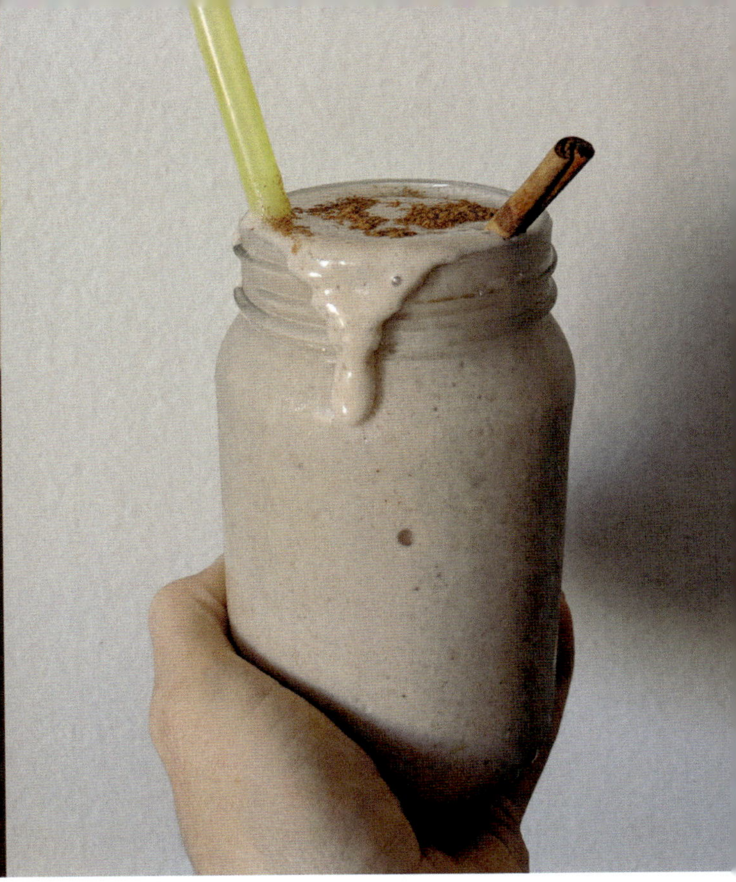

PIÑA COLADA SMOOTHIE

A yummy way to get your yellow and white phytonutrients. Pineapple smoothie is a super simple, sweet, and refreshing treat to enjoy anytime of day.

Servings: 3 tall glasses

INGREDIENTS:

- 12 oz. pineapple, frozen
- 4–5 bananas, frozen
- 2 cups vanilla coconut milk

STEPS:

1. Peel and freeze bananas and pineapple ahead of time.
2. Combine ingredients in a blender.
3. Blend until smooth and well combined.
4. Pour into three tall glasses to share.
5. Enjoy!

DELICIOUS WITH: Garnish with dried coconut flakes or a lime wedge.

THE CINNAMON BANINI

Bananas and tahini (ground sesame seeds) make the perfect pair in this creamy smoothie with a dash of cinnamon spice.

Servings: 1 tall glass, ~340 calories

INGREDIENTS:

- 2 bananas, frozen
- 1.5 cups almond milk
- 1 tbsp. tahini
- 1 tsp. cinnamon

STEPS:

1. Peel and freeze bananas ahead of time.
2. Place ingredients into your blender.
3. Blend until smooth and well combined.
4. Pour into a tall glass.
5. Enjoy!

DELICIOUS WITH: Cinnamon sprinkle, a tahini drizzle, a sprinkle of sesame seeds, banana slices, or a sprinkle of coconut flakes.

Banana + Tahini = The Banini

My first decade of making smoothies was actually fairly boring. My standard smoothies were peanut butter with banana and maybe some cacao (or cocoa) thrown in, and a basic blueberry-banana smoothie. Just before I turned 30, my smoothie creativity was ignited by the simple addition of tahini to my banana smoothie in place of peanut butter. Meet the "Banini." The idea for the combo came from a friend, and then many variations of the combo came through my experimenting. Now I almost never have basic banana and peanut butter smoothies and enjoy creating new tasty smoothie recipes using combinations of just fruits and seeds.

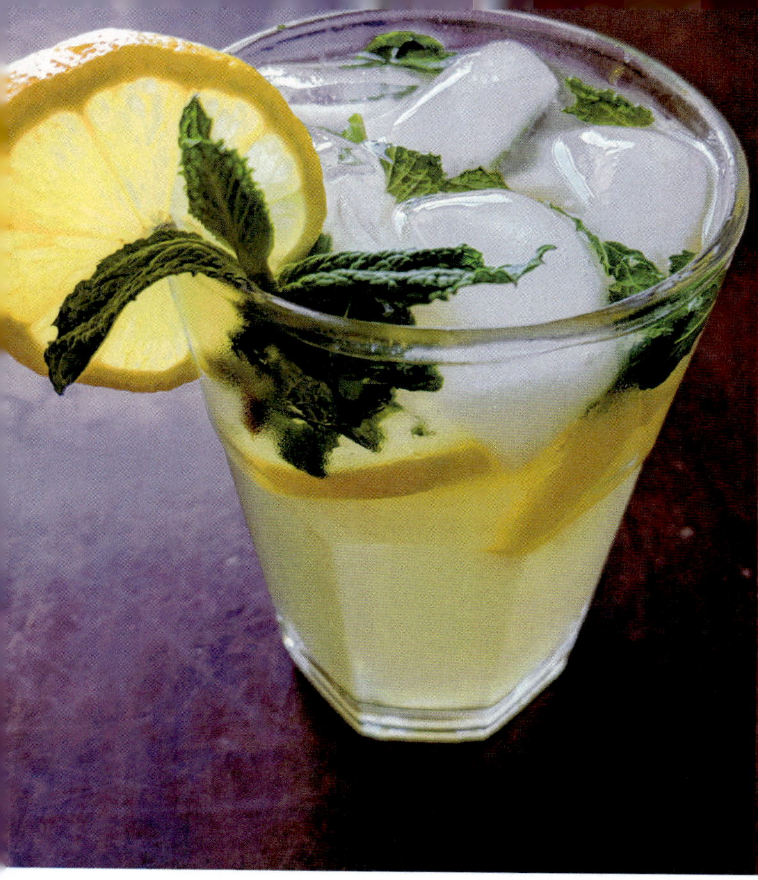

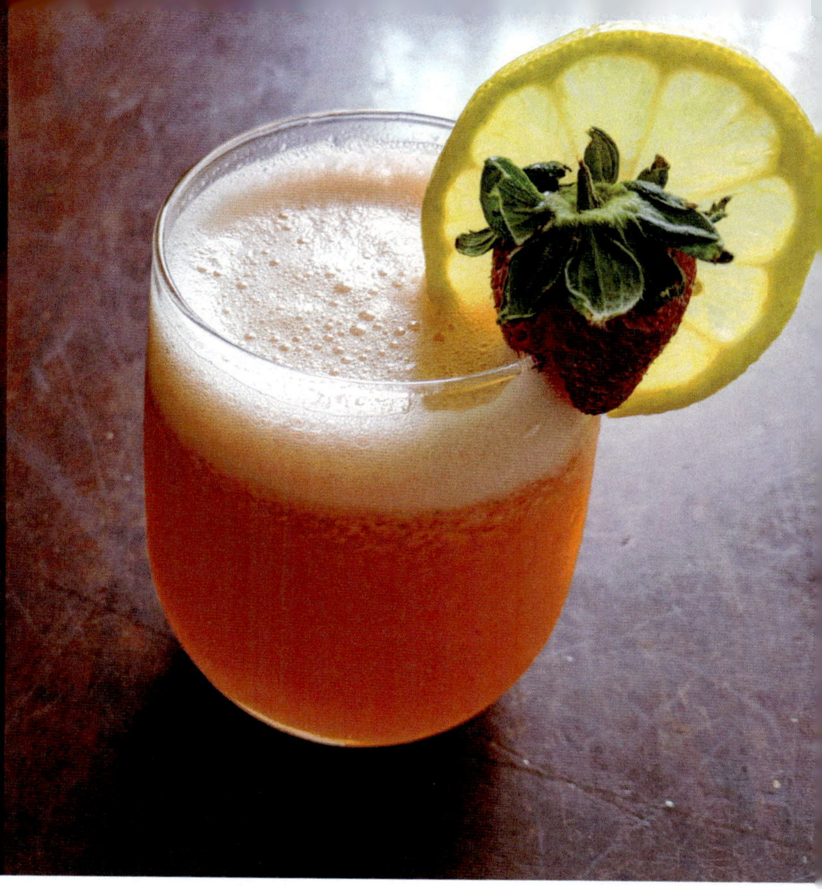

FRESH MINT LEMONADE

Cool, minty-fresh lemonade nourishes the body.

SERVINGS: 4 1-cup servings

INGREDIENTS:

- 1/4 cup mint leaves (handful), fresh
- 5 lemons
- 3 tbsp. agave syrup
- 1 liter of water + ice (to desired potency)

STEPS:

1. Cut lemons in half, juice, and strain out seeds.
2. Add lemon juice to pitcher with agave.
3. Use hands to "crush" mint leaves, helping release their flavorful substances and add to pitcher.
4. Add water to desired potency, stir, and serve over ice.[1]

1. Marinate this lemonade in the fridge for a while to enhance its minty goodness.

STRAWBERRY LEMONADE

Luscious lemonade with the added goodness of strawberries.

SERVINGS: 4 1-cup servings

INGREDIENTS:

- 1 lb strawberries (~3 cups)
- 5 lemons (juiced)
- 3 tbsp. agave syrup
- 1 liter of water + ice (to desired potency)

STEPS:

1. Cut lemons in half, juice, and strain out seeds.
2. Add lemon juice to blender with strawberries, water, and agave.
3. Blend until well combined and pour into serving pitcher or directly into glasses.
4. Serve over ice and garnish with a lemon slice and a fresh strawberry. Enjoy!

For the Love of Lemons

Here's just a few of the reasons to love the fruit of the lemon tree.

- The smell of lemons are naturally pleasing to frugivores like us humans—why do you think so many soaps and lotions use their scent?! Science shows that the scent of lemons can boost worker productivity and alertness.
- Lemons in water promote hydration and deliver a healthy dose of nutrients.
- Each lovely lemon contains over 100 nutrients including vitamins, minerals, and protective phytonutrients.
- Lemon scent is effective at combating nausea and vomiting.
- Lemon juice helps freshen the breath.
- Each lemon packs 30 mg of vitamin C—necessary for healthy immune function and so many other important jobs, like producing the collagen that holds our bodies together and keeps us looking fresh.

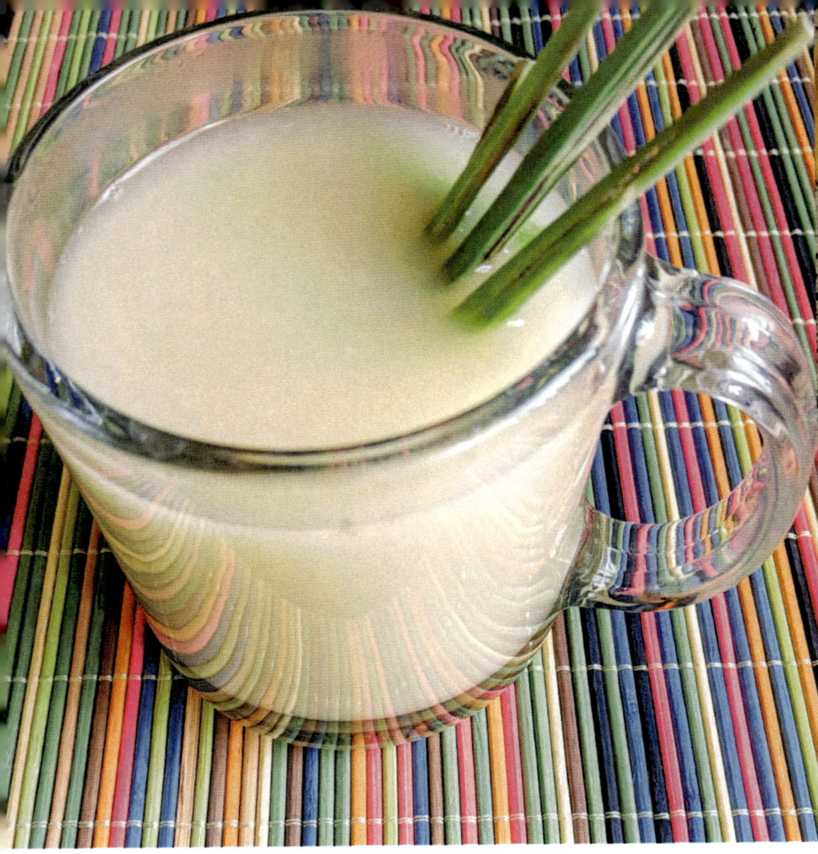

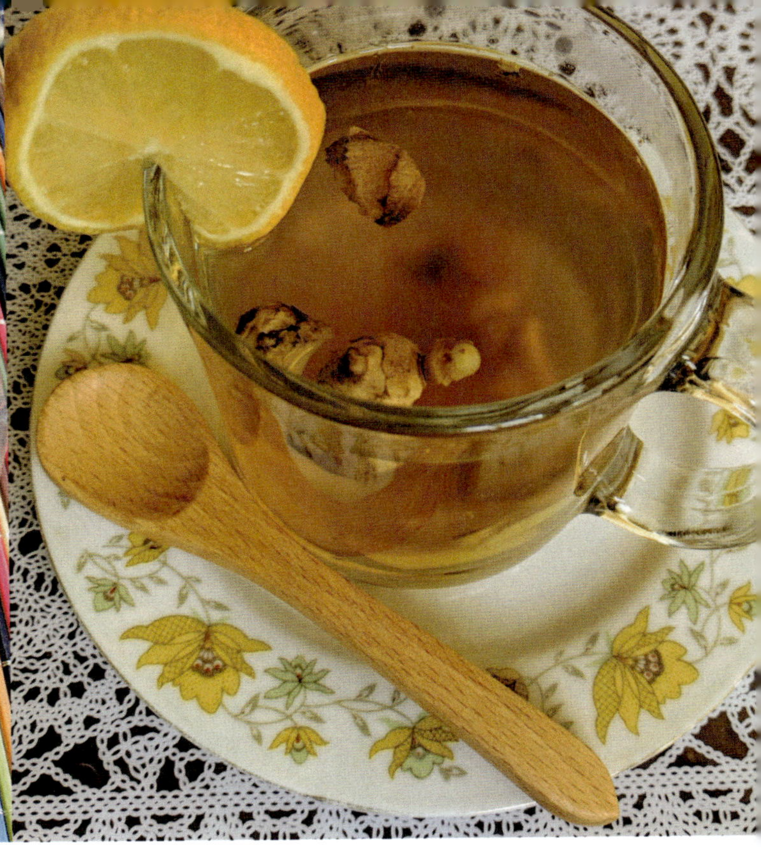

LEMONGRASS TEA

This nutritious and aromatic sweet tea is made from grass.

SERVINGS: 2

INGREDIENTS:

- 2 lemongrass shoots
- 2 cup water
- 1 cup coconut milk, unsweetened
- 1 tsp. agave nectar

STEPS:

1. Rinse lemongrass to remove any debris.
2. Chop lemongrass into small pieces.
3. Add chopped lemongrass to small pot with water and bring to a low boil. Cover pot.
4. Allow tea to brew while covered on low heat for about 10 minutes or until it becomes a pale yellow-green color.
5. Reduce heat to low and add coconut milk and agave. Stir.
6. Serve tea warm or allow to cool and refrigerate to enjoy cold lemongrass tea.

GINGER ROOT TEA

A fragrant spicy tea that warms your insides.

SERVINGS: 2

INGREDIENTS:

- 1/4 cup fresh ginger root, chopped
- 4 cups water
- 3 tbsp. agave nectar
- optional: lemon slice

STEPS:

1. Chop ginger. Slice into pieces 1/4 inch thick. You do not need to remove the skin.
2. Add ginger to small sauce pan and warm on medium heat until simmering.
3. Allow pot to simmer for about 10 minutes. Remove pot from heat and stir in agave.
4. Allow ginger to steep another 10 minutes before serving.
5. Scoop tea into mug with chunks of ginger included. Add a slice of lemon or lemon wedge to your tea if desired. Enjoy!

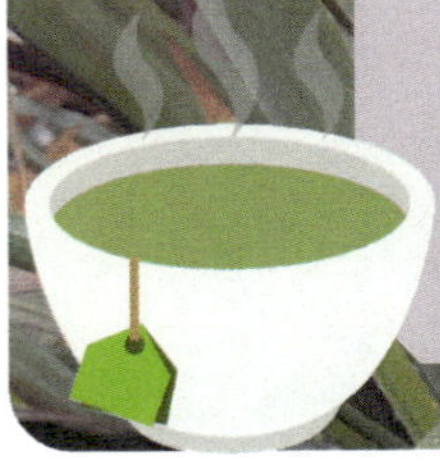

Where To Find Lemongrass

Lemongrass is a regular part of Asian cuisine and so your best luck for finding affordable fresh lemongrass is to visit your local Asian food market. If you aren't so lucky to have one nearby that carries this fragrant grass, you might still find lemongrass in the produce section of your local grocery. You may also find frozen prepared lemongrass in the freezer section of your grocery. If all else fails, I have an affordable source of lemongrass listed in the Food Products section of the Healing With Plants store—HealingWithPlants.us/store—purchase it online with ease and let Amazon deliver it straight to your door.

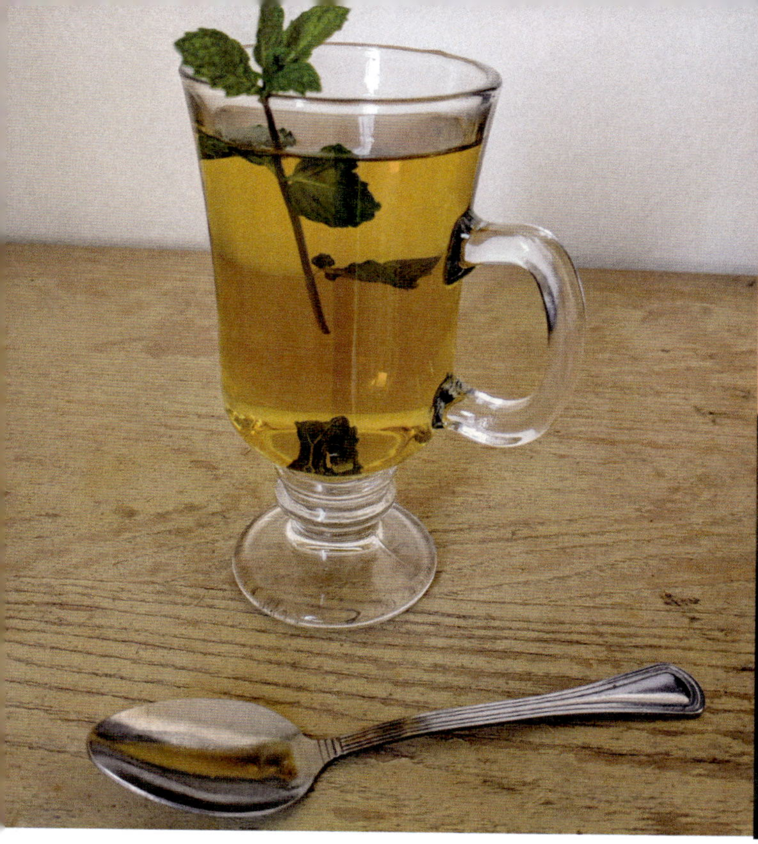

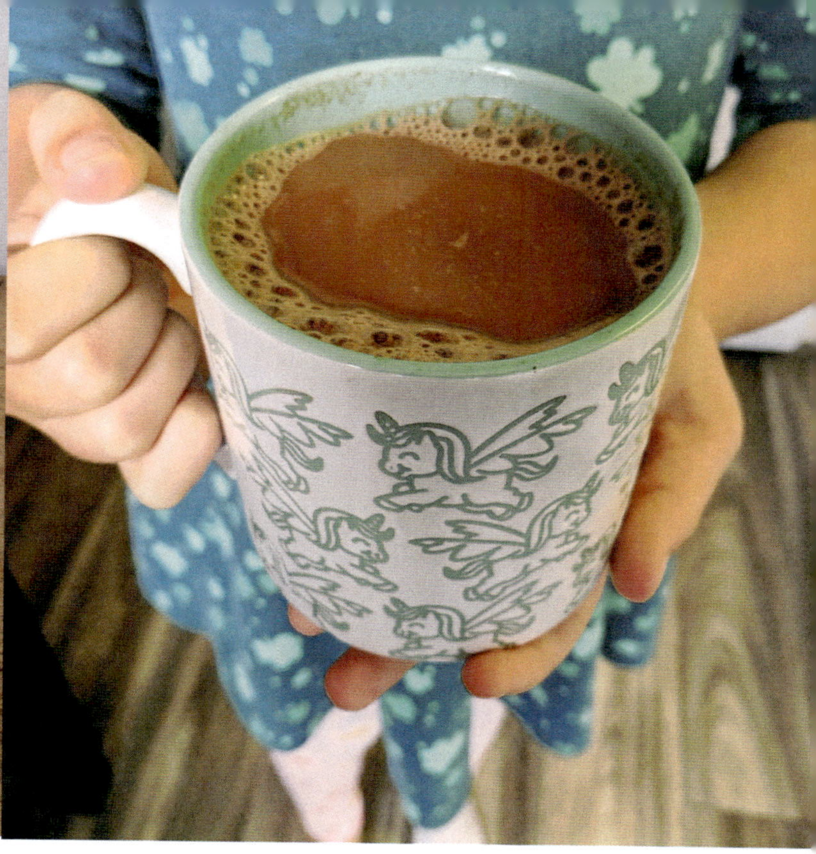

MINT TEA

A refreshing tea that is a good stomach healer.

SERVINGS: 2

INGREDIENTS:

- 4 cups water
- 4 tbsp. mint leaves, packed
- optional: plant milk (almond, coconut, oat, soy, rice, hemp)
- optional: agave nectar

STEPS:

1. Remove fresh mint leaves from stem and pack 4 tablespoons full for two 2-cup servings.
2. Add water and mint leaves to pot and bring to a low simmer.
3. When water starts to boil slightly, before it reaches a rolling boil, turn off heat.
4. Allow tea to steep for about 8 minutes before serving.
5. Enjoy! Add a teaspoon of agave or a splash of plant milk if desired.

MOM'S HOT COCOA

Creamy and wholesome liquid chocolate to warm your heart in any weather.

SERVINGS: 2 1-cup servings

INGREDIENTS:

- 1 cup water
- 1 cup vanilla almond milk
- 1 tbsp. cocoa powder
- 1 tbsp. agave nectar

STEPS:

1. Add all ingredients to a small saucepan and place on the stovetop.
2. Bring contents of pot to a low simmer. Do not allow mixture to boil.
3. Simmer on low heat until the cocoa is steamy.
4. Remove pot from heat, stir, and allow to sit for a few minutes before serving.
5. Pour and enjoy!

"The Stomach Healer"

Mint, in its many varieties, has long been known as "the stomach healer" for its many medicinal properties that aid digestion and support a healthy tummy. I made this glass, pictured above, for my son when he had an upset stomach. He drank it and then told me, "*Mom, it's a miracle! My stomach feels better!*"—it's mint's medicinal magic!

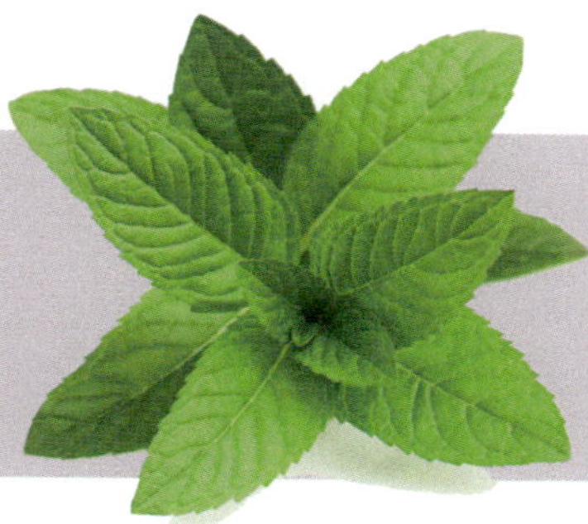

INGREDIENT INDEX

Eat the Rainbow

Made in the USA
Columbia, SC
21 May 2021

38340174R00084